Springer
New York
Berlin
Heidelberg
Hong Kong
London
Milan
Paris
Tokyo

Handbook of Evidence-Based Critical Care

Paul Ellis Marik, MD, FCCM, FCCP

Professor of Critical Care and Medicine
Department of Critical Care
University of Pittsburgh Medical School
Pittsburgh, Pennsylvania

With 50 Illustrations

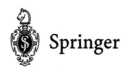 Springer

Paul Ellis Marik, MD
University of Pittsburgh Medical School
Department of Critical Care
640 A Scaife Hall
3550 Terrace Street
Pittsburgh, PA 15261
USA
pmarik@zbzoom.net

Library of Congress Cataloging-in-Publication Data
Marik, Paul Ellis.
    Handbook of evidence-based critical care / Paul Ellis Marik.
        p.cm.
    Includes bibliographical references and index.
    ISBN 0-387-95153-9 (softcover : alk. paper)
    1. Critical care medicine. 2. Evidence-based medicine.
    I. Title.
    RC86.7 .M367 2001
    616′.028–dc21   00-045039

Printed on acid-free paper.

Production managed by MaryAnn Brickner; manufacturing supervised by
Erica Bresler.
Typeset by Best-set Typesetter Ltd., Hong Kong.
Printed and bound by R.R. Donnelley and Sons, Harrisonburg, PA.
Printed in the United States of America.

9 8 7 6 5 4 3 2

ISBN 0-387-95153-9   SPIN 10900512

Springer-Verlag   New York   Berlin   Heidelberg
A member of BertelsmannSpringer Science+Business Media GmbH

To My Girls,
Kathryn, Emma, Claire, and Laura,
who have enriched my life

Learning without thinking is useless. Thinking without learning is dangerous.

—Confucius

A Note to the Reader

The author and publisher have made every attempt to check information and dosages for accuracy. Because information and science of pharmacology is continually advancing, our knowledge base continues to expand. Therefore, we recommend that the reader check all information and all product information for changes, especially changes in dosages or administration before administering any medication.

Contents

1

What Is Evidence-Based Medicine, and How Does It Apply to Critical Care?

Before medicine developed its scientific basis of pathophysiology, clinical practice was learned empirically from the events of daily experience in diagnosing and treating the maladies patients presented. Students learned as apprentices to clinicians, observing the phenomena of disease, the skill of diagnosis and treatment, and the outcomes of different remedies. Sir William Osler's classic textbook of medicine was based almost entirely on his *"personal experience correlated with the general experience of others."* With advances in our understanding of human physiology and the pathophysiologic basis of disease, these remedies fell by the wayside and treatment became based on modalities of treatment that were shown to interrupt or otherwise modify the disease process. Until recently, it was considered sufficient to understand the disease process in order to prescribe a drug or other form of treatment. However, when these treatment modalities were subjected to randomized, controlled clinical trials (RCTs) examining clinical outcomes and not physiological processes, the outcome was not always favorable. The RCT has become the reference in medicine by which to judge the effect of an intervention on patient outcome, because it provides the greatest justification for conclusion of causality, is subject to the least bias, and provides the most valid data on which to base all measures of the benefits and risk of particular therapies. Numerous ineffective and harmful therapies have been abandoned as a consequence of RCTs, while others have become integral to the care of patients and have become regarded as the standard of care. Intuition, anecdotes, common sense, personal biases, and clinical experience can no longer be used to justify clinical decisions or therapeutic policies. Every decision that the clinician makes must be based on sound scientific evidence (a collection of anecdotes is not scientific evidence).

Many RCTs are, however, inconclusive or provide conflicting results. In this situation, systematic reviews that are based on meta-analysis of published (and unpublished) RCTs are clearly the best strategy for appraising the available evidence. While meta-analyses have many limitations, they provide the best means of determining the significance of the *treatment effect* from inconclusive or conflicting RCTs. Furthermore, as a result of publication bias, positive studies are more likely to be published and usually in more prestigious journals than negative studies. A clinician may base his/her therapeutic decisions on these select RCTs, which may then lead to inappropriate patient care. It is therefore important that common medical interventions be systematically reviewed and the strength of the evidence (either positive or negative) be evaluated. Although over 250,000 RCTs have been performed, for many clinical problems, there are no RCTs to which we can refer to answer our questions. In these circumstances, we need to base our clinical decisions on the *best evidence available* from experimental studies, cohort studies, case series, and systematic reviews.

As critical care medicine has evolved into a discrete specialty that crosses anatomical and other artifical boundaries and deals with an enormous array of human conditions, it has become evident that, to achieve the best outcomes for our very complex patients, all our clinical decisions should be based on the *best available evidence*. The complexity of the critically ill patient together with the vast armamentarium of therapeutic options available make it essential that we critically evaluate established and emerging clinical practices. Bone throwing, bloodletting, and other forms of hocus-pocus have no role in modern critical care.

The *Handbook of Evidence-Based Critical Care* is not a reference text but presents a practical *evidence-based approach* to the management of critically ill ICU patients. Due to the vast number of therapeutic interventions that ICU physicians make daily, the topics are presented as narrative summaries of the *best available evidence* rather than as systematic reviews of each and every intervention. While all attempts have been made to be current, due to the exponential growth of medical knowledge, some of the information presented may already be outdated when this book comes to print. The reader therefore should keep up-to-date with the current medical literature. In keeping with the goal of providing an evidence-based approach to critical care, selected references are provided to support the more controversial topics.

Critical care medicine can only be practiced by close observation of the patient *at the bedside*, by contemplation, and by the integration of a large database of evidence-based medicine together with a good deal of humility.

2

House Officers' Housekeeping Guidelines

Intensive care units embody the miraculous advances of modern medicine. An ICU provides an environment where high-quality, compassionate, physiologically orientated, and evidence-based medicine can be practiced. The ICU is an exciting and challenging place to work and provides a remarkable learning environment. The keys to a successful rotation in the ICU are (1) teamwork and (2) a systematic, disciplined, and organized approach to patient care.

■ ADMISSION HISTORY AND PHYSICAL EXAMINATION

It is essential that a detailed and systematic history and physical examination be performed on all patients admitted to the ICU. This should include past medical and surgical history, current medications, as well as details of the current illness. It is essential that the patient's code status and the presence of advanced directives be established on admission to the ICU. The initial physical examination frequently serves as the baseline reference, and it should include a basic neurological examination (including reflexes, motor power, evaluation of mental status, and funduscopic examination). Following the history, physical examination, and review of the available laboratory data and chest radiograph, a differential diagnosis and a management plan should be formulated.

■ DAILY EXAMINATION

It is essential that a thorough physical examination be performed daily. The following features should be documented:

General

Overall condition of patient
The presence of all invasive lines, tubes, and devices
Vital signs: temperature, including maximum 24-hour temperature, blood pressure, pulse (rate and rhythm), and respiration rate
The presence of all pulses and the adequacy of peripheral perfusion
Limb symmetry and swelling (presence of venous thrombosis)
Presence of rashes and decubitus ulcers

Heart

Heart sounds and murmurs

Chest

Symmetry of air entry (i.e., presence of breath sounds) and presence of rhonchi or crackles

Abdomen

The presence of distention and tenderness (especially right upper quadrant)
The type of enteral feeds, evidence of reflux, and the gastric residual volumes
Presence of diarrhea

CNS

A focused neurological examination is essential, particularly in patients receiving hypnotic/sedative agents, and should include the following:
Level of consciousness and response to commands
Pupillary size and response
Eye movements
Limb movements; spontaneous and in response to noxious stimuli (pain)
Presence of deep tendon reflexes

The Ventilator

The ventilator is an extension of the patient and it is therefore essential that the following features be recorded:

Mode of ventilation (assist control, synchronized intermittent mandatory ventilation, pressure-controlled ventilation, etc.)
Set rate
Patient rate
Tidal volume
Fraction of inspired oxygen
Positive end-expiratory pressure
Peak and plateau airway pressure

Importance of the Daily Neurological Examination

Critically ill patients in the ICU are at risk of developing serious neurological complications including ICU psychosis, "septic" encephalopathy, critical illness polyneuropathy, entrapment neuropathies, compartment syndromes, cerebral edema, intracerebral hemorrhages (related to coagulopathies), cerebral ischemia (related to hemodynamic instability), and cerebral embolism. These conditions can be detected and diagnosed only by physical examination. Furthermore, these conditions may frequently be masked in patients who are sedated. It is therefore essential that the motor and eye response to a noxious stimulus (pain) as well as the deep tendon reflexes be recorded in all sedated patients. If the patient does not respond to a noxious stimuli, the sedation must immediately be stopped, to facilitate further neurological evaluation.

Laboratory Tests and Chest Radiographs

All ICU patients require a daily complete blood count (hemoglobin, white cell count, and platelet count) and urea and electrolyte tests. (If a patient does not require these tests, he/she probably does not need to be in the ICU!) Oxygenation should be assessed in all patients (usually by pulse oximetry—blood gasses when appropriate). All other laboratory tests should be ordered on merit; standing laboratory tests are not cost-effective. It is not cost-effective to perform a complete blood count and urea and electrolytes testing more frequently than every 24 hours unless special circumstances dictate. In patients receiving large volumes of fluid (e.g., those with diabetic ketoacidosis or hypernatremia), serum Na^+ and K^+ may be tested every 2 to 4 hours. In patients who are bleeding, a hematocrit should be followed no more frequently than every 8 hours (it takes 72 hours for the hematocrit to stabilize following blood loss). Almost all intubated patients require a daily chest radiograph. In all other patients, chest radiographs should be ordered when indicated.

Presenting on Daily Rounds

Producing a succinct and complete summary of a patient's status represents an important skill that all clinicians must master. Due to the large volume of data, together with the rapid turnover of high acuity patients, clear, succinct, and logical presentation are essential in the ICU.

The following approach is suggested:

1. Begin your presentation with the patient's name, sex, and age. List the primary medical problems responsible for ICU admission (e.g., pneumonia with respiratory failure; upper gastrointestinal bleed with hypotension); then, list significant secondary medical problems (e.g., myocardial infarction, diabetes mellitus, chronic obstructive pulmonary disease, chronic renal failure, etc.).

2. Outline the events of the past 24 hours.

3. Record the current physical findings:
   Blood pressure, pulse rate, respiration rate (patient rate/ventilator set rate)
   Current and maximal temperature in the last 24 hours
   24-hour urine output and fluid balance
   General
   Chest
   Heart
   Abdomen
   Central nervous system

4. Ventilator settings and most recent blood gas (pH, P_{CO_2}, P_{O_2}, H_{CO_3}, saturation) or oxygen saturation

5. Relevant laboratory results

6. Review of medications

7. Assessment and plan

■ KEY POINTS

1. ICU patients are at a high risk for deep venous thrombosis (DVT), and therefore all ICU patients require DVT prophylaxis (i.e., subcutaneous heparin, subcutaneous low-molecular-weight heparin, compression stockings alone or in combination).

2. All ICU patients should be evaluated for risk factors for stress ulceration, and high-risk patients should receive stress ulcer prophylaxis.
3. All intubated patients require a nasogastric (NG) tube. The orogastric route is preferred. NG tubes provide access to the gastrointestinal tract for feeding, allow measurement of the residual volumes, and allow decompressions of the stomach to minimize the risk of aspiration. Small-bore tubes have no advantages over standard NG tube unless feeding is being given into the small intestine.
4. Determine the adequacy of venous access.
5. Don't forget to feed the patient; absent bowel sounds do not preclude enteral feeding.
6. Communicate with the patient's nurse and respiratory therapist.
7. Keep the family informed.
8. If you don't understand something, *ask*!

Part 1

The Respiratory System

3

Airway Management: Endotracheal Intubation

■ INDICATIONS FOR INTUBATION

- Acute or impending respiratory failure
- Upper airway obstruction
- Airway trauma
- Inhalational injury
- Upper airway bleeding
- Loss of airway reflexes and airway protection
    Central nervous system diseases
    Stupor and coma
    Massive upper gastrointestinal (GI) bleeding
- Apnea
- Flail chest

■ ROUTE OF INTUBATION

Endotracheal intubation can be accomplished by either the orotracheal or nasotracheal route. Each has its specific advantages and disadvantages. In general, orotracheal intubation is preferred because it is rapid, more frequently successful, and allows a larger tube to be used. Blind nasotracheal intubation, however, is often preferred in the conscious patient, because it affords greater patient comfort, is usually well tolerated, and does not require anesthesia. Furthermore, the tube is more stable, is easier to secure, and mouth care is easier.

Patients who are nasally intubated are at a high risk of developing sinusitis. Almost all patients with a nasotracheal tube in situ will develop opacification of the paranasal sinuses within 3 days. Many of these patients will subsequently develop bacterial sinusitis. Therefore, if intubation for longer than 3 days is anticipated, patients should be intubated orally.

Contraindications to nasotracheal intubation include

- Apnea
- A bleeding diathesis
- Nasal polyps

It has been taught that patients with a suspected or proven basal skull fracture should not be intubated nasally, due to the possibility of intracranial placement of the endotracheal tube. However, this complication is exceedingly rare and probably related to poor technique.

Patients with suspected or confirmed cervical spine injuries should be intubated with extreme caution, with every effort taken to avoid hyperextension of the neck. Intubation may be performed by either the oral or nasal route, preferably by an experienced intubator. If the orotracheal route is used, the intubator's assistant must provide "inline traction" to prevent excessive extension of the neck. Intubation can also be achieved using a flexible bronchoscope/laryngoscope (by those experienced with the technique).

■ ENDOTRACHEAL TUBE SELECTION

The internal diameter of endotracheal tubes is usually measured in millimeters. Tubes are available in 0.5-mm increments from 2.5 mm. Selection of the correct size tube is of the utmost importance. The resistance to airflow varies with the fourth power of the radius of the tube. Selecting an inappropriately small tube increases the work of breathing. Furthermore, small tubes (<7.5 to 8.0 mm) will prohibit bronchoscopic procedures being performed through the endotracheal tube. Intubation with an inappropriately large tube may damage the larynx and vocal cords. In general, the larger the patient, the larger the endotracheal tube that should be used. Adult females should generally be intubated with a size 7.5- or 8.0-mm tube and adult males with an 8.0- or 8.5-mm tube.

■ ANESTHESIA FOR INTUBATION

When orotracheal intubation is attempted, it is crucial that the patient be adequately sedated to avoid fighting and airway trauma. If sedation alone does not result in adequate relaxation, an intravenous anesthetic induction agent alone or with a short-acting neuro-muscular blocking agent can be used. It should be appreciated that both sedative and induction agents may precipitate severe hypoten-sion, particularly in elderly patients and patients whose intravascular volume is depleted.

Sedation may be achieved using incremental doses of midazolam (2 to 5 mg) and/or fentanyl (100 μg). However, these agents may not achieve the level of anesthesia required for intubation, and they are difficult to titrate, with escalating doses frequently resulting in pro-found hypotension postintubation. The newer intravenous anesthetic agents therefore (alone or together with a neuromuscular blocking agent) have particular utility in emergent intubations. Etomidate (0.2 to 0.4 mg/kg) is a carboxylated imidazole hypnotic agent that has a rapid and predictable onset of action with a short duration of action. The most distinctive property of etomidate as compared with other rapid-acting agents is its minimal effect on cardiovascular parameters. Propofol is an intravenous sedative-hypnotic agent used for the induc-tion and maintenance of anesthesia or sedation. Intravenous injection propofol produces hypnosis rapidly with minimal excitation, usually within 40 seconds from the start of an injection. The major cardio-vascular side effect of propofol is arterial hypotension (particularly in volume-depleted patients). However, this can be minimized if the drug is titrated to effect. For induction, propofol should be titrated (approximately 40 mg every 10 seconds) against the response of the patient until the clinical signs show the onset of anesthesia.

Traditionally, neuromuscular blockade has been achieved with suc-cinylcholine (1 to 2 mg/kg), though newer agents such as rocuronium may have added benefits. Rocuronium is a steroidal nondepolarizing muscle relaxant that, in a dose of 0.9 to 1.2 mg/kg, has a duration of onset similar to succinylcholine. Rocuronium is devoid of significant hemodynamic effects. The use of paralytic agents in patients who cannot be ventilated with a bag and mask may result in a fatal outcome if intubation is unsuccessful. Therefore, paralytic agents should be used only by experienced intubators.

Etomidate and propofol have no analgesic properties and do not blunt the sympathetic response to endotracheal intubation; this is particularly important in head-injured patients (to prevent surges in intracranial pressure). Lidocaine in doses of 1.5 to 2.0 mg/kg is com-monly utilized in this setting. However, a number of studies have demonstrated this drug to be ineffective in reducing the sympathetic response during endotracheal intubation. Esmolol is a short-acting beta-blocker that has been demonstrated to consistently blunt the heart rate and blood pressure response to airway stimulation. Fentanyl (50 to 100 μg) has also been used during rapid-sequence intubation to attenuate the sympathetic response.

Hypotension is common following intubation and is best treated with volume replacement. Phenylephrine (Neo-Synephrine) is useful in patients who do not respond rapidly to fluids: Dilute 1 mL of phenylephrine (10 mg/mL) with 9 mL of saline, and give 1/2- to 1-mL boluses.

■ ENDOTRACHEAL INTUBATION

With the intubator standing behind the head of the bed, the initial step is to establish an airway by placing the finger of one hand under the mandible and lifting upward and backward (extending the patient's neck), or by using the index fingers of both hands, to lift the mandible from the angle of the jaw. The ability to ventilate and oxygenate the patient with a bag and mask must then be established. Care should be taken not to generate excessive pressure when ventilating by bag and mask. Airway pressure exceeding 25 mm Hg is likely to overcome the resistance of the gastroesophageal sphincter and fill the patient's stomach with gas. This will increase the risk of regurgitation and gastric aspiration. When ventilation is effective, the chest rises with each squeeze of the bag. The patient should be preoxygenated in this way with 100% oxygen before intubation. Arterial oxygen saturation should be monitored continuously by pulse oximetry.

When an airway has been established and the patient adequately ventilated, preparation can now be made for intubation. It is vitally important to assemble *all* the necessary equipment, drugs, and personnel at the bedside before attempting intubation. All the equipment must be inspected for completeness and tested for function.

As a general rule no, more than two attempts, by a single operator, should be made to intubate the trachea.

If the second attempt is unsuccessful, continue to ventilate the patient with 100% oxygen until more experienced help becomes available. Further attempts at intubation increase the risk of airway trauma and make subsequent attempts even more difficult.

■ OROTRACHEAL INTUBATION

- The intubator should wear protective gloves and a mask to protected him/herself from potentially infectious agents that may be transmitted during intubation.
- Perhaps the most important aspect of this technique is the correct positioning of the patient. The intubator should stand at the head of the bed. The patient must be in the supine position with the height of the bed adjusted to achieve a comfortable

position for the intubator. The patient's head should then be placed in the "sniffing" position, with the neck flexed and the head slightly extended. This is best achieved by placing a rolled bath towel under the occiput. It should always be assumed that the patient has a full stomach, and Sellick's maneuver (pressure applied to the cricoid cartilage) should be performed to prevent aspiration of regurgitated stomach contents into the trachea.

- The laryngoscope is grasped in the left hand while the patient's mouth is opened with the gloved right hand. The laryngoscope blade is inserted on the right side of the mouth and advanced to the base of the tongue, pushing the tongue to the left. If a straight blade is used, it should be extended below the epiglottis. If the curved blade is used, it is inserted in the vallecula.

- With the blade in place, the operator should lift the handle of the laryngoscope forward in a plane of 45 degrees to the horizontal to expose the vocal cords. It is essential to keep the left wrist stiff and use the arm and shoulder to lift the laryngoscope. It is important to use a lifting action rather than use the patient's teeth as a fulcrum to extend the head.

- The endotracheal tube is then held in the right hand and inserted into the right corner of the patient's mouth in a plane that intersects with the laryngoscope blade at the glottis. This angle avoids the problem of the endotracheal tube obscuring the view of the cords.

- The endotracheal tube is advanced through the vocal cords until the cuff just disappears from sight. If difficulty is encountered in advancing the tube through the cords or when only the posterior portion of the cords is visible, it may be useful to use the introducing stylet. The soft metal stylet should be bent into the shape of a hockey stick.

- ***Orotracheal intubation should not be performed if the cords cannot be visualized. This is not a blind procedure.*** If the vocal cords cannot be visualized using a curved blade, a straight blade may facilitate visualization. In addition, firm cricoid pressure may bring the vocal cords into view.

- The cuff is then inflated with just enough air to prevent a leak during ventilation.

- The patient should be bagged with a CO_2 detector to confirm endotracheal placement of the endotracheal tube.

- The chest should be auscultated to ensure bilateral breath sounds.

- The tube should then be tied in position. The incisors should be at the 23-cm mark in men and 21 cm in women.

- A portable chest radiograph should be obtained to confirm the position of the endotracheal tube and to exclude any complications that may have occurred during intubation.

■ NASOTRACHEAL INTUBATION

- The nares should be anesthetized with topical anesthesia and a vasoconstrictor then applied.
- A 7.5 endotracheal tube is generally used. Warming the tube in hot water softens the tube and may allow for a less traumatic intubation.
- The endotracheal tube should be well lubricated. It is then inserted through the nares and gently advanced until breath sounds can be heard (with the intubator's ear near the end of the tube). The endotracheal tube is now positioned just above the cords. *Note*: The tube should be advanced gently. Using excessive force can cause severe upper aiway trauma, including naso-pharyngeal lacerations and rupture.
- As the patient takes a breath (and the vocal cords abduct), the tube is advanced through the cords and secured in position. If resistance is felt when advancing the tube, gentle flexion of the neck may correctly align the larynx.
- No more than two attempts at nasotracheal intubation should be made before the oral route is used.

■ DIFFICULT INTUBATION

The following features may suggest that intubation will be difficult:

- Short neck–chin-to-larynx distance (thyromental) less than three finger widths
- Obesity
- Protruding incisors
- Limited opening of mouth: interdental gap less two finger widths
- Limited neck extension
- High arched palate

However, many patients with none of these features may be difficult to intubate. The most accepted method to ease intubation involves direct visualization of the oral pharynx with the patient sitting and the tongue protruded. This type of assessment can rarely be made in an emergent situation.

■ FAILED INTUBATION

In those rare instances when an experienced intubator fails endotracheal intubation, fiberoptic bronchoscopic intubation may be successful. In the emergent situation, either a cricothyroidotomy or an emergent tracheostomy can be performed.

■ COMPLICATIONS ASSOCIATED WITH INTUBATION

Complications During Intubation

- Arterial hypotension
- Upper airway trauma, including perforation or laceration of the pharynx, hypopharynx, and larynx
- Mainstem intubation
- Regurgitation with aspiration
- Arrhythmias and cardiorespiratory arrest
- Bleeding
- Esophageal intubation
- Cranial intubation

Delayed Complications

- Sinusitis, otitis media, and pneumonia
- Tube blockage or kinking

Late Complications

- Tracheomalacia
- Subglottic or tracheal stenosis
- Tracheo–esophageal fistula
- Vocal cord paralysis

4

Noninvasive Positive-Pressure Ventilation

The recent introduction of noninvasive positive-pressure ventilation (NPPV) and its successful and widespread use in the management of chronic ventilatory failure have resulted in its application in selected patients with acute respiratory failure. NPPV has now become a treatment option for some patients who would otherwise be managed by intubation or perhaps would not have received mechanical ventilation at all.

The advantages of NPPV include improved patient comfort, reduced need for sedation, and avoidance of the complications of endotracheal intubation, including upper airway trauma, sinusitis, otitis, and nosocomial pneumonia. Furthermore, airway defense mechanisms and speech and swallowing are left intact, and the patient remains alert and communicative. NPPV has been used successfully to treat acute respiratory failure in postoperative patients and in those with pulmonary edema, chronic obstructive pulmonary disease (COPD), and obstructive sleep apnea. NPPV has also been used to facilitate weaning. NPPV also appears to be particularly effective in patients with an exacerbation of COPD who are alert and cooperative.

Bott and colleagues reported the first prospective, randomized clinical trial of NPPV compared with conventional therapy in patients with an acute exacerbation of COPD. In this study, nasal ventilation was more effective than conventional therapy in lowering the Pa_{CO_2} and reversing acidosis. Furthermore, there was a significant reduction in mortality with NPPV (9% vs. 30%; $P = 0.01$). A number of other studies have been reported that have demonstrated that NPPV reduces the need for intubation and is well tolerated in patients with acute respiratory failure who are otherwise "stable." Meduri and colleagues recently reported their experience using NPPV in patients with status asthmaticus. NPPV using a face mask was highly effective in improving gas exchange, with only 2 of 17 patients requiring intubation.

The most common complication with the use of NPPV is facial trauma. The problem of skin necrosis, particularly over the bridge of the nose, makes it difficult for patients to be ventilated continuously for more than 1 to 2 days. Retention of secretions and gastric distension may be problematic in some patients.

Several interfaces and ventilator modes have been used to deliver NPPV to patients with acute respiratory failure, including facial masks covering both the nose and mouth and nasal masks. NPPV can be delivered using a conventional ventilator using volume- or pressure-limited ventilation or specialized noninvasive ventilators. The BiPAP ventilator is a variable-flow generator that permits independent control of inspiratory (IPAP) and expiratory (EPAP) pressures and provides nasal pressure support ventilation. It can augment spontaneous breaths by virtue of a sensitive trigger and increase flow to compensate for leaks around the mask and through the open mouth.

■ INDICATIONS FOR NPPV

Hypercapnic Respiratory Failure

- Severe dyspnea at rest
- Respiratory rate > 25 breaths/min
- Use of accessory muscle of respiration
- Acute respiratory acidosis (pH < 7.30)
- An alert and cooperative patient

Hypoxemic Respiratory Failure

- Respiratory rate > 30 breaths/min
- $PaO_2/FiO_2 < 200$
- Increased use of accessory muscle or $Paco_2$ retention
- Alert and cooperative patient

■ CONTRAINDICATIONS TO NPPV

- Hemodynamic or electrocardiographic instability
- Patient at risk for aspiration
- Inability to clear copious secretions
- Obtunded or uncooperative patient

■ FACE MASK MECHANICAL VENTILATION USING A VENTILATOR

There are a number of advantages and disadvantages of noninvasive ventilation using a ventilator (e.g., Puritan Bennett 7200). The advantages of the 7200 with a full face mask are

- The ability to set higher levels of pressure-support ventilation (PSV) if required. BiPAP machines are usually limited to 20 cm H_2O of PSV, and that is only if no positive end-expiratory pressure PEEP is applied.
- The ability to set a specific FIO_2 at any range. On the BiPAP machine, O_2 must be bled into the system and the FIO_2 can fluctuate greatly, depending on the minute ventilation.
- The alarm system is superior to that on the BiPAP machine. In apnea ventilation, an alarm will sound, whereas in the timed mode on BiPAP, no apnea warning is given.

The biggest disadvantage of using the ventilator for NPPV is its inability to compensate for air leaks; this the BiPAP machine does well. This means that when using the 7200 in the PSV mode, if there is the slightest leak in the mask (the mask may not fit the contour of the face, or a nasogastric tube may prevent the mask from fitting tightly on the face), then the patient will not be able to cycle the ventilator into exhalation, causing inspiratory flow to continue for 5 seconds. This will cause dyssynchrony between the patient and ventilator.

If you have a leak in the mask that cannot be sealed and you must use the 7200, the problem can be minimized by using the pressure control mode instead of pressure support. It would be beneficial to have a ventilator with graphic capabilities. By examining the *pressure vs. time* graph, you can determine the length of the patient's inspiratory time. You can then set the specific inspiratory time in pressure control so that the machine stops giving flow at approximately the same time that the patient is done inspiring. It would be better to have the inspiratory time set slightly shorter than the patient's inspiratory time rather than longer, as any sudden decrease in the patient's inspiratory time will cause the patient to exhale against flow from the machine.

In summary, using noninvasive ventilation with the 7200 (or equivalent), start with PSV of 8 to 15 cm H_2O, start with 3 cm H_2O continuous positive airway pressure (CPAP) to keep the mask from becoming a CO_2 reservoir; and increase the CPAP as needed. Use flow-by. If the device has no flow-by, set the pressure sensitivity as low as possible without the ventilator "chattering." If you have a leak that cannot be sealed, try pressure-controlled ventilation (PCV) in the assist control (A/C) mode with 8 to 15 cm H_2O pressure and an

inspiratory time of 1 second. Using the pressure/time waveform, estimate the patient's inspiratory time by measuring the length of time of
negative pressure and make your adjustments.

A protocol for noninvasive face mask mechanical ventilation is outlined below. However, similar guidelines can be used for BiPAP nasal
ventilation.

■ PROTOCOL FOR NONINVASIVE FACE MASK MECHANICAL VENTILATION

Procedure for Patient Setup

- Explain to the patient what you are doing and what to expect.
- Set up the ventilator by the bedside.
- Keep the head of the patient's bed at ≥ 45-degree angle.
- Turn on the ventilator, and dial in the settings.
- Do not strap the mask on, but hold the mask gently over the patient's face until the patient becomes comfortable with it.
- After the patient has become comfortable with the mask, strap the face mask on using the rubber head strap, making sure that the strap fits above and below the patient's ears to minimize air leak without causing discomfort.
- After placing the patient on the ventilator, the humidification system should be connected, *but do not turn on the heater*.
- Connect the patient to the bedside pulse oximeter for continuous O_2 saturation monitoring.
- Assess the patient's respiratory rate, heart rate, level of dyspnea, O_2 saturation, blood pressure, minute ventilation and exhaled tidal volume (Vt.) Monitor for abdominal distention and for production of secretions.

Initial Ventilator Settings

- Initial ventilatory setting should be CPAP mode with PSV (10 to 20 cm H_2O) titrated to achieve a respiratory rate < 25 breaths/min and Vt ≥ 7 mL/kg.
- If a significant leak around the mask prevents the use of PSV, the patient should be placed on PCV mode.
- Ventilator settings should be adjusted based on arterial blood gasses (ABGs).

■ WEANING PATIENTS FROM NPPV

Titrate PSV to 5 cm H_2O, based on the patient's tolerance and ABGs, at which point the patient should be weaned from NPPV by removal of the face mask for short periods of time to patient tolerance and objective findings. Patients should be placed on supplemental O_2 by nasal cannula or face mask while off NPPV. The weaning procedure is similar to T-piece weaning trials.

■ SELECTED REFERENCES

1. Abou-Shala N, Meduri GU. Noninvasive mechanical ventilation in patients with acute respiratory failure. *Crit Care Med.* 1996;24:705–715.
2. Bott J, Conway JH, Ward EM, et al. A randomized controlled study of nasal intermittent positive pressure ventilation in acute exacerbations of chronic obstructive airways disease. *Lancet.* 1993;341:1555–1557.
3. Kramer N, Meyer TJ, Meharg J, Cece RD, Hill NS. Randomized, prospective trial of noninvasive positive pressure ventilation in acute respiratory failure. *Am J Respir Crit Care Med.* 1995;151:1799–1806.
4. Meduri GU, Cook TR, Turner RE, Cohen M, Leeper KV. Noninvasive positive pressure ventilation in status asthmaticus. *Chest.* 1996;110:767–774.
5. Patrick W, Webster K, Ludwig L, Roberts D, Wiebe P, Younes M. Noninvasive positive-pressure ventilator in acute respiratory failure. *Am J Respir Crit Care Med.* 1996;153:1005–1011.
6. Wysocki M, Tric L, Wolf MA, Millet H, Herman B. Noninvasive pressure support ventilation in patients with acute respiratory failure. A randomized comparison with conventional therapy. *Chest.* 1995;107:761–768.

5

Mechanical Ventilation 101

■ TYPES OF VENTILATORS

Ventilators have traditionally been classified according to the cycling method (cycling from inhalation to exhalation). However, modern ventilators have microprocessors, which allow them to function in many different modes with enormous versatility.

- *Volume cycled.* The ventilator delivers fresh gas until the preselected volume of gas is delivered. The rise in alveolar pressure is proportional to pulmonary compliance and the volume of gas delivered.
- *Pressure cycled.* Inspiration continues until a predetermined peak airway pressure is reached. The tidal volume is variable (from breath to breath) and depends on
     Pulmonary compliance
     Respiratory rate
     Inspiratory time and flow rate
- *Time cycled.* Inspiration continues for a preset interval, with exhalation beginning when this time interval has elapsed, regardless of airway pressure or volume delivered.

■ MODES OF VENTILATION (Figure 5-1)

Controlled mechanical ventilation (CMV). The respiratory rate and tidal volume are preset. The patient cannot trigger the ventilator or move air through the ventilator circuit. The minute volume is therefore dependent on the preset respiratory rate and tidal volume. The CMV mode of ventilation is used only in paralyzed patients.

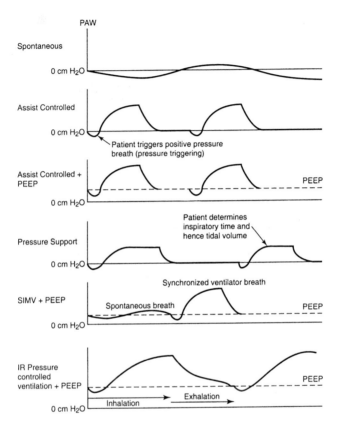

Figure 5-1. "Idealized" waveforms of common modes of ventilation. (IR = inverse ratio; PAW = Airway pressure.)

Assist control (AC). In the AC mode, the ventilator senses an inspiratory effort by the patient and responds by delivering a preset tidal volume. The trigger threshold is the negative force that the patient must generate to trigger the ventilator (see below). This trigger threshold can be adjusted, determining how hard the patient must work to trigger the ventilator. The trigger threshold is usually set at −2 cm H_2O. To prevent hypoventilation, a control mode backup rate is set on the ventilator. If the time between two spontaneous inspiratory efforts is greater than the interval corresponding to the backup rate, a breath of the same tidal volume is delivered.

Synchronized intermittent mandatory ventilation (SIMV). In the SIMV mode, the patient breathes spontaneously through the ventilator circuit at a tidal volume and rate that he/she determines according to need. The patient however, must open (trigger) a demand valve to breathe through the circuit, increasing the work of breathing. At regular intervals, the ventilator delivers breaths based on a preset tidal volume and rate, which are synchronized with the patient's respiratory efforts. The degree of respiratory support is determined by the SIMV rate. SIMV theoretically has a number of advantages over AC ventilation:

- Mean airway pressure is less, limiting the hemodynamic effects of positive pressure ventilation and reducing the risk of barotrauma.
- Hyperventilation and respiratory alkalosis are less likely.
- Patients may maintain respiratory muscle strength.
- Patients may tolerate SIMV better than AC, requiring less sedation.

Pressure-controlled ventilation (PCV). This is a form of AC ventilation; however, following patient or automatic triggering, the ventilator delivers a pressure-limited breath. The pressure above end-expiratory pressure is set, and the ventilator delivers a breath until this pressure is reached. As the pressure difference falls with progression of inspiration, the flow rate has a decelerating pattern. This inspiratory waveform has been shown to result in a more homogeneous distribution of gas flow in patients with acute respiratory distress syndrome (ARDS). The tidal volume varies being dependent upon the set pressure, the compliance of the respiratory system, and the inspiratory time.

Pressure-support ventilation (PSV). PSV was developed to reduce the work of spontaneous breathing in the SIMV/continuous positive airway pressure (CPAP) mode. Each time the patient inhales, the ventilator delivers a pressure-limited breath, which continues for as long as the patient inhales. PSV compensates for the inherent impedance of the ventilator circuit and endotracheal tube, enabling the patient to establish a more natural breathing pattern. A PSV of between 5 and 10 cm H_2O will overcome the resistance of the ventilator circuit and endotracheal tube.

■ PEEP

- PEEP provides *positive end-expiratory pressure* above atmospheric pressure. The mean airway pressure increases in proportion to the level of PEEP. In patients with pulmonary edema, PEEP shifts the pressure–volume inflation curve toward normal, increasing compliance, recruiting alveoli, and increasing functional residual capacity (FRC). It is thought that PEEP redistributes lung water.

- PEEP is "good" for left ventricular function
  - Decreases preload.
  - Decreases afterload.
  - Improves pulmonary compliance and therefore decreases work of breathing.
- PEEP is "bad" for right ventricular (RV) function
  - Increases RV afterload; RV may acutely fail in patients with severe pulmonary hypertension and patients with RV infarction.
- *Physiologic PEEP*: Some intensivists use "physiological" or prophylactic PEEP (5 cm H_2O) to prevent atelectasis. Although recommended, no data exists to support or refute this practice.
- Indications for PEEP:
  - Cardiogenic pulmonary edema
  - Acute lung injury and ARDS
  - Postoperative patients (decreased FRC)
- Contraindications:
  - Bullous lung disease and emphysema
  - Raised intracranial pressure
  - Unilateral lung disease (relative contraindication)
- *Best PEEP*: The level of PEEP that should be used is "Best PEEP." In patients with large intrapulmonary shunts, increasing the FIO_2 will not increase the PaO_2. However, excessive PEEP will overinflate compliant lungs and increase V/Q mismatching as well as reduce cardiac output. *A PEEP trial should be performed daily to determine the lowest level of PEEP that provides adequate arterial saturation and the maximal oxygen delivery*.
- *PEEP valve*: When using > 5 cm H_2O PEEP, a PEEP valve should be used when suctioning the patient. Disconnecting the endotracheal tube will result in a loss of PEEP, a rapid reduction in the FRC, and alveolar flooding.
- Detrimental effects of PEEP include
  - Reduced venous return and cardiac output
  - Increased intracranial pressure
  - Reduction in hepatic and renal blood flow
  - Barotrauma
  - Increased intra-abdominal pressure
  - Fluid retention
  - Increased inspiratory workload
  - Increased extravascular lung water
  - Alveolar overdistention and reduction in PaO_2
  - Ileus
- *Auto-PEEP*: As with spontaneous ventilation, exhalation during mechanical ventilation is a passive event and continues until the

FRC is achieved. In patients with airflow limitation (asthma and chronic obstructive pulmonary disease) and in patients ventilated with reversed inspiration/expiration (I/E) ratios, a positive pressure breath may be initiated before exhalation is complete. This process leads to air trapping and intrinsic PEEP or auto-PEEP. Auto-PEEP is common in mechanically ventilated patients. Auto-PEEP increases intrathoracic pressure, thereby exacerbating the effects of positive-pressure ventilation. In patients with severe airflow limitation, severe auto-PEEP may develop. Patients may present with hemodynamic collapse similar to that of a tension pneumothorax. Auto-PEEP is treated by disconnecting the patient from the ventilator to "vent" the trapped air, and then changing the I/E ratio, allowing more time for exhalation. The presence of auto-PEEP cannot be detected unless the exhalation port venting to the atmosphere is occluded at end expiration (using a one-way valve). Some ventilators have an expiratory hold valve, enabling the auto-PEEP to be measured directly.

See Chapter 12; ventilatory strategies in ARDS (setting up PEEP and PCV).

■ INSPIRATORY WAVEFORMS

Most ventilators offer at least three different types of inspiratory flow patterns in the SIMV and AC modes of ventilation. These include

- A square wave: The inspiratory flow rises rapidly to a preset level and then stays at that level until the end of inspiration.
- A sinusoidal wave: The flow gradually increases and then decreases toward the end of inspiration.
- A descending ramp wave: The flow increases very rapidly and then decreases gradually until the end of inspiration. This pattern most closely mimics the normal inspiratory pattern.

In addition, the inspiratory wave can be modified by adjusting the inspiratory flow rate and inspiratory time and by providing an inspiratory pause (i.e., changing the I/E ratio).

■ INSPIRATORY-TO-EXPIRATORY RATIO

Some ventilators allow the operator to set the I/E ratio directly. Other ventilators allow adjustment of the I/E ratio by altering the flow rate, respiratory rate, and inspiratory time (including an inspiratory pause). For most adults, a normal I/E ratio of 1:2 or 1:3 is used. In patients with chronic obstructive lung disease and asthma, longer I/E ratios are necessary to allow the lungs time to exhale to resting FRC and to avoid hyperinflation.

Patients who are hypoxemic secondary to ARDS require increased mean airway pressure to increase the FRC and to allow more surface area for gas transfer to occur. This is achieved using both PEEP and inverse ratio ventilation. In addition, studies have demonstrated that prolonging inspiration can result in a more homogeneous distribution of ventilation within abnormal lungs. When the I/E ratio is increased to 1:1 or more, the inspiratory pressure is maintained for a longer period of time; however, the peak inspiratory pressure does not increase.

■ VENTILATOR TRIGGER VARIABLES

With most commonly used modes of mechanical ventilation (AC, SIMV, PSV) and CPAP, a set trigger sensitivity has to be reached before the ventilator delivers flow. Pressure and flow triggering are the most commonly used trigger variables.

With pressure triggering, a set negative pressure must be attained for the ventilator to deliver fresh gas into the inspiratory circuit (both a spontaneous breath [CPAP and SIMV] or a patient-triggered ventilator breath). This is usually set at $-2\,cm\ H_2O$. The higher (more negative) the trigger sensitivity, the harder the patient has to work to trigger a breath.

With flow triggering, two variables need to be set; the base flow rate and the flow sensitivity. The base flow consists of fresh gas that circulates continuously within the inhalation and exhalation circuit. The base flow for adults can be set between 5 and 20 L/min. The flow sensitivity can be set at a minimum of 1 L/min to one half the base flow. The initial demand for flow is satisfied by the base flow, while at the same time, generating the inspiratory flow signal according to the set flow sensitivity.

In both the healthy subject and the intubated patient, the inspiratory muscle work has been demonstrated to be significantly higher with pressure-triggered CPAP (without PSV) than with flow-triggered CPAP. However, pressure support of 5 cm H_2O has been demonstrated to reduce the inspiratory muscle work of pressure-triggered CPAP to a level comparable with that of flow-triggered CPAP.

■ MONITORING VENTILATED PATIENTS

- All patients receiving mechanical ventilation should be monitored by pulse oximetry.
- Arterial blood gas analysis should be performed during the initial ventilator adjustments and then when clinically indicated. The arterial saturation as measured by pulse oximetry provides adequate information for managing most ventilated patients. Patients with CO_2 retention and patients with complex metabolic derangements generally require regular arterial blood gasses. It is not necessary to perform an arterial blood gas analysis after every ventilator change.
- All the ventilator parameters, including peak airway pressure, should be recorded on the patient's flowchart hourly.
- The following formulas are useful in evaluating patients in respiratory failure:

  Age-predicted Pao_2 = Expected $Pao_2 - 0.3(age - 25)$ [expected Pao_2 at sea level is 100 mg/Hg]

  As a rough rule of thumb: Expected $Pao_2 \approx Fio_2$ (%) $\times 5$

  $AaDo_2 = (Fio_2 \times [BP - 47]) - (Pao_2 + Paco_2)$, where BP = barometric pressure

  The Pao_2/Fio_2 ratio is a better indicator of the degree of intrapulmonary shunting than the $AaDo_2$.

  $Vd/Vt = (Paco_2 - PEco_2) / Paco_2$ ($N = 0.2$–0.4)

■ SUDDEN INCREASE IN AIRWAY PRESSURE AND/OR FALL IN ARTERIAL SATURATION

Causes

- Blocked endotracheal tube
- Herniated endotracheal tube cuff
- Tension pneumothorax
- Kinked endotracheal tube
- Tube migration (right mainstem bronchus)
- Mucous plug with lobar atelectasis
- Patient biting down on tube
- Patient ventilator synchrony

Management

- Bag patient with 100% oxygen.
- Check position of endotracheal tube.

- Suction through endotracheal tube: If unable to pass catheter, then reintubate.
- Listen for tension pneumothorax: place chest drain if silent and deviated trachea.
- Urgent chest X-ray.
- If the most likely cause is patient/ventilator synchrony, increasing the sedation may alleviate the problem. A patient should never be paralyzed until the cause has been determined.

■ WHEN TO PERFORM A TRACHEOSTOMY IN THE VENTILATED PATIENT

No clear data aid in the timing and indications of tracheostomy. The complication and infection rate appear to be similar when comparing long-term (up to 6 weeks) endotracheal intubation with tracheostomy. Indications (relative) for tracheostomy include

- When prolonged endotracheal intubation is anticipated (i.e., >14 days)
- Patients with neurological diseases who are unable to protect their airway
- For bronchial toilet in patients who are unable to clear secretions
- Laryngeal edema from intubation

6

Weaning/Liberation from Mechanical Ventilation

■ GENERAL CONCEPTS

Weaning is the process by which a patient is removed from the ventilator. This process has also been referred to as *separation*, *liberation*, *withdrawal*, and *divorce from* the ventilator, as well as *discontinuation of* mechanical ventilation. The currently popular term is *liberation from mechanical ventilation*.

Studies suggest that physicians do not initiate weaning early enough and that more than 40% of the time that a patient receives mechanical ventilation is spent trying to wean the patient from the ventilator. The process of weaning, therefore, contributes significantly to a patient's length of stay and morbidity in the ICU. Furthermore, it is likely that the duration and outcome of weaning from mechanical ventilation are influenced by the weaning strategy chosen.

A number of studies have demonstrated that clinical judgment alone does not accurately predict whether mechanical ventilation can be discontinued successfully; the positive and negative predictive values of these assessments are only 50% and 67%, respectively. It has recently been demonstrated that screening patients daily to identify those who can breathe spontaneously will promote earlier weaning from mechanical ventilation. In addition, weaning protocols have been shown to be highly effective and reduce the length of the weaning process. This approach is favored.

The factors that need to be evaluated when considering weaning a patient from mechanical ventilation include the patient's underlying disease process, the reasons for intubation and mechanical ventilation in the first instance, the patient's level of consciousness, ability to protect his/her airway, pulmonary mechanics, and oxygenation defect. In many patients, ventilatory assistance need not be decreased gradually; mechanical ventilation and artificial airways can simply be removed (liberated). According to this thesis, patients can simply be removed from the ventilator once the disease process that led to intubation and mechanical ventilation has improved or resolved; a prolonged weaning process is therefore not required. However, in a proportion of patients, resuming spontaneous breathing without mechanical assistance is poorly tolerated. This is particularly so for patients with neuromuscular disorders and patients with advanced chronic lung disease with respiratory muscle dysfunction. These patients may benefit from conventional ventilator weaning, which should be considered as a respiratory muscle conditioning program. Short intervals of conditioning should be interspersed with generous rest periods, with patients resting at night.

Effect of Weaning on Oxygen Consumption and Cardiac Function

It has been demonstrated that oxygen consumption increases by about 15% when critically ill patients are switched from assist-control mechanical ventilation to spontaneous breathing continuous positive airway pressure (CPAP). The increased oxygen consumption is likely due to the increased mechanical load and the inefficiency of the respiratory muscles. This increased oxygen consumption must be met by an increased oxygen delivery. In patients who are unable to increase oxygen delivery, this may result in tissue hypoxia in vital organs due to a redistribution of blood flow. Mohsenifar and colleagues demonstrated the development of gastric intramucosal acidosis in patients who failed to be weaned from mechanical ventilation.

Positive-pressure ventilation (PPV) decreases left ventricular preload as well as left ventricular afterload. Therefore, PPV may improve left ventricular performance. Removing PPV results in both an increased cardiac demand and an increased workload on the heart. In patients with coronary artery disease (CAD), this may result in myocardial ischemia and pulmonary edema (which further increases pulmonary workload). Chatila et al. detected electrocardiographic evidence of cardiac ischemia in 10% of patients with a history of CAD who were being weaned. Evidence of myocardial ischemia was associated with a failure to wean in 22% of these patients. In patients with significant cardiac disease, T-tube weaning is not recommended, due to the significant increased work of breathing with this technique. Antianginal medication, inotropes, and diuretics may be useful in preventing both myocardial ischemia and failure, when weaning patients with CAD from the ventilator.

It should be recalled that the endotracheal tube provides the greatest resistance in the ventilator circuit (inversely related to radius).

During T-tube breathing, the already fatigued muscles have to work against an increased workload (the endotracheal tube), causing further fatigue. CPAP and flow-by reduce this work to some degree. In addition, there is a loss of laryngeal positive end-expiratory pressure (PEEP) with a reduction of (FRC) when using a T-tube. Patients should not be left on a T-bar for longer than 2 hours due to the increased work of breathing and respiratory muscle fatigue that can occur with this technique.

The Cuff Leak Test

The cuff leak test is performed in patients suspected of having laryngeal edema. The cuff of the endotracheal tube is deflated; if there is no laryngeal edema, the patient should be able to breathe around the tube. A patient with a positive cuff leak test (i.e., no leak) has approximately a 30% chance of developing postextubation stridor; however the risk is negligible in patients with a negative cuff leak test. The cuff leak test should be performed before extubation in the following circumstances:

- Traumatic intubation
- Prolonged intubation; i.e., longer than 5 to 7 days
- Patients with head and neck trauma
- Head and neck surgery
- Patients with previous failed extubation accompanied by stridor
- Patients with airway edema (e.g., angioedema)

Treatable Causes of Failure to Wean

- Hypophosphatemia.
- Hypokalemia.
- Hypomagnesemia.
- Hypocalcemia (ionized).
- Pulmonary edema.
- Inadequately treated angina.
- Anemia. In most ICU patients, a hematocrit >25 is adequate; however, patients with chronic obstructive pulmonary disease (COPD) may benefit from a hematocrit >30.
- Malnutrition.
- Overfeeding with excessive carbohydrate (increased CO_2 production). Change enteral feed to a formula with a higher fat content.

■ LIBERATION FROM MECHANICAL VENTILATION: AN APPROACH PROTOCOL

A number of different approaches to ventilator liberation have been reported; these are, however, largely variations on the same theme. The most popular method is described. According to this approach: (1) *All* ICU patients are screened daily by the respiratory therapist to determine if they are suitable for attempts at liberation. (2) Suitable patients then undergo a 3-minute T-tube trial, (3) followed by a 30-minute to 2-hour T-tube trial in those who pass the 3-minute test.

Step 1. Screening of Patients*

Candidates for the 3-minute spontaneous breathing trial

- Improvement or resolution of the underlying cause of respiratory failure
- Adequate gas exchange
    Non-COPD: a Pao_2 > 60 mm Hg with an Fio_2 of ≤0.4
        Pao_2/Fio_2 > 150)
    COPD: pH > 7.30, Pao_2 > 50 mm Hg with an Fio_2 of ≤0.35
- PEEP ≤5 cm H_2O
- Alert and cooperative patient
- Temperature <38°C
- No requirement for vasopressor agents
- Minimal or no sedative agents required
- Minute ventilation <15 L/min and respiratory rate <30
- Adequate cough during suctioning
- Heart rate <100 beats/min
- Systolic blood pressure >90 or <180 mm Hg

Step 2. Three-Minute T-tube/CPAP Trial

Patients who meet all the above criteria then undergo a 3-minute T-tube trial/CPAP. The Fio_2 is set at the same level as that used during mechanical ventilation. Alternatively, the patient may remain connected to the ventilator with flow-by and CPAP of 5 cm H_2O.

---

* *Note*: These are screening criteria; some patients who fail to meet these criteria may be candidates for the "3-minute trial" if approved by the ICU medical team.

Patients must fulfill all of the following criteria during the 3-minute T-tube/CPAP trial to progress to Step 3. The trial must be monitored by pulse oximetry and electrocardiography.

- Respiratory rate/tidal volume (liters) <105
- Respiratory rate >8 and <35
- Spontaneous tidal volume ≥4cc/kg
- Arterial saturation >90%
- Heart rate <140 or heart rate change (either direction) <20%; no arrhythmia

The trial must be stopped immediately when the patient fails to meet any of these criteria.

Step 3. Trial of Liberation

Patients with severe cardiac or pulmonary disease or patients who have been ventilated for longer than about 7 days may be better candidates for pressure support weaning (Step 3b); all other patients can be weaned by T-tube (Step 3a). All patients must be monitored with pulse oximetry and electrocardiography. The blood pressure should be measured every 30 minutes (in the absence of invasive hemodynamic monitoring). The tube feeds should be stopped at this point in time. Intravenous glucose must be given to prevent hypoglycemia.

Step 3a. T-Tube Weaning Trial

Patients continue to breathe through the T-piece/CPAP circuit. The Fio_2 may be increased up to 50%. The trial is terminated when

- Respiratory rate >35/min
- Arterial saturation <90
- Heart rate >140 or heart rate change (either direction) >20% or arrhythmias
- Systolic blood pressure >180 or <90
- Increased anxiety and diaphoresis

Should the patient tolerate the T-piece trial for 2 hours (some studies have used 30 minutes), then the patient may be extubated. The trial is repeated daily in those patients who fail to tolerate this spontaneous breathing trial. The time to liberation is not shortened by repeating the spontaneous breathing trial multiple times per day. The ICU team must be notified if the patient passes this phase of the liberation process and if an order is obtained to extubate the patient. Orogastric tubes, if present, should be removed to reduce the risk of aspiration. If gastric access is required, a nasogastric tube should be placed.

Step 3b. Pressure Support Weaning Trial

The level of pressure support is adjusted until the respiratory rate is ≤25. The level of pressure-support ventilation (PSV) is then gradually reduced as tolerated by the patient. The rate at which the PSV is reduced will depend on the patient's underlying disease and physiologic reserve. When one or more signs of poor tolerance appear, the level of PSV is increased back to the preceding level. When the patient can tolerate a PSV of 8 cm H_2O (or less) for ≥2 hours, the patient is then extubated. Orogastric tubes, if present, should be removed to reduce the risk of aspiration. If gastric access is required, a nasogastric tube should be placed.

■ TRADITIONAL WEANING

Several modes of partial ventilatory support have been proposed with the aim of gradually decreasing the level of mechanical assistance to eventually wean the patient from the ventilator. These methods include synchronized intermittent mandatory ventilation (SIMV), PSV, and a combination of the two. Several studies have been performed comparing the efficacy of SIMV, T-piece, and PSV weaning. No technique has proven superior to T-piece weaning.

SIMV weaning (with or without PSV) is performed by progressively reducing the SIMV rate until the patient is on CPAP. Once on CPAP, the endotracheal tube is removed. Studies suggest that this technique results in the longest duration of weaning, probably because the SIMV rate is reduced slowly.

PSV efficiently reduces the workload imposed on the respiratory muscles. Monitoring the respiratory rate and the use of accessory muscles allows the physician to find a satisfactory workload for the patient, avoiding excessive loading on the one hand and total rest of the respiratory muscles on the other. This technique allows the respiratory muscles to recover and progressively increase their strength. The level of assistance can be gradually decreased until it only compensates for the additional work imposed by the endotracheal tube and the demand valve of the ventilator (PSV of 5 to 10 cm H_2O), at which time tracheal extubation can be performed.

■ EARLY EXTUBATION FOLLOWED BY NONINVASIVE POSITIVE-PRESSURE VENTILATION IN COPD

Nava and colleagues reported a novel method of weaning COPD patients who required mechanical ventilation for respiratory failure.

These authors provided intensive medical management for 48 hours, followed by extubation at 48 hours, regardless of the patient's respiratory parameters. These early extubated patients were then treated with noninvasive positive-pressure ventilation until their respiratory function returned to baseline. The authors reported a high success rate with a shortened length of ICU stay, lower mortality, and decreased complication rate using this approach.

■ SELECTED REFERENCES

1. Brochard L, Rauss A, Benito S, et al. Comparison of three methods of gradual withdrawal from ventilatory support during weaning from mechanical ventilation. *Am J Respir Crit Care Med.* 1994;150:896–903.
2. Chatila W, Ani S, Guaglianone D, Jacob B, Amoateng-Adejepong Y, Manthous CA. Cardiac ischemia during weaning from mechanical ventilation. *Chest.* 1996;109:1577–1583.
3. Ely EW, Baker AM, Dunagan DP, et al. Effect on the duration of mechanical ventilation of identifying patients capable of breathing spontaneously. *N Engl J Med.* 1996;335:1864–1869.
4. Esteban A, Frutos F, Tobin MJ, et al. A comparison of four methods of weaning patients from mechanical ventilation. Spanish Lung Failure Collaborative Group. *N Engl J Med.* 1995;332:345–350.
5. Esteban A, Alia I, Tobin MJ, et al. Effect of spontaneous breathing trial duration on outcome of attempts to discontinue mechanical ventilation. *Am J Respir Crit Care Med.* 1999;159:512–518.
6. Esteban A, Alia I, Gordo F, et al. Extubation outcome after spontaneous breathing trials with T-tube or pressure support ventilation. The Spanish Lung Failure Collaborative Group. *Am J Respir Crit Care Med.* 1997; 156:459–465.
7. Hurford WE, Favorito F. Association of myocardial ischemia with failure to wean from mechanical ventilation. *Crit Care Med.* 1995;23:1475–1480.
8. Manthous CA, Schmidt GA, Hall JB. Liberation from mechanical ventilation. A decade of progress. *Chest.* 1998;114:886–901.
9. Mohsenifar Z, Hay A, Hay J, Lewis MI, Koerner SK. Gastric intramucosal pH as a predictor of sucess or failure in weaning patients from mechanical ventilation. *Ann Intern Med.* 1997;119:794–798.
10. Nava S, Ambrosino N, Clini E, et al. Noninvasive mechanical ventilation in the weaning of patients with respiratory failure due to chronic obstructive pulmonary disease. A randomized, controlled trial. *Ann Intern Med.* 1998; 128:721–728.
11. Wesley E, Baker AM, Dunagan DP, et al. Effect on the duration of mechanical ventilation of identifying patients capable of breathing spontaneously. *N Engl J Med.* 1996;335:1864–1869.

7

Acute Exacerbation of Chronic Obstructive Pulmonary Disease

Patients with chronic obstructive pulmonary disease (COPD) who acutely decompensate may benefit from admission to the ICU. Patients with COPD admitted to an ICU for an acute exacerbation of COPD have a hospital mortality between 10% and 25% with a 1-year mortality of about 40%. However, the need for mechanical ventilation appears not to influence either short- or long-term outcome; therefore, the need for mechanical ventilation should not be used as a reason for not offering respiratory support. Noninvasive positive-pressure ventilation (NPPV) is a viable alternative to endotracheal intubation in patients with a COPD exacerbation, and depending on the circumstances, this may be instituted on a general medical floor, a step-down unit, or in a medical ICU. NPPV should be considered in patients with severe COPD who have indicated their preference for the limitation of life-sustaining therapy.

■ COMMON PRECIPITATING EVENTS

Precipitating factors must be determined in patients with COPD who present with an acute deterioration in respiratory status. While chest infection is the most common precipitating factor, other readily treatable factors (e.g., atrial fibrillation, cardiac failure) should actively be investigated, including the following:

- Upper respiratory tract infection
- Chest infection: acute bronchitis or pneumonia
- Pneumothorax
- Pleural effusion
- Pulmonary embolus
- Heart failure

- Arrhythmias
- Atelectasis/mucous plugging

Lower airway colonization by bacteria is common in patients with stable COPD. *Hemophilus influenzae* (nontypable), *S. pneumonia* and *Moraxella catarrhalis* are the most common colonizing organisms. Approximately 20% of exacerbations of COPD are associated with viral infections; influenza, parainfluenza, and respiratory syncytial virus are the most common etiological agents. Recent studies using invasive diagnostic testing suggest that between 50% and 70% of exacerbations of COPD are related to bacterial infection. However, it is not possible to differentiate clinically those patients whose exacerbation of COPD is caused by a bacterial infection. *Hemophilus influenzae*, *S. pneumonia*, *M. catarrhalis*, and *Chlamydia pneumoniae* were the most common pathogens; however, gram-negative rods (including *Pseudomonas aeruginosa*) were isolated in a few patients. Gram stain and culture should therefore be performed in all patients admitted to the ICU with an exacerbation of COPD (not to diagnose infection but to isolate the potential pathogens).

■ TREATMENT

- Correct hypoxia; this usually requires only small increases in Fio_2 A high Pao_2 may cause an increase in CO_2; the mechanisms of this phenomenon are complex and include an increase in V/Q mismatching, the Haldane effect, and possibly a suppression of the "hypoxic drive." Patients with severe COPD developed chronic compensatory mechanisms for a low Pao_2 and therefore do not require a "normal" Pao_2; a Pao_2 between 50 and 60 mm Hg is usually well tolerated.
- An elevated $Paco_2$ is acceptable as long as the patient is alert and cooperative and the arterial pH >7.2.
- Empiric antibiotics are usually given even in the absence of clinical features of infection. Levofloxacin, azithromycin, and ceftriaxone are suitable choices. The antibiotics may need to be changed, guided by a postintubation tracheal aspirate culture and sensitivity result or results from lower respiratory tract sampling methods.
- Inhaled bronchodilators are usually given to all patients even if the patient does not have measurable reversible airway disease. Beta-2 agonists and ipratropium bromide should be used.
- A short course of intravenous corticosteroid has been shown to be beneficial even in patients with no demonstrable airway obstruction. Treatment with systemic glucocorticoids has been demonstrated to result in a moderate improvement in clinical

outcomes among patients hospitalized for an exacerbation of COPD.

- Recent studies have clearly demonstrated that in patients with an acute exacerbation of COPD, NPPV can reduce the need for endotracheal intubation, the length of hospital stay, and the in-hospital mortality rate. NPPV should be considered in all patients who are alert and cooperative and able to tolerate NPPV (see Chapter 4).
- Subcutaneous heparin.
- Treat cardiac failure, electrolyte disturbances, etc.
- Chest physiotherapy; directed at coughing and deep breathing, with chest percussion for atelectasis.
- Do not use sedative drugs unless the patient is on a ventilator.

Indications for NPPV

- Respiratory rate >30 breaths/min
- Pao_2 <45 to 50 mm Hg (RA)
- $Paco_2$ >45 to 50 mm Hg
- pH <7.32

Indications for Endotracheal Intubation

- Somnolence/decreased level of arousal
- Unable to protect airway
- Unable to deal with pulmonary secretions
- Failed trial of NPPV

■ SELECTED REFERENCES

1. Grossman RF. The value of antibiotics and the outcomes of antibiotic therapy in exacerbations of COPD. *Chest.* 1998;113:249S–255S.
2. Monso E, Ruiz J, Rosell A, et al. Bacterial infection in chronic obstructive pulmonary disease. A study of stable and exacerbated outpatients using the protected specimen brush. *Am J Respir Crit Care Med.* 1995;152:1316–1320.
3. Niewoehner DE, Erbland ML, Dupree RH, et al. Effect of systemic glucocorticoids on exacerbations of chronic obstructive pulmonary disease. Department of Veterans Affairs Cooperative Study Group. *N Engl J Med.* 1999;340:1941–1947.
4. Pela R, Marchesani F, Agostinelli C, et al. Airways microbial flora in COPD patients in stable clinical conditions and during exacerbations: a bronchoscopic investigation. *Monaldi Arch Chest Dis.* 1998;53:262–267.
5. Schentag JJ, Tillotson GS. Antibiotic selection and dosing for the treatment of acute exacerbations of COPD. *Chest.* 1997;112:314S–319S.
6. Soler N, Torres A, Ewig S, et al. Bronchial microbial patterns in severe exacerbations of chronic obstructive pulmonary disease (COPD) requiring mechanical ventilation. *Am J Respir Crit Care Med.* 1998;157:1498–1505.

8

Acute Severe Asthma

The response to initial treatment is an important predictor of a patient's course. Patients whose peak expiratory flow rates increase significantly within 2 hours of bronchodilator therapy in the emergency department have a lower incidence of hospital admission and are unlikely to require admission to the ICU.

■ INDICATIONS FOR ADMISSION TO THE ICU

- Difficulty talking due to breathlessness
- Altered level of consciousness
- Inability to lie supine
- Forced expiratory volume in 1 second (FEV_1) and/or peak flow <40% predicted
- Pulsus paradoxus >18 mm Hg
- Pneumothorax or pneumomediastinum
- Pao_2 <65 mm Hg on 40% O_2
- $Paco_2$ >40 mm Hg
- Patient tiring
- Poor (or no) response to initial bronchodilator therapy (<10% increase in peak expiratory flow rate)

The classic signs of wheezing correlate poorly with the degree of airflow limitation. Severely obstructed patients may have a silent chest if there is insufficient alveolar ventilation and airflow for wheezes to occur. In these patients, the development of wheezes generally indicates improved airflow. Localized wheezing or crackles on chest auscultation may represent mucous plugging or atelectasis, but they should prompt consideration of pneumonia, pneumothorax, endo-bronchial lesions, or a foreign body.

Initial Treatment

- Oxygen mask
- Beta-2 agonist by nebulization every 15 to 20 minutes initially, then 1 to 4 hourly
- Corticosteroids: methylprednisolone 60 mg IV q6h
- Ipratropium bromide nebulization, q2–4h, has synergistic bron-chodilatory activity with beta-2 agonists
- Theophylline (use controversial): use if no ischemic heart disease, FEV_1 and/or peak flow <30% predicted, and/or altered level of consciousness

  Theophylline has a narrow therapeutic index; therefore, the serum level should be monitored in all critically ill patients.

  If the patient is receiving maintenance theophylline, obtain a baseline theophylline level before starting theophylline.

  Loading dose is 5 mg/kg given over 30 minutes (if not on main-tenance theophylline).

  Maintenance dose of 0.4 to 0.8 mg/kg/h:

    0.4 mg/kg/h in patients with chronic obstructive pulmonary disease (COPD), heart failure, and liver dysfunction

    0.6 mg/kg/h in nonsmoking asthmatics

    0.8 mg/kg/h in asthmatics who smoke

  Aim for theophylline level of 10 to 15 μg/mL

  In refractory patients, a level of 15 to 20 μg/mL may offer some therapeutic advantage. The dose–response curve for theo-phylline is curvilinear. The level at which toxicity occurs is variable, however, and therefore all patients should be monitored for signs of toxicity.

- Do not use sedative drugs unless the patient is on a ventilator. If the patient has a large psychosomatic component to his/her asthma and sedative drugs are deemed necessary, use small doses and observe closely in an ICU.
- Keep the patient well hydrated.

Larger and more frequent doses of beta-agonists are needed in acute severe asthma because the dose–response curve and duration of activity of these drugs are affected adversely by the degree of bron-choconstriction. Recent data suggest that in both nonintubated and intubated patients metered dose inhalers combined with a spacing device are just as effective as nebulizers, and they are quicker and cheaper to use (four to six puffs of albuterol every 20 minutes).

Subcutaneously administered epinephrine or terbutaline sulphate has no advantage over inhaled beta-agonists. Subcutaneous therapy should be considered, however, in patients not responding to inhaled beta-agonists. Furthermore, the available data do not support the routine use of intravenous beta-agonists in the treatment of patients with severe asthma. Several studies have demonstrated inhaled therapy to be equal to or better than intravenous (IV) therapy in treating airflow obstruction and less likely to cause cardiac toxicity. However, IV beta-agonists may be considered in patients who have not responded to inhaled therapy and have life-threatening disease.

The role of theophylline and its pathophysiological mechanism of action in asthma is unclear. An analysis of the trials that have evaluated the use of theophylline in the emergency room treatment of asthma leads one to conclude that the evidence is inadequate to either support or reject the use of theophylline in this setting. However, it is possible that theophylline benefits patients in ways distinct from bronchodilation such as through anti-inflammatory or effects on respiratory muscle function. Phosphodiesterase inhibitors decrease tumor necrosis factor α mRNA in response to stimuli such as endotoxin; this may partly explain the drug's anti-inflammatory action. The available data do not support the routine use of magnesium in the treatment of severe asthma. However, magnesium can be considered in patients who have failed standard therapy (2 g in 10 mL dextrose in water over 5 minutes, followed by 4 g in 200 mL dextrose in water over 2 hours; halve the dose in patients with renal dysfunction). Because respiratory tract infections that trigger asthma are usually viral, there is no role for the routine use of antibiotics.

■ OTHER THERAPEUTIC OPTIONS

- IV beta-2 agonists.
- Subcutaneous epinephrine 0.3 mL 1:1000 solution (drug of choice in anaphylactoid asthma). Epinephrine should be avoided in patients with a history of ischemic heart disease and/or hypertension.
- Heliox is a blend of helium and oxygen (80:20, 70:30, or 60:40), with a gas density approximately one third that of air. In normal subjects, Heliox reduces airway resistance (raw) by about 40% and increases maximum expiratory flows by about 50%. Heliox may be useful in buying time and avoiding intubation in acute attacks of asthma. In mechanically ventilated patients with severe asthma, Heliox (60:40) has been demonstrated to reduce peak inspiratory pressure and $Paco_2$ by up to 50%.
- Mechanically ventilated patients with severe bronchospasm in whom mechanical ventilation has become extremely difficult (cannot get air in or out) may benefit from halothane or enflu-

rane anesthesia. This procedure should be performed only in the operating room by an experienced anesthesiologist. Halothane/enflurane anesthesia can dramatically reduce bronchospasm even in patients with slow-onset asthma. It is important to ensure that the patient is well hydrated (to minimize halothane-induced hypotension). The concentration of halothane is gradually increased as blood pressure allows and maintained at anesthetic concentrations until ventilation improves and airway pressures decrease. The halothane should be weaned slowly to prevent recurrence of bronchospasm.

- In patients in extremis, extracorporeal lung assist has proven to be lifesaving. Both percutaneous venoarterial and venovenous bypass have been reported in patients with refractory status asthmaticus.

■ COMPLICATIONS OF ACUTE ASTHMA

- Pneumothorax
- Pneumomediastinum, pneumopericardium
- Myocardial infarction
- Mucous plugging
- Atelectasis
- Theophylline toxicity
- Electrolyte disturbances: hypokalemia, hypophosphatemia, hypomagnesemia
- Lactic acidosis
- Myopathy

■ NONINVASIVE POSITIVE-PRESSURE VENTILATION IN STATUS ASTHMATICUS

Patients with severe asthma have a significant increase in both inspiratory and expiratory indexes of airway obstruction and considerable dynamic compliance. Inspiratory muscle failure and increased physiologic dead space lead to ventilatory failure. Endotracheal intubation is associated with a high rate of complications and results in increased airway resistance. In patients with COPD with acute respiratory failure, noninvasive positive-pressure ventilation (NPPV) has been demonstrated to be very effective in reducing the work of breathing, in oxygenation, and in the need for intubation. Several studies have demonstrated that in severe asthma, continuous positive airway pressure (CPAP) mask causes (1) bronchodilation and decreases airway resistance, (2) reexpands atelectasis and promotes removal of secretions, (3) rests the diaphragm and inspiratory muscles and may offset intrinsic positive end-expiratory pressure (iPEEP), and (4) decreases the adverse hemodynamic effects of large negative peak and mean inspiratory pleural pressures. Meduri et al. have demonstrated that NPPV can safely be applied to patients with severe asthma and hypercarbia whose condition has failed to improve with aggressive medical management. In their series, only 2 of 17 patients required intubation. It may be reasonable to try NPPV before intubation in alert cooperative patients (see guidelines on NPPV, Chapter 4). NPPV should not be attempted in patients who are rapidly deteriorating or are somnolent or confused.

Indications for Intubation

Endotracheal intubation is not curative, is associated with significant morbidity, and can increase the degree of airway narrowing and inflammation. The timing of intubation is essentially one of clinical judgment. A high $Paco_2$ in itself is not an indication for intubation if the patient is alert and cooperative and the arterial pH is >7.2. The following are indications for intubation and mechanical ventilation:

- Altered consciousness
- Pao_2 <50 mm Hg on a rebreathing mask
- Rising $Paco_2$ with a falling pH
- Anaphylactic asthma with rapidly deteriorating clinical course
- Patient fatigue

Intubating an asthmatic patient can be extremely difficult and should be performed by an operator with extensive experience in upper airway management. It should be remembered that it may be impossible to ventilate a severe asthmatic with an Ambubag (air will follow the path of least resistance and go into the stomach). A blind nasal intubation is reasonably safe when performed by an operator experienced in this technique (beware nasal polyps). Orotracheal intubation will invariably require rapid-sequence anesthesia.

Ketamine—an IV general anesthetic agent with sedative, analgesic, anesthetic, and bronchodilating properties—has been used successfully for the emergent intubation of patients with severe asthma. The usual dose of ketamine, 1 to 2 mg/kg, generally provides 10 to 15 minutes of general anesthesia without significant respiratory depression. Ketamine increases laryngeal reflexes and does not block laryngeal reflexes; thus, particular care must be taken to avoid laryngospasm and aspiration.

Mechanical Ventilation

Mechanical ventilation of patients with severe asthma is fraught with difficulties. Severe airflow obstruction results in a prolonged expiratory time with incomplete exhalation even at low ventilator rates. This results in progressive dynamic hyperinflation and the development of auto-PEEP (i-PEEP), until a new equilibrium is reached at some volume above functional residual capacity (FRC). This equilibrium occurs because increasing lung volume increases both the lung elastic recoil pressure driving expiratory flow and reduced airway resistance by expansion of the small airways in parallel with lung volume. If conventional tidal volumes and rates are used, significant i-PEEP will develop. i-PEEP acts as an inspiratory threshold load and contributes to the increased work of breathing. Furthermore, i-PEEP may be associated with severe hemodynamic compromise. These effects are compounded by the fact that the minute ventilation required for normocapnia is increased to approximately 16 ± 3 L/min in patients with severe asthma. These changes will result in increased morbidity and morality if patients are ventilated to achieve normocapnia.

The use of PEEP (extrinsic PEEP) in patients with asthma is controversial. PEEP has been demonstrated to reduce the work of breathing and dyspnea in patients with severe COPD and acute respiratory failure. Because flow is limited in the small airways, low levels of pressure applied downstream from the compression site may alter its anatomic location without causing a proportional rise in alveolar pressure. PEEP that is set at a level below iPEEP might then dilate collapsed or severely narrowed airways, enabling decompression of the alveolar units they serve. In addition, this will narrow the gradient between end-expiratory alveolar pressure (total PEEP) and the pressure in the central airways. This would then reduce the effort required to trigger the ventilator. However, PEEP has been demonstrated to increase lung volumes and alveolar pressures with a concomitant fall in venous return and hypotension. A practical method of identifying those patients who may benefit from PEEP may be to observe the response of the ventilator cycling pressures to small increments of PEEP. If little change in peak dynamic and static cycling pressures occurs after PEEP, then extensive dynamic collapse is unlikely and PEEP may be helpful. The level of PEEP should not be set higher than the level of the original i-PEEP. On the other hand, if the cycling pressures increase in direct relationship to the level of applied PEEP, additional hyperinflation will develop.

It is rarely a problem to oxygenate the patient with severe asthma; the problem is one of achieving adequate alveolar ventilation. The goals of ventilatory therapy include the following:

- Keep the peak airway pressure <50 cm H_2O.
- Maintain arterial pH > 7.2.
- Limit iPEEP to <5 to 10 cm H_2O.
- If the patient is not paralyzed, the synchronized intermittent mandatory ventilation mode with no or very low pressure support is recommended. The assist-control ventilation should not be used, because it can lead the patient to generate excessive minute ventilation, resulting in excessive iPEEP.
- The setting of the inspiratory flow rate remains controversial, with both high and low flow rates being recommended. The weight of evidence appears to favor a high inspiratory flow. However, in patients with severe airway obstruction, a prolonged inspiratory time may be required; a high flow rate will result in excessive pressures in these patients.

Initial Ventilator Settings

- Fio_2 60% to 80%
- Rate 8 to 12/min, depending on the degree of airway obstruction
- Peak flow 80 to 100 L/min
- Tidal volume 6 to 8 mL/kg

The iPEEP and the exhaled tidal volumes must be measured in all patients to avoid significant air trapping. A low I/E ratio (long expiration) should always be used. Permissive hypoventilation should be used in patients with severe airway obstruction; the arterial pH, however, should be kept above 7.20. Sodium bicarbonate boluses may make matters worse (increased intracellular CO_2 and acidosis) due to the fixed CO_2 elimination and should be avoided.

- Atelectasis should be treated by aggressive chest physiotherapy. Bronchoscopy is potentially dangerous in intubated asthmatic patients.
- Maintain adequate rehydration and maintain preload.
- Propofol is a very useful sedative drug and may be used in combination with a benzodiazepine and/or fentanyl to avoid the use of a paralytic agent. The combination of high-dose corticosteroids and neuromuscular blocking agents has been reported to lead to a severe necrotizing myopathy. If neuromuscular blocking drugs are required, their activity needs to be closely monitored and the drug stopped as soon as feasible (see guidelines on the use of neuromuscular blocking agents). Avoid pancuronium, which causes histamine release and is vagolytic.
- Monitor for barotrauma.

■ SELECTED REFERENCES

1. Corbridge TC, Hall JB. The assessment and management of adults with status asthmaticus. *Am J Respir Crit Care Med.* 1995;151:1296–1316.
2. Marii J. Should PEEP be used in airflow obstruction. *Am Rev Respir Dis.* 1989;140:1–3.
3. McFadden. Dosages of corticosteroids in asthma. *Am Rev Respir Dis.* 1993; 147:1306–1310.
4. Meduri GU, Cook TR, Turner RE, Cohen M, Leeper KV. Noninvasive positive pressure ventilation in status asthmaticus. *Chest.* 1996;110:767–774.
5. Petrof BJ, Legare M, Goldberg P, Milic-Emili J, Gottfried SB. Continuous positive airway pressure reduces work of breathing and dyspnea during weaning from mechanical ventilation in severe chronic obstructive pulmonary disease. *Am Rev Respir Dis.* 1990;141:281–289.
6. Tuxen DV. Detrimental effects of positive end-expiratory pressure during controlled mechanical ventilation of patients with severe airflow obstruction. *Am Rev Respir Dis.* 1989;140:5–9.
7. Tuxen D, Lane S. The effects of ventilatory pattern on hyperinflation, airways pressures, and circulation in mechanical ventilation of patients with severe airflow obstruction. *Am Rev Respir Dis.* 1987;136:872–879.
8. Weinberger M, Hendeles L. Theophylline in asthma. *N Engl J Med.* 1996; 334:1380–1388.

9

Severe Community-Acquired Pneumonia

In the United States, community-acquired pneumonia (CAP) in adults results in approximately 600,000 hospital admissions annually and ranks as the sixth leading cause of death. Of those patients with CAP hospitalized, between 18% and 36% require treatment in an ICU. The mortality of these patients is about 35%. While approximately 20% of patients admitted to the ICU with CAP are in septic shock, the mortality of these patients may be as high as 60%.

Poor Prognostic Factors and Indications for Admission to the ICU

- Age >60 years
- $30 <$ white blood cell count $< 4 \times 10^9$/L
- Blood urea nitrogen >20 mg/dL
- Pao_2 <60 mm Hg (room air)
- Multilobe involvement
- Respiratory rate >30/min
- Diastolic blood pressure <60 mm Hg
- Platelet <80,000 $\times 10^9$/L

Noninfectious diseases masquerading as CAP should be excluded, namely

- Bronchiolitis obliterans organizing pneumonia (BOOP)
- Eosinophilic pneumonia
- Hypersensitivity pneumonia
- Drug-induced pneumonitis: methotrexate, nitrofurantoin, gold, amiodarone
- Pulmonary vasculitis
- Pulmonary embolism/infarction
- Pulmonary malignancy

- Radiation pneumonitis
- Tuberculosis

A knowledge of the spectrum of pathogens (and their sensitivity profiles) implicated in severe CAP is important, because initial broad-spectrum empiric therapy, directed at the known spectrum of likely pathogens, is associated with an improved outcome, while identification of a specific etiologic pathogen with targeted antimicrobial therapy has not been shown to improve outcome (Figure 9-1). Indeed, Leroy and colleagues demonstrated that ineffective initial antimicrobial therapy was an independent predictor of mortality in patients with severe CAP. A review of those studies that have investigated the etiological diagnosis in patients with severe CAP have isolated a pathogen in approximately 60% of patients, with the infection being polymicrobial in about 17% of patients. In these studies, the most common pathogen was pneumococcus (15% to 46%), followed by *Legionella* species (0% to 23%), *Staphylococcus aureus* (0 to 22%), *Hemophilus influenzae* (0 to 14%), and gram-negative bacilli (4% to 25%). There is controversy as to whether *Legionella* is uniformly present in all settings, or if it has specific geographic and epidemiologic foci. Moine and colleagues diagnosed *Legionella* infection in only 3% of patients with

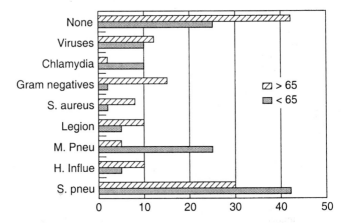

Figure 9-1. Spectrum of pathogens associated with community-acquired pneumonia stratified by age.

severe CAP, while Leroy et al., in a study of 299 patients, failed to diagnose *Legionella* in a single case. The role of *Pseudomonas aeruginosa*, *Acinetobacter baumannii*, and enteric gram-negatives in severe CAP is unclear. Indeed, it has been previously commented that "*CAP is not caused by certain organisms even in abnormal hosts, including Proteus, Enterobacter, or Pseudomonas.*" However, Torres et al. isolated *P. aeruginosa* in 5 of 42 (12%) patients with CAP. Similarly, other studies have found *Pseudomonas* to be an important pathogen in patients with severe CAP. It appears that *Proteus, Enterobacter, Pseudomonas, Acinetobacter*, and other gram-negatives are more common in alcoholic patients with severe CAP. It should also be noted that the prevalence of *Legionella* and gram-negative bacteria increase with advancing age and underlying co-morbidities.

■ MICROBIOLOGICAL DIAGNOSIS

- Bronchoscopy and protected specimen brush sampling (or lavage) *before* commencing antibiotic therapy is probably the most sensitive and specific diagnostic method. This is, however, extremely invasive and not routinely indicated.
- Sputum Gram stain and culture has a sensitivity of about 20%, with a specificity of over 90%. This is a cheap test and should be performed in all patients with pneumonia who have a productive cough. If the patient is not productive, therapy should not be withheld until a specimen can be obtained.
- Blood cultures are positive in about 20% of patients with pneumococcal pneumonia and in <10% of patients with gram-negative pneumonia. Blood cultures should be drawn in all but the mildest cases of pneumonia.
- *Legionella* urinary antigen, serology and direct fluorescent antibody (DFA) on bronchoscopic specimens.
- Serology for *Chlamydia pneumonia*.

■ OTHER LABORATORY TESTS

Patients with previously undiagnosed human immunodeficiency virus (HIV) infection may develop severe CAP. The Centers for Disease Control currently recommends testing for HIV infection in patients between the ages of 15 and 55 years who present with CAP. Abnormalities in liver function tests and electrolytes (especially phosphate) are common in patients with severe pneumonia; these tests are therefore warranted in all patients with severe CAP.

■ ANTIBIOTIC TREATMENT

The empiric antibiotic treatment of CAP and severe CAP is somewhat controversial and problematic. The current guidelines of the American Thoracic Society and Infectious Disease Society of America differ somewhat and do not take into account the rapidly changing resistence patterns of *Streptococcus pneumoniae*. As *S. pneumoniae* is the major pathogen implicated in CAP, it is essential that the local sensitivity patterns be known before deciding on empiric treatment protocols for CAP.

Currently in the United States, approximately 30% of pneumococci are of intermediate resistance, and 16% to 20% show high-grade penicillin resistance. Most disturbing is the fact that 30% of total isolates are resistant to macrolides (67% of high-grade isolates). The isolates with high-grade penicillin resistance are also usually resistant to amoxicillin-clavulanic acid, cefuroxime, and ceftriaxone. Currently in the United States, all penicillin isolates are reported to be susceptible to levofloxacin and vancomycin. As a result of these data, macrolides can no longer be considered the empiric antibiotic of choice in CAP and severe CAP. Furthermore, unless the local sensitivity patterns differ from the national patterns, levofloxacin should be considered the empiric agent of choice for both CAP and severe CAP. The addition of nafcillin should be considered in patients with a prior history of an upper respiratory tract infection during the influenza season and ceftazidime in alcoholic patients.

■ PERSISTENT TEMPERATURE ON ANTIBIOTIC TREATMENT

A common misconception is that the patient's temperature should settle within 24 hours of commencing antibiotic therapy. It has been demonstrated that it may take up to 72 hours for the temperature to normalize in a patient with pneumococcal pneumonia. However, in a patient with a widely swinging temperature, it would be prudent to exclude a complication within this time frame. The following are the major reasons for a failure to respond to antimicrobial agents:

- Wrong antibiotic: wrong spectrum or drug resistance
- Wrong dosage
- Viral, fungal, or opportunistic pathogen
- Superadded complication
    Complicated pleural effusion/empyema
    Endocarditis
    Purulent pericarditis
    Septic arthritis
    Meningitis, etc.

Complicated Pleural Effusion/Empyema

When pleural fluid is detected in a patient with pneumonia, a diagnostic thoracocentesis should always be performed to rule out pleural space infection (except if the effusion is very small). Pleural fluid studies differentiate between a benign parapneumonic effusion and an early empyema (complicated pleural effusion). Drainage is necessary when the pleural fluid is grossly purulent or if pleural fluid studies show any of the following:

- pH < 7.2 (most sensitive indicator)
- Glucose <40 mg/dL
- White cell count >10,000/mL

Chest tube drainage alone often fails because the fluid is loculated with fibrinous adhesions, necessitating surgical drainage. However, chest tube drainage together with the intrapleural instillation of streptokinase (250,000 IU daily for 3 days) has been demonstrated to aid the treatment of pleural infections by improving pleural drainage without causing systemic fibrinolysis or local hemorrhage and by reducing the requirement for surgery.

■ SELECTED REFERENCES

1. Bartlett JG, Breiman BR, Mandell LA, File TM. Community-acquired pneumonia in adults: Guidelines for management. *Clin Infect Dis*. 1998;26:811–838.
2. Davies RJ, Traill ZC, Gleeson FV. Randomised controlled trial of intrapleural streptokinase in community acquired pleural infection. *Thorax*. 1997;52:416–421.
3. Guidelines for the initial management of adults with community-acquired pneumonia: diagnosis, assessment of severity and initial antimicrobial therapy. *Am Rev Respir Dis*. 1993;148:1418–1426.
4. Harwell JI, Brown RB. The drug-resistant pneumococcus. Clinical relevance, therapy and prevention. *Chest*. 2000;117:530–541.
5. Henke CA, Leatherman JW. Intrapleurally administered streptokinase in the treatment of acute loculated nonpurulent parapneumonic effusions. *Am Rev Respir Dis*. 1992;145:680–684.
6. Leroy O, Santre C, Beuscart C, et al. A five-year study of severe community-acquired pneumonia with emphasis on prognosis in patients admitted to an intensive care unit. *Intensive Care Med*. 1995;21:24–31.
7. Leroy O, Vandenbussche C, Coffinier C, et al. Community-acquired aspiration pneumonia in intensive care units. Epidemiological and prognosis data. *Am J Respir Crit Care Med*. 1997;156:1922–1929.
8. Moine P, Vercken JB, Chevret S, Gajdos P. Severe community-acquired pneumococcal pneumonia. The French Study Group of Community-Acquired Pneumonia in ICU. *Scand J Infect Dis*. 1995;27:201–206.
9. Niederman MS. Severe community-acquired pneumonia: what do we need to know to effectively manage patients? *Intensive Care Med*. 1996;22:1285–1287.

10. Rudin ML, Michael JR, Huxley EJ. Community-acquired acinetobacter pneumonia. *Am J Med*. 1979;67:39–43.
11. Thornsberry C, Hickey ML, Kahn J, Mauritz Y, Sahm DF. Surveillance of antimicrobial resistance among respiratory tract pathogens in the United States, 1997 to 1998. *Drugs*. 1999;58(suppl 2):361–363.
12. Torres A, Serra-Bataille J, Ferrer A et al. Severe community-acquired pneumonia epidemiology and prognostic factors. *Am Rev Respir Dis*. 1991;144: 312–318.

10

Ventilator-Associated Pneumonia

Ventilator-associated pneumonia (VAP) occurs in approximately 25% of patients undergoing mechanical ventilation. The impact of VAP on patient outcome has been much debated; however, Fagon and colleagues reported an attributable mortality of 27%. The optimal management of patients with suspected VAP requires confirmation of the diagnosis and identification of the responsible pathogen(s) to provide appropriate antimicrobial therapy. The diagnosis of VAP remains one of the most difficult clinical dilemmas in critically ill mechanically ventilated patients. Many conditions may either obscure or give rise to a clinical picture similar to that of pneumonia in the mechanically ventilated patient. A fever, pulmonary infiltrate, and purulent tracheobronchial secretions are almost diagnostic of pneumonia in a previously healthy nonintubated patient. However, this constellation of features, while suggestive, is not diagnostic of pneumonia in mechanically ventilated patients. Using multivariate analysis, Fagon and colleagues demonstrated that no combination of clinical, laboratory, or radiographic findings could accurately predict which patients had VAP.

A number of invasive and minimally invasive techniques have been reported to aid in the diagnosis of VAP. The number of methods currently available attests to the fact that no single method is ideal. The optimal technique(s) for diagnosis of VAP remains unclear, and a uniformly agreed upon gold standard for the diagnosis is lacking. Bronchoscopic protected specimen brushing (PSB) with quantitative culture has, however, become recognized as the standard with which to compare other techniques.

The impact of diagnostic tests for VAP on patient outcome is controversial. Using a decision analysis method, Sterling and co-authors demonstrated that invasive or semi-invasive microbiological diagnostic techniques improved the outcome of patients with suspected VAP.

However, three independent studies have demonstrated that the most important factor affecting outcome in patients with VAP is the early initiation of appropriate antibiotic therapy. In the study by Luna et al., the mortality of patients who were changed from inadequate antibiotic therapy to appropriate therapy based on the results of a bronchoalveolar lavage (BAL) was comparable to the mortality of those patients who continued to receive inadequate therapy. Recently, Fagon and colleagues performed a large, multicenter randomized, controlled clinical trial, in which patients with suspected VAP were randomized to an invasive (bronchoscopic PSB/BAL) or noninvasive strategy. The patients in the invasive group received fewer antibiotics and had a lower 28-day mortality (30.9 vs. 38.8%). This study provides convincing evidence in favor of an invasive (or semi-invasive) strategy in the diagnosis of VAP. It is important to note that an invasive (or semi-invasive) diagnostic approach will result in a change in antibiotics in about 25% of patients with pneumonia and allow the discontinuation of antibiotics in those patients who are proven not to have pneumonia. This will result in significant cost savings and have an impact on the selection of resistant organisms.

Culture of endotracheal aspirates (sputum culture) is routinely requested for ICU patients, even for those patients without pulmonary infiltrates. These patients are frequently treated with antibiotics based on the results of the sputum culture. However, the specificity of sputum culture in the diagnosis of VAP is only approximately 50% (the same as flipping a coin but infinitely more expensive). Because of the lack of specificity of sputum culture, quantitative culture of endotracheal aspirates has been proposed as a simple and noninvasive method of diagnosing VAP. The operating characteristics of this technique are, however, unclear, with some studies showing a poor sensitivity, specificity, and predictive values, while others have demonstrated good characteristics. Furthermore, when quantitative culture of endotracheal aspirates correctly identifies patients with pneumonia, it is frequently difficult to determine which microorganisms present in the culture are responsible for the pneumonia.

Several factors limit the routine use of bronchoscopic-directed PSB and/or BAL in the clinical setting; bronchoscopy is expensive (about $1000), time-consuming, and not readily available in many ICUs. Delay in obtaining specimens by bronchoscopy may delay institution of appropriate antibiotic therapy. Furthermore, bronchoscopy is not without risks in patients requiring high levels of positive end-expiratory-pressure and high fractional inspired oxygen concentrations. Recently, a number of studies have examined the utility of nonbronchoscopic PSB as well as nonbronchoscopic BAL in the diagnosis of VAP. These studies have found that results obtained from these "blind" techniques are comparable to those obtained with the bronchoscope. Furthermore, studies have shown that respiratory therapists can safely and reliably perform these procedures in patients with respiratory failure requiring mechanical ventilation.

■ RECOMMENDED APPROACH TO THE PATIENT WITH SUSPECTED VAP

Patients with suspected *Pneumocystis carinii* pneumonia and/or neutropenic patients should undergo formal bronchoscopy with PSB and BAL. Tracheal aspirates are suitable specimens in patients with suspected tuberculosis. *Postintubation* tracheal aspirate culture may be useful for the diagnosis of CAP and exacerbation of chronic obstructive pulmonary disease. Patients with suspected VAP should undergo invasive or semi-invasive lower respiratory tract sampling.

Indications for Invasive or Semi-invasive Lower Respiratory Tract Sampling

1. Patient intubated for >48 hours
2. *New or progressive* pulmonary infiltrate on the chest radiograph (clear chest radiograph precludes diagnosis of pneumonia and performance of PSB)
3. At least two of the following clinical criteria:
   Fever ≥38.3°C (≥101°F)
   Leukocytosis (>10 × 10^9/L)
   Purulent tracheal secretions

Empiric Antibiotics Until Culture Data Available

The choice of empiric antibiotics is extremely important in determining the outcome of patients with VAP, and it should be based on local epidemiological data as well as national/international data. A consistent pattern of pathogens has been reported in the literature in patients with VAP. The most common pathogen is *Staphylococcus aureus* followed by *Pseudomonas aeruginosa* and then *Enterobacter* spp., *Streptococcus pneumonia, Hemophilus influenzae, Escherichia coli, Klebsiella* spp., and *Acinetobacter baumannii. P. aeruginosa* and *A. baumannii* are more common in patients intubated >4 days, while *S. pneumonia* and *H. influenzae* are more common in patients intubated for ≤ 4 days. Anaerobes have been shown to be unimportant in most patients with VAP. The following generic guidelines are based on the above cited information:

Empiric Antibiotic Coverage

> *Vancomycin or oxacillin* (or equivalent if MRSA is not endemic) *and* *gram-negative coverage* (double cover if *Pseudomonas* is endemic in the ICU) or *levofloxacin* (if MRSA is not endemic): For example, vancomycin or oxacillin *plus* ceftazidime or ciprofloxacin or imipenem or piperacillin/tazobactam.

Kollef and colleagues demonstrated that a scheduled change of antibiotic class for the treatment of suspected or proven gram-negative infections in the ICU can reduce both the incidence of VAP and the incidence of VAP attributed to antibiotic-resistant gram-negative bacteria.

In patients with positive and borderline positive cultures, the antibiotic regimen *must be* tailored according to the sensitivities of the pathogen(s) isolated. In patients with negative cultures, the decision to continue or stop the antibiotics should be made by the patients' attending physicians based on their assessment of the risk of stopping antibiotics. However, it is recommended that unless VAP is strongly suspected, antibiotics be stopped and patients recultured if a strong index of suspicion for VAP still exists.

Nosocomial Cytomegalovirus Infection in Nonimmunocompromised ICU Patients (See Chapter 44)

■ SELECTED REFERENCES

1. Bello S, Tajada A, Chacon E, et al. "Blind" protected specimen brushing versus bronchoscopic techniques in the aetiolological diagnosis of ventilator-associated pneumonia. *Eur Respir J*. 1996;9:1494–1499.
2. Chastre J, Trouillet JL, Fagon JY. Diagnosis of pulmonary infections in mechanically ventilated patients. *Semin Respir Infect*. 1996;11:65–76.
3. Fagon JY, Chastre J, Hance AJ, Montravers P, Novara A, Gibert C. Nosocomial pneumonia in ventilated patients: a cohort study evaluating attributable mortality and hospital stay. *Am J Med*. 1993;94:281–288.
4. Fagon JY, Chastre J, Hance AJ, Domart Y, Trouillet JL, Gibert C. Evaluation of clinical judgement in the identification and treatment of nosocomial pneumonia in ventilated patients. *Chest*. 1993;103:547–553.
5. Fagon JY, Chastre J, Wolff M, et al. Invasive and non-invasive strategies for management of suspected ventilator-associated pneumonia. *Ann Intern Med*. 2000;132:621–630.
6. Kollef MH, Ward S. The influence of mini-BAL cultures on patient outcomes. Implications for the antibiotic management of ventilator-associated pneumonia. *Chest*. 1998;113:412–420.
7. Kollef MH, Bock KR, Richards RD, Hearns ML. The safety and diagnostic accuracy of minibronchoalveolar lavage in patients with suspected ventilator-associated pneumonia. *Ann Intern Med*. 1995;122:743–748.

8. Kollef MH, Vlasnik J, Sharpless L, Pasque C, Murphy D, Fraser V. Scheduled change of antibiotic classes: a strategy to decrease the incidence of ventilator-associated pneumonia. *Am J Respir Crit Care Med*. 1997; 156:1040–1048.

9. Luna CM, Vujacich P, Niederman MS, et al. Impact of BAL data on the therapy and outcome of ventilator-associated pneumonia. *Chest*. 1997;111:676–685.

10. Marik PE, Brown WJ. A comparison of bronchoscopic vs blind protected specimen brush sampling in patients with suspected ventilator-associated pneumonia. *Chest*. 1995;108:203–207.

11. Marik PE, Careau P. A comparison of mini-bronchoalveolar lavage and blind-protected specimen brush sampling in ventilated patients with suspected pneumonia. *J Crit Care*. 1998;13:67–72.

12. Rello J, Gallego M, Mariscal D, Sonora R, Valles J. The value of routine microbial investigation in ventilator-associated pneumonia. *Am J Respir Crit Care Med*. 1997;156:196–200.

13. Sterling TR, Ho EJ, Brehm WT, Kirkpatrick MB. Diagnosis and treatment of ventilator-associated pneumonia—impact on survival. A decision analysis. *Chest*. 1996;18:1025–1034.

11

Aspiration Syndromes

Aspiration is defined as the misdirection of oropharyngeal or gastric contents into the larynx and lower respiratory tract. An assortment of pulmonary syndromes may occur following aspiration depending on the quantity and nature of the aspirated material, the frequency of aspiration, as well as the nature of the host's defense mechanisms and the host's response to the aspirated material. The most important syndromes include (1) aspiration pneumonitis, or Mendelson's syndrome, which is a chemical pneumonitis caused by the aspiration of gastric contents, and (2) aspiration pneumonia, an infectious process caused by the aspiration of oropharyngeal secretions colonized by pathogenic bacteria. While there is some overlap between these two syndromes, they are distinct clinical entities (Table 11-1). Other aspiration syndromes include airway obstruction, lung abscess, exogenous lipoid pneumonia, chronic interstitial fibrosis, and *Mycobacterium fortuitum* pneumonia.

Risk factors for aspiration include

- Depressed level of consciousness, including seizures, drug overdose, cerebrovascular accident (CVA)
- Swallowing dysfunction, e.g., **post-stroke**, neuromuscular disorders
- Esophageal strictures
- Small bowel obstruction
- Alcoholics

The approach to a patient with witnessed or suspected aspiration depends on the following:

- What is aspirated
- How much is aspirated
- The patient's local and systemic defense mechanisms

Table 11-1. Contrasting features of aspiration pneumonitis and aspiration pneumonia.

	Aspiration Pneumonitis	Aspiration Pneumonia
Mechanism	Aspiration of sterile gastric contents	Aspiration of colonized oropharyngeal material
Pathophysiology	Acute lung injury due to acidic and particulate gastric material	Acute pulmonary inflammatory response to bacteria and bacterial products
Bacteriology	Initially sterile, may develop bacterial superinfection	Gram-positive cocci and gram-negative rods, ? anaerobic bacteria
Major predisposing factor(s)	Markedly depressed level of consciousness	Dysphagia, gastric dysmotility
Age group	Any age, usually young	Usually elderly
Aspiration witnessed	May be witnessed	Usually not witnessed
Typical presentation	Patient with a history of depressed level of consciousness who develops a pulmonary infiltrate and respiratory symptoms	Institutionalized patient with dysphagia who develops clinical features of pneumonia and an infiltrate in a dependent bronchopulmonary segment
Clinical features	May be asymptomatic or vary from a nonproductive cough to tachypnea, bronchospasm, bloody/frothy sputum, and respiratory distress 2–5h after aspiration	Tachypnea, cough, and clinical sign of pneumonia

- The patient's level of consciousness
- The patient's oral hygiene and oropharyngeal flora

The interaction of the factors listed above will determine the nature of the aspiration syndrome:

■ MENDELSON'S SYNDROME/ASPIRATION PNEUMONITIS

These syndromes are defined as acute lung injury following the aspiration of regurgitated gastric contents. They occur in patients with a marked disturbance of consciousness such as drug overdose, seizures, massive cerebrovascular accident, and anesthesia. Mendelson's syndrome is characterized by a severe chemical pneumonitis and rapidly progressive acute respiratory distress syndrome (ARDS). The aspiration pneumonitis syndrome is caused by the aspiration of gastric contents whose pH and volume are insufficient to cause the Mendelson's syndrome. These patients develop a noninfectious, self-limited pneumonitis.

The volume and pH of the aspirated fluid are important pathogenetic factors. As little as 20 mL of gastric fluid with a pH <2.5 is sufficient to cause Mendelson's syndrome. However, the stomach contains a variety of other substances in addition to acid. Several experimental studies have revealed that aspiration of small, particulate food matter from the stomach may cause pulmonary damage, even if the pH of the aspirate is >2.5.

Steroids have not be proven to improve the outcome of patients with Mendelson's syndrome/aspiration pneumonitis. Gastric acid prevents the growth of bacteria, and therefore the contents of the stomach are normally sterile. Bacterial infection, therefore, does not play a significant role in the early stages of acute lung injury following aspiration of gastric contents. Bacterial superinfection may occur at a later stage; however, the incidence of this complication has not been studied. While common practice, the prophylactic use of antibiotics in patients with suspected or witnessed aspiration is not recommended. Similarly, the use of antibiotics shortly after an aspiration episode in a patient who develops a fever, leukocytosis, and a pulmonary infiltrate is discouraged, as it may select for more resistant organisms in a patient with an uncomplicated chemical pneumonitis. However, empiric antimicrobial therapy is appropriate in patients who aspirate gastric contents in the setting of small bowel obstruction or in other circumstances associated with colonization of gastric contents (see "Chemical Pneumonitis/Pneumonia Syndrome," later in this chapter). Antimicrobial therapy should be considered in

Table 11-2. Empiric antibiotic recommendations for the most common aspiration syndromes.

Clinical Situation	Antibiotic	Usual Dose*
Aspiration pneumonitis		
Signs/symptoms > 48 hours	Levofloxacin or Ceftriaxone	500 mg daily[†] 1–2 g daily
Small bowel obstruction or antacids/antisecretory therapy	As above and Ciprofloxacin or Piperacillin/tazobactam or Ceftazidime	400 mg q12h 3.375 g q6h 2 g q8h
Aspiration pneumonia		
Community acquired	Levofloxacin or ceftriaxone	As above
Chronic care facility	Levofloxacin Piperacillin/tazobactam Ceftazidime	500 mg daily[†] 3.375 g q6h 2 g q8h
Severe periodontal disease, putrid sputum and/or alcoholics	Piperacillin/tazobactam or Imipenem or	3.375 g q6h 500 mg q8h 1 g q6h
	Levofloxacin/ciprofloxacin/ ceftriaxone +	As above
	Clindamycin or Metronidazole	600 mg q8h 500 mg q8h

* In patients with normal renal function.
[†] By slow infusion over 60 minutes.

patients with aspiration pneumonitis that fails to resolve within 48 hours. Empiric therapy with broad-spectrum agents is recommended (Table 11-2). Antimicrobials with anaerobic activity are not routinely required.

■ ASPIRATION PNEUMONIA

Aspiration pneumonia syndrome results from the aspiration of oropharyngeal contents that have been colonized by pathogenic bacteria. This syndrome occurs in patients with dysphagia, predominantly post-CVA patients. In patients with aspiration pneumonia, unlike the case of aspiration pneumonitis, the episode of aspiration is generally not witnessed. The diagnosis is therefore inferred when a patient with known risk factors for aspiration has an infiltrate in a characteristic bronchopulmonary segment. In patients who aspirate in the recumbent position, the most common sites of involvement are the posterior segments of the upper lobes and the apical segments of the lower lobes. In patients who aspirate in the upright or semirecumbent position, the basal segments of the lower lobes are favored. The usual picture is that of an acute pneumonic process, which runs a course similar to that of a typical community-acquired pneumonia. Untreated, however, these patients appear to have a higher incidence of cavitation and lung abscess formation.

Although anaerobic bacteria are frequently isolated from the oropharyngeal flora, their pathogenetic role in aspiration pneumonia is unclear. Anaerobic bacteria have traditionally been considered common pulmonary pathogens and believed to play a major role in aspiration pneumonia. These data are based on a handful of studies conducted in the 1970s, when transtracheal aspiration was used for the collection of "uncontaminated" respiratory secretions. Consequently, antimicrobials with anaerobic coverage have been recommended in patients with aspiration pneumonia. However, recent studies suggest that, while anaerobes are quantitatively important oropharyngeal commensals, they are relatively unimportant pulmonary pathogens in patients with aspiration pneumonia. The bacteriology of these syndromes reflects the aerobic organisms that are likely to colonize the patients at the time of aspiration, with pneumococcus and *Hemophilus influenzae* being common in "community aspiration" and enteric gram-negatives in patients with nosocomial aspiration syndromes (including small bowel obstruction). These studies imply that antimicrobial agents with anaerobic coverage may no longer be required in the treatment of these patients. Furthermore, penicillin G and clindamycin, the traditional antimicrobials of choice in patients with aspiration pneumonitis, provide inadequate antimicrobial coverage in most patients with aspiration pneumonia. Antibiotics such as ceftriaxone or levofloxacin are probably adequate for most patients with aspiration pneumonia. Anaerobic coverage may be indicated in patients with poor oral dentition and patients with putrid sputum (see Table 11-2).

■ CHEMICAL PNEUMONITIS/PNEUMONIA SYNDROME

Colonization of the gastric contents by potentially pathogenic organisms may occur when the gastric pH is increased by the use of antacids, H_2-blockers, or proton pump inhibitors. In addition, gastric colonization by gram-negative bacteria occurs in patients receiving gastric enteral feedings, as well as in patients with gastroparesis and small bowel obstruction (colonization of gastric contents is common in ICU patients). Aspiration of gastric contents in these circumstances is likely to result in a pulmonary inflammatory process from both bacteria and gastric particulate matter.

■ LUNG ABSCESS

Lung abscess usually occurs in patients with an altered level of consciousness and poor oral hygiene. Patients who are suspected to have aspirated under such circumstances should be treated with antibiotics, such as clindamycin, penicillin, or ampicillin/sulbactam.

■ ASPIRATION OF UNDIGESTED FOOD

Aspiration of undigested food occurs in patients who vomit and are unable to protect their airway. This syndrome requires endotracheal intubation with suctioning. Flexible and/or rigid bronchoscopy may be required. These patients are at risk of developing pneumonia/abscess and should be treated with antibiotics.

■ FOREIGN BODY ASPIRATION

Foreign body aspiration is most common in children but may occur in adults with depressed level of consciousness. These patients require rigid bronchoscopy and may require a thoracotomy.

■ MICROASPIRATION

Microaspiration of oropharyngeal contents in hospitalized patients is the leading cause of nosocomial pneumonia.

■ ASPIRATION IN CRITICALLY ILL PATIENTS

Critically ill patients are at an increased risk of oropharyngeal and gastric aspiration with the development of aspiration pneumonia/pneumonitis. In mechanically ventilated patients, this syndrome is called ventilator-associated pneumonia (see Chapter 10). A number of factors increase the risk of aspiration including supine position, gastroparesis, and nasogastric intubation. Gastroesophageal reflux occurs in critically ill patients even in the absence of nasogastric tubes and enteral feedings; up to 30% of patients who are kept in the supine position are estimated to have gastroesophageal reflux. Significant gastrointestinal dysmotility, ranging from moderate delay in gastric emptying to marked gastric paresis, has been described in critically ill patients with a variety of clinical conditions such as burns, sepsis, trauma, surgery, and shock. High gastric residuals volumes secondary to gastroparesis with gastric distention leading to regurgitation increase the risk for aspiration of gastric contents. Postpyloric feeding may have advantages in these patients.

After tracheal extubation, patients are especially at risk of aspiration because of the residual effects of sedative drugs; the presence of nasogastric tubes; and swallowing dysfunction related to alterations of upper airway sensitivity, glottic injury, and laryngeal muscular dysfunction. Alteration in the swallow reflex can be detected in patients who have been intubated for as short as 24 hours. This abnormality usually recovers within 48 hours. I recommend withholding feeding for at least 6 hours after extubation (in case reintubation is required), followed by a pureed and then soft diet for at least 48 hours. A formal swallow evaluation is suggested in cases of traumatic intubations and in patients with anatomical or functional abnormalities of the upper airway.

■ SELECTED REFERENCES

1. de Larminat V, Montravers P, Dureuil B, Desmonts JM. Alteration in swallowing reflex after extubation in intensive care unit patients. *Crit Care Med.* 1995;23:486–490.
2. Knight PR, Rutter T, Tait AR, Coleman E, Johnson K. Pathogenesis of gastric particulate lung injury: a comparison and interaction with acidic pneumonitis. *Anesth Analg.* 1993;77:754–760.
3. Leder SB, Cohn SM, Moller BA. Fiberoptic endoscopic documentation of the high incidence of aspiration following extubation in critically ill trauma patients. *Dysphagia.* 1998;13:208–212.
4. Marik PE, Careau P. The role of anaerobes in patients with ventilator-associated pneumonia and aspiration pneumonia. A prospective study. *Chest.* 1999;115:178–183.
5. Marik PE. Aspiration pneumonitis and pneumonia: a clinical review. *N Engl J Med.* 2000;(in press).
6. Mier L, Dreyfuss D, Darchy B, et al. Is penicillin G an adequate initial treatment for aspiration pneumonia? A prospective evaluation using a protected specimen brush and quantitative cultures. *Intensive Care Med.* 1993;19: 279–284.
7. Schwartz DJ, Wynne JW, Gibbs CP, Hood CI, Kuck EJ. The pulmonary consequences of aspiration of gastric contents at pH values greater than 2.5. *Am Rev Respir Dis.* 1980;121:119–126.
8. Tolep K, Getch CL, Criner GJ. Swallowing dysfunction in patients receiving prolonged mechanical ventilation. *Chest.* 1996;109:167–172.

12

Acute Respiratory Distress Syndrome

■ DEFINITION, CAUSES, AND ASSESSMENT OF SEVERITY

The adult respiratory distress syndrome (ARDS) was initially described by Petty and Ashbaugh as a syndrome characterized by diffuse pulmonary infiltrates, with decreased pulmonary compliance and hypoxemia. It has been recognized, however, that ARDS is a spectrum varying from mild acute lung injury (ALI) at one end to ARDS at the other. The diagnosis of ARDS should be reserved for patients with ALI who have severe disease (see criteria below). The outcome of ALI is largely dependent on both the severity of ALI and the causative factors. It should be emphasized that in most cases ALI is a multisystem disease; the microcirculatory changes that occur in the lung occur in all the organs; the pathophysiological derangements, however, are most evident in the lung.

Definition of Acute Lung Injury

ALI is a condition involving

1. An oxygenation defect with bilateral alveolar infiltrates
2. A patient who has suffered an acute catastrophic event
3. A pulmonary capillary wedge pressure ≤18 mm Hg or no clinical evidence of an elevated left atrial pressure

ALI: A patient is defined as having ALI when the Po_2/Fio_2 (fraction of inspired oxygen) ≤300, regardless of the amount of positive end-expiratory pressure (PEEP).

ARDS: A patient is said to have ARDS when the $Po_2/Fio_2 \leq 200$, regardless of the amount of PEEP.

Causes of ALI

ALI may result from either direct or indirect lung injury. It is likely that the severity of ALI and the outcome are related to the causation of ALI. The common causes include the following:

Direct Lung Injury

- Pneumonia
- Aspiration pneumonitis
- Smoke inhalation
- Chemical inhalation
- Drowning

Indirect Lung Injury

- Sepsis and sepsis syndrome
- Polytrauma
- Pancreatitis
- Drug induced (heroin, tricyclic antidepressants, etc.)
- Fat embolism
- Post-transfusion
- Burns

■ MANAGEMENT OF THE ACUTE PHASE

The management of ARDS is essentially supportive: cardiorespiratory and nutritional support, the prevention of further lung injury, and the prevention of complications while waiting for the acute inflammatory response to resolve and lung function to improve.

Ventilation Strategy

The chest radiographs of patients with ARDS classically show widespread involvement of all lung fields. It was therefore assumed that ARDS was a homogeneous process. However, high-resolution computed tomographic scans performed in patients with ARDS have demonstrated areas of normal, consolidated, and overinflated lung. The large area of consolidated and collapsed lung is predominantly distributed in the dependent areas and participates minimally in gas exchange. The normal lung is usually anterior and often markedly overdistended. In addition, in the early stages of ARDS, consolidated lung units can be recruited with the application of modest distending pressures. Consequently, patients with ARDS typically have three functionally distinct lung zones, namely

1. That portion of the lung that is diseased and not recruitable
2. That portion of the lung that is diseased but recruitable
3. That portion of the lung that is normal

Because a significant portion of the lung is consolidated and not recruitable, only a small amount of aerated lung receives the total tidal volume; ARDS leads to "baby lungs." The use of traditional tidal volumes (12 to 15 mL/kg) in these patients will result in high inspiratory pressures with overdistention of the normally aerated lung units. A growing body of experimental evidence has demonstrated that mechanical ventilation that results in high transpulmonary pressure gradients and overdistention of lung units will cause acute lung injury, characterized by hyaline membranes, granulocytic infiltration, pulmonary hypertension, and increased pulmonary and systemic vascular permeability. Animal studies have demonstrated that a transpulmonary pressure in excess of 35 cm H_2O will lead to alveolar damage. These studies have demonstrated that ventilation with low tidal volumes preserves pulmonary ultrastructure. Furthermore, it has been postulated that the cyclic opening and closing of lung units (recruitment and derecruitment) in patients with ARDS who are ventilated with insufficient PEEP may further potentiate this iatrogenic lung injury. It has therefore been suggested that ventilatory strategies that avoid regional or global overdistention of lung units and also avoids end-expiratory alveolar collapse may limit the degree of lung injury in ARDS.

A relative form of "lung rest" using low tidal volume mechanical ventilation has therefore been advocated. This may be achieved with low-volume, volume-cycled ventilation with a decelerating inspiratory flow or pressure-controlled ventilation (PCV). The decelerating waveform with both these techniques results in a more laminar flow at the end of inspiration, resulting in a more even distribution of ventilation in patients who have markedly different resistance values from one region of the lung to another. PCV, however, has the advantage that the clinician can precisely titrate the lung-distending pressure and the inspiratory time, allowing the peak airway pressure to be accurately determined and maintained. In addition, in volume-controlled ventilation, the clinician must set the peak flow. As patient demand changes, so must the rate of flow. The clinician must be meticulous about meeting the patient's flow demand by adjusting the flow as conditions change. In PCV the clinician does not set the peak flow but rather the inspiratory pressure. The machine will constantly adjust flow so that the inspiratory pressure is maintained during the entire set inspiratory time.

The Acute Respiratory Distress Syndrome Network recently completed a randomized, controlled clinical trial (RCT) in which patients with ARDS were randomized to receive traditional volume-controlled ventilation (an initial tidal volume of 12 mL/kg and a plateau pressure of ≤50 cm H_2O) or low tidal volume ventilation (an initial tidal volume of 6 mL/kg and a plateau pressure of ≤30 cm H_2O). The trial was stopped after the enrollment of 861 patients because mortality was lower in the group treated with lower tidal volumes (31.0% vs. 39.8%, $P = 0.007$). This study has provided convincing evidence that a strategy that avoids alveolar overdistention in ARDS improves outcome. PCV has yet to be carefully compared in an RCT with volume-cycled ventilation in patients with ARDS in terms of morbidity, length of mechanical ventilation, and ultimate patient outcome. Furthermore, it is unlikely that such a trial will be performed; however, from the foregoing, it is likely that ventilation strategies that achieve the same end points (i.e., prevent alveolar overdistention and limit airway pressures) will have similar outcomes. However, it is likely that the cyclic opening and collapse of diseased alveoli are more important than alveolar overdistention in potentiating the lung injury in ARDS. Therefore, it may be more important to achieve an adequate level of PEEP than to tightly limit the plateau pressure to <30 cm H_2O. In the face of adequate PEEP, a plateau pressure of 35 to 40 cm H_2O may be acceptable. This strategy, however, is untested.

Achieving Adequate/Best PEEP

PEEP appears to be protective against ventilator-induced lung injury in animal studies, perhaps by recruiting more aerated lung and preventing shear forces produced during repetitive opening of closed airways or alveoli. Low tidal volume ventilation has been demonstrated to cause a decline in compliance in healthy subjects as well as in patients in respiratory failure. It has been suggested that, the smaller the tidal volume, the higher the PEEP level needed to optimize lung mechanics. It is generally believed that PEEP set <10 cm H_2O will probably keep healthy alveoli open at end exhalation but will not be enough to distend diseased airways. These airways will then continually open and collapse throughout the ventilator cycle. The goal is to set PEEP at a level that does not overdistend healthy alveoli but at the same time does not let diseased airways collapse. The term the *open lung approach* has been used to describe this method of ventilation. It has been reported that in patients with ARDS a mean PEEP level of 15 cm H_2O is required to keep the airways "open" at end expiration.

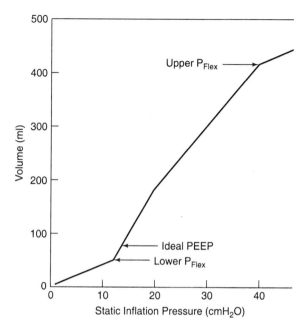

Figure 12-1. Static pressure/volume curve. *Source*: Marik PE, Krikorian J. Pressure-controlled ventilation in ARDS: a practical approach. *Chest.* 1997;112:1102–1106.

Best PEEP can be estimated by plotting a static pressure–volume curve measuring airway pressure at each incrementally higher tidal volume. This curve classically demonstrates an upper and lower inflection point (Figure 12-1). PEEP should be set above the lower inflection point such that the sum of the PEEP and the inspiratory pressure should be <35 cm H_2O (a plateau pressure up to 40 may be acceptable) or the upper inflection point. If an inflection point is not present on the pressure/volume curve, or if it is not possible to perform this maneuver, the initial PEEP should be set between 10 and 15 cm H_2O.

Pressure-Controlled Ventilation

To prevent alveolar overdistention and reduce the transpulmonary pressure gradients, the inspiratory pressure is set such that the peak

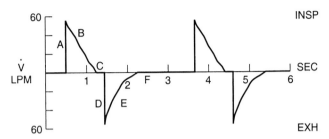

Figure 12-2. Flow vs. time waveform. *Source*: Marik PE, Krikorian J. Pressure-controlled ventilation in ARDS: a practical approach. *Chest.* 1997;112:1102–1106.

inspiratory pressure is less than 35 cm H_2O (i.e., applied PEEP + inspiratory pressure <35 cm H_2O) when possible and always less than 40 cm H_2O. An inspiratory pressure of 20 cm H_2O (plus PEEP of 10 cm H_2O) with a respiratory rate of 16 breaths/min are convenient starting points.

The inspiratory and expiratory times (or I/E ratio) and respiratory rate are best determined by analyzing the flow vs. time waveform (Figure 12-2). Flow will initially enter the lung rapidly because the ventilator attempts to reach the set airway pressure as quickly as it can (Point A, Figure 12-2). Airways that are open and have the least resistance will receive the greatest amount of gas flow and reach equilibrium with the preset pressure more quickly than airways with greater resistance. As the open airways fill and the lung pressure reaches equilibrium with the preset pressure, flow will decelerate as the airways with higher resistance continue to fill with gas (Point B, Figure 12-2). Flow into the lung will continue until one of two events occur: (1) The preset pressure reaches equilibrium throughout all lung units (indicated by the flow pattern decelerating to zero), or (2) the preset inspiratory time ends inspiration before pressure has equilibrated throughout all lung units (indicated by the flow pattern not reaching zero). When inspiratory flow reaches zero, it means the pressure in the lung is equal to the pressure set on the ventilator (Point C, Figure 12-2). It is essential that adequate inspiratory time be given so that all the airways, both healthy and diseased, have time to reach the preset pressure level. In ARDS, much of the airway bed may take a relatively long time to open. Therefore, it may be necessary to lengthen the inspiratory time, sometimes to the point that the inspiratory time is longer than the expiratory time. If air trapping is not present, this approach will increase mean airway pressure without increasing maximal end expiratory pressure In patients with ARDS, oxygenation is primarily a function of mean airway pressure. This

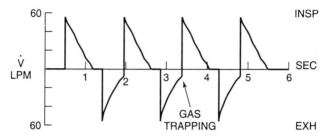

Figure 12-3. Flow vs. time waveform demonstrating air trapping. *Source*: Marik PE, Krikorian J. Pressure-controlled ventilation in ARDS: a practical approach. *Chest*. 1997;112:1102–1106.

strategy will therefore increase alveolar ventilation and improve oxygenation.

The inspiratory time can be lengthened in two ways: (1) If the ventilator will allow for the adjustment of inspiratory time, then simply increase the inspiratory time until the inspiratory flow reaches zero (recommended method). (2) If the ventilator will allow adjustment of the I/E ratio, then reducing the "E" part of the ratio will increase "I." If flow reaches zero and there is a long inspiratory pause, this is an indication that inspiratory time is too long. There is little benefit in having a prolonged inspiratory pause. Setting inspiratory time longer than that which is required to open recruitable airways increases the likelihood of significant auto-PEEP, with its attendant hemodynamic complications.

To evaluate the adequacy of the expiratory time, the flow vs. time waveform (see Figure 12-2) needs to be studied again. This waveform shows whether the patient has enough time to exhale to the preset PEEP level before the ventilator gives the next breath. In Figure 12-2, point D represents the beginning of exhalation. When exhalation begins, gas will exit the lungs quickly at first because a large pressure gradient exists between the lungs and the atmosphere. As gas continues to exit the lungs, the pressure gradient will become smaller and flow will decelerate (Point E, Figure 12-2). Exhalation will continue until one of two events occurs: (1) The pressure in the lung reaches atmospheric pressure plus the set PEEP pressure (Point F, Figure 12-2), or (2) the set inspiratory time mandates that inhalation begin before exhalation of the previous breath is complete, thus causing auto-PEEP. Figure 12-3 demonstrates gas trapping as inhalation begins before expiratory flow is allowed to reach zero. If gas trapping is evident on the flow vs. time waveform, either the respiratory rate or inspiratory time should be reduced, allowing time for complete exhalation and thereby minimizing auto-PEEP. The respiratory rate and inspiratory time should both be independently and sequentially reduced, to determine which maneuver affects ventilation the least.

It is essential that the level of auto-PEEP be measured in all patients receiving PCV. There are no data that intrinsic PEEP has any advantage over extrinsic (i.e., applied) PEEP. However, the unrecognized development of auto-PEEP may result in hemodynamic compromise, leading to the inappropriate use of fluid and vasopressor therapy.

The flow vs. time waveform should be monitored regularly. As the patient's pulmonary mechanics change, the inspiratory time and respiratory rate may need to be altered. Once the patient's condition has stabilized, attempts should be made to reduce the level of PEEP (and FIO_2).

Permissive Hypercapnia

The strategy to reduce volume-induced lung injury by using small tidal volumes may lead to CO_2 retention. The term *permissive hypercapnia* has been used to the describe this ventilatory strategy. Hypercapnic acidosis is generally well tolerated by ARDS patients, especially when it develops gradually over 1 to 2 days. The intracellular acidosis is corrected rapidly during sustained hypercapnia, whereas the extracellular acidosis may persist for much longer. The lowest pH that can be safely tolerated is unknown; however, a pH >7.2 is generally recommended. Some patients, however, have tolerated a pH as low as 7.05 without obvious adverse effects. It has been suggested that bicarbonate should be used to correct the pH. However, the administration of bicarbonate may paradoxically increase intracellular acidosis. Permissive hypercapnia should not be used in patients with acute intracranial pathology, as this may cause a precipitous increase in intracranial pressure. Furthermore, in patients with ischemic heart disease, arrhythmias, and patients requiring high doses of inotropic drugs, hypercapnia should be allowed to develop gradually.

Prone Ventilation

A number of case series and experimental data have demonstrated an improvement in gas exchange, with a decrease in shunt perfusion, in patients with ARDS who were ventilated in the prone position. It has been postulated that the observed improvement in oxygenation in the prone position results from better removal of secretions, redistribution of perfusion (Q) along a gravitational gradient to less injured lung regions, increased functional residual capacity, and change in regional diaphragm motion.

Oxygenation improves in about 70% of patients when turned from the supine to the prone position. However, the degree of improvement is highly variable, with some patients showing no improvement or even a deterioration in oxygenation. Three different responses have been observed in patients with improved oxygenation in the prone position who are turned back to the supine position: (1) Some patients return to basal supine oxygenation; (2) some patients display better oxygenation than in the original supine position, although the values are lower than in the prone position; and (3) some patients display improved oxygenation compared to both the previous supine and prone positions. However, when the patient is turned several times, the effect of the maneuver may change with time.

Ventilation in the prone position is not widely practiced in the management of patients with severe ARDS. This maneuver may be lifesaving. Furthermore, contrary to expectations, it is not particularly difficult to nurse patients in this position. However, neuromuscular paralysis with its attendant risks are probably mandatory in such patients. Therefore, meticulous care must be used in positioning the arms to avoid peripheral nerve injury. I recommend placing a neck roll under the patient's shoulders and turning the head to one side. Furthermore, multifunction electrode pads that allow for defibrillation, cardioversion, and pacing should be placed on the patient and connected appropriately before turning the patient into the prone position. This may allow for cardiopulmonary resuscitation to be performed in the prone position.

Other Ventilatory Strategies

Extracorporeal CO_2 removal with apneic oxygenation (extracorporeal membrane oxygenation, ECMO) has been used to avoid additional ventilator-induced lung injury in patients with severe ARDS. However, ECMO is very labor intensive, is expensive, is associated with additional complications, and *has not been shown to reduce mortality*. Similarly, intravascular membrane oxygenation devices have shown some utility in the treatment of ARDS; these devices remain experimental at this time. Partial liquid ventilation has found some success in pediatric patients; however, the role of this mode of ventilation in adult patients has yet to be determined.

Hemodynamic Support

The optimal fluid strategy in patients with ARDS is a hotly debated subject, with a *"wet lung"* and a *"dry lung"* camp. These two approaches have not yet been compared in an adequately powered RCT. In the absence of such data, I recommend that the lowest intravascular volume (or pulmonary capillary wedge pressure) that maintains an adequate cardiac output *and renal perfusion* should be achieved. A volumetric pulmonary artery catheter may be particularly useful in patients with ARDS to "optimize hemodynamics" (see Chapter 18). Inotropic agents may be required to maintain an adequate cardiac output and perfusion pressure (mean arterial pressure >75 to 80 mm Hg). If hemodynamics allow, the patient should be kept in a negative fluid balance. Once hemodynamic stability is achieved, the patient should be actively diuresed (until the serum urea nitrogen climbs to approximately 30 mg/dL). In patients with ALI, the higher the pulmonary capillary hydrostatic pressure, the greater the degree of capillary leak (and the greater the intrapulmonary shunt). It has been suggested that iatrogenically increasing oxygen delivery (DO_2) to predetermined levels may improve the outcome of patients with ARDS. Little evidence supports this strategy. Oxygen transport should be titrated to tissue demands (see Chapter 48).

Other Supportive Measures

- Gastrointestinal prophylaxis (see Chapter 25).
- Deep venous thrombosis prophylaxis (see Chapter 13).
- Early enteral nutrition with an immune-enhancing formula is recommended (see Chapter 49).
- To facilitate low-volume ventilation, deep hypnosis and in some instances neuromuscular blockade may be required (see Chapter 48).

■ PULMONARY INFECTION IN ARDS

- Patients with ALI/ARDS have a high incidence of "secondary" pulmonary infection. Pulmonary sepsis should therefore be aggressively diagnosed and treated (see Chapter 10, "Ventilator-Associated Pneumonia").
- Nosocomial cytomegalovirus infection in nonimmunocompromised ICU patients (see Chapter 44).

Experimental Treatment Modalities

- *Inhaled nitric oxide* acts as a selective pulmonary vasodilator when inspired at concentrations of 5 to 80 ppm. The rapid binding of nitric oxide to hemoglobin prevents systemic vasodilation. In patients with ARDS, inhaled nitric oxide will go preferentially to well-ventilated alveolar units, thereby diverting pulmonary blood flow away from the poorly ventilated alveoli to the better-ventilated alveoli, with the net effect of decreasing intrapulmonary shunting. While inhaled nitric oxide has been demonstrated to improve oxygenation and pulmonary hypertension in a proportion of patients, this therapy has yet to be shown to improve outcome. Patients may become nitric oxide dependent, with hemodynamic embarrassment when the drug is temporarily discontinued.

- *Corticosteroids*: Prospective, multicenter, placebo-controlled studies have demonstrated that high-dose corticosteroids administered early in the course of ALI/ARDS are of no benefit. Patients treated with corticosteroids are at an increased risk of developing complications.
- *Experimental therapeutic modalities*: The use of antioxidants, inhibitors of thromboxane and leukotrienes (nonsteroidal anti-inflammatory drugs, ketoconazole, etc.), prostaglandin E_1, pentoxifylline, anticytokines, and exogenous surfactant, as well as many other therapeutic modalities, have not been proven to be of benefit in patients with ARDS and therefore cannot be recommended.

■ MANAGEMENT OF CHRONIC PHASE OF ARDS

Patients who after 10 to 14 days of aggressive supportive therapy require high levels of ventilatory support ($FIO_2 \geq 50\%$) are candidates for corticosteroid therapy. Corticosteroids should be considered only if lower respiratory tract sampling can be performed to diagnose and treat pulmonary sepsis. Some authors recommend an open lung biopsy before commencing corticosteroid therapy, to obtain histologic evidence of the fibroproliferative phase of ARDS and to exclude infection.

Before embarking on corticosteroid therapy, all possible sites of sepsis should be aggressively investigated and treated; i.e., intravascular and urinary catheters should be changed, protected lower respiratory tract sampling performed, blood cultures performed, etc. Once corticosteroids are commenced, vascular catheters should be changed, and surveillance cultures and protected lower respiratory tract sampling should be performed every fourth day.

■ SELECTED REFERENCES

1. Amato MBP, Barbas CSV, Medeiros DM, et al. Beneficial effects of the "Open lung approach" with low distending pressures in acute respiratory

distress syndrome: a prospective randomized study on mechanical ventilation. *Am J Respir Crit Care Med.* 1995;152:1835–1846.

2. Humphrey H, Hall J, Sznajder I, Silverstein M, Wood L. Improved survival in ARDS patients associated with a reduction in pulmonary capillary wedge pressure. *Chest.* 1990;97:1176–1180.

3. Marik PE, Krikorian J. Pressure-controlled ventilation in ARDS: a practical approach. *Chest.* 1997;112:1102–1106.

4. Meduri GU, Belenchia JM, Estes RJ, et al. Fibroproliferative phase of ARDS. Clinical findings and effects of corticosteroids. *Chest.* 1991;100:943–952.

5. Meduri GU, Headley S, Golden E, et al. Effect of prolonged methylprednisolone therapy in unresolving acute respiratory distress syndrome. A randomized controlled trial. *JAMA.* 1998;280:159–165.

6. Ventilation with lower tidal volumes as compared with traditional tidal volumes for acute lung injury and the acute respiratory distress syndrome. *N Engl J Med.* 2000;342:1301–1308.

7. Ware LB, Matthay MA. The acute respiratory distress syndrome. *N Engl J Med.* 2000;342:1334–1349.

13

Thromboembolism in the Intensive Care Unit

Deep venous thrombosis (DVT) and pulmonary emboli are in reality one and the same disease, thromboembolic disease, as a large proportion of patients with DVT have "asymptomatic" PE. Critically ill ICU patients have many of the risk factors that increase the risk of DVT, including prolonged venous stasis caused by bed rest, cardiac failure, dehydration, obesity, and advanced age. Consequently, routine DVT prophylaxis is recommended in all ICU patients; i.e., every ICU patient should receive DVT prophylaxis. Patients with femoral venous catheters may be at an increased risk of thromboembolism, and DVT prophylaxis is therefore particularly important in this group of patients. For practical purposes, it is convenient to group the patients according to the risk of DVT (Table 13-1). It should be appreciated that the improper use and/or application of intermittent compression devices will result in ineffective prophylaxis. Routine screening for DVT is not cost-effective in ICU patients who are receiving DVT prophylaxis. However, a high index of suspicion for DVT should exist with a low threshold for performing venous Doppler ultrasonography. Recently, aspirin has been demonstrated to have utility in DVT prophylaxis. However, the role of this agent in ICU patients who are at an increased risk of gastric stress ulceration is unclear.

■ DIAGNOSIS OF PULMONARY EMBOLISM

The diagnosis of pulmonary embolism (PE) is one of the more challenging dilemmas in clinical medicine. While pulmonary angiography is the gold standard with which to compare other methods, angiog-

Table 13-1. DVT prophylaxis according to risk profile.

Risk Group	Patients	Prophylaxis
Moderate risk	All patients except those listed below	LDH, 5000 U SQ q12h or external pneumatic compression (EPC)
Moderate- to high-risk ICU patients	Obesity (body mass index > 30) Deep sedation/paralysis Neuromuscular disorders, e.g., Guillain-Barré syndrome Acute spinal cord injury Polytrauma Urological surgery Burns ? femoral catheters	EPC + LDH or LMWH; enoxaprin sodium 40 mg SQ daily
High-risk ICU patients	Total hip replacement Total knee replacement Hip fracture surgery	LMWH; enoxaprin sodium 40 mg SQ q12h or low-intensity (INR 2.0–3.0) oral anticoagulation, or adjusted dose heparin to upper limit of normal range

(EPC = external pneumatic compression; INR = international normalized ratio; LDH = low-dose heparin; LMWH = low-molecular-weight heparin; SQ = subcutaneous.)

Table 13-2. Probability of pulmonary embolus based on clinical suspicion and V/Q scan result.

Lung Scan Interpretation	Prescan Clinical Suspicion	
	Any	high
High probability	0.87	0.96
Intermediate probability	0.30	0.66
Low probability	0.14	0.40
Normal	0	0.04

raphy is invasive, costly, not readily available in most hospitals, and associated with significant complications. A radionuclide perfusion (+/– ventilation scan) should be performed in all patients, even those patients with DVT (baseline V/Q scan important). The interpretation of the V/Q scan result depends on the scan results as well as the index of clinical suspicion for pulmonary embolism (Table 13-2). In patients with indeterminate/intermediate probability scans or low probability scan with a high clinical suspicion, the following tests maybe considered:

D-Dimer

A negative D-dimer (<500 ng/mL) has a negative predictive value of about 90%. The specificity of the test is only 45%. Therefore, a negative D-dimer is useful in excluding thromboembolic disease; however, a positive D-dimer has little diagnostic value.

Contrast-Enhanced Helical or Electron Beam Computed Tomography

Contract-enhanced helical computed tomography (CT) allows visualization of PE involving the central pulmonary arteries (main through segmental branches). Most PEs involve the central pulmonary arteries; only 6% of PE in the PIOPED study involved subsegmental pulmonary arteries. When compared with conventional pulmonary angiography, helical CT has a sensitivity of approximately 72% and specificity of 95%. The sensitivity and specificity of central PE have been reported to be 94%. The role of helical CT in the diagnosis of PE is uncertain. In institutions where experience and skill with this diagnostic modality are available, this technique is of value in diagnosing central PE. Spiral CT also has the advantage of imaging of the lung parenchyma (a useful adjunct to exclude parenchymal causes of dyspnea and hypoxemia).

■ TREATMENT OF THROMBOEMBOLIC DISEASE

Immediate anticoagulation with heparin is the treatment of choice in all patients unless heparin is absolutely contraindicated (see below). Unfractionated heparin (UH) has until recently been considered the treatment of choice. However, with increasing experience with low-molecular-weight heparin (LMWH), this class of drugs is emerging as the drug of choice. LMWHs have a number of practical and therapeutic advantages over UH. The disadvantage of LMWHs include their long half-life and difficulty in monitoring the degree of anticoagulation.

UH binds to plasma proteins, endothelial cell surfaces, macrophages, and acute-phase reactants. This contributes to heparin resistance, which may occur shortly after initiation of anticoagulant therapy during the acute thromboembolic state, when acute-phase reactant proteins are increased. In contrast, LMWH has decreased binding to these proteins; therefore when LMWHs are given on a weight-adjusted basis, the anticoagulant response is predictable and reproducible (enoxaparin 1 mg/kg subcutaneously, q12h). This obviates the need for diligent laboratory monitoring (frequent partial thromboplastin time [PTT] tests). Anticoagulant monitoring is not required in most patients receiving LMWH. However, as LMWH is renally excreted, monitoring of anti-factor Xa may be required in high-risk patients with renal impairment. Furthermore, in comparison with UH, LMWH has a substantially higher bioavailability after subcutaneous injection (90% vs. 30%) and a longer plasma half-life (4 to 6 hours vs. 0.5 to 1 hour). LMWH is therefore ideally suited to twice-daily subcutaneous administration. Furthermore, because LMWH has a lower propensity to react with platelet factor 4, it is associated with a lower incidence of heparin-induced thrombocytopenia syndrome. In patients with acute DVT with PE or in patients with acute DVT without PE, the recommended dose of enoxaparin sodium injection is 1.0 mg/kg (up to 80 mg) every 12 hours administered subcutaneously.

Anticoagulation With UH

The dose of UH should be titrated to maintain a PTT of 2 to 2.5 times normal for 5 to 7 days. The single most common error in heparin therapy is underdosing (which leads to recurrent pulmonary emboli).

- Heparin 10,000 U bolus followed by
- 1250 U/h (heparin 25,000 U in 500 mL dextrose in water infused at 25 mL/h)
- PTT in 6 hours

Chronic Anticoagulation

Coumadin 5 mg/day should be started 3 to 5 days after initiation of treatment with heparin. Heparin and coumadin therapy should overlap for 3 days. The dose of coumadin should be adjusted to achieve an International Normalized Ratio (INR) of 2.0 to 3.0 and given for at least 3 months and possibly for as long as 24 months (after the first episode) and lifelong after the second episode.

Thrombolytic Therapy

Thrombolytic therapy should be considered in patients with acute massive pulmonary embolus who are hemodynamically unstable

Table 13-3. Thrombocytics approved for pulmonary embolus.

Drug	Regimen
Streptokinase	250,000 over 30 min followed by 100,000 U/h for 24 h
Urokinase	4400 U/kg over 10 min followed by 4400 U/kg/h for 12–24 h
recombinant tissue plasminogen activator (rt-PA)	100 mg over 2 h

(hypotension, oliguria) and who have no contraindication to thrombolysis. In hemodynamically stable patients, thrombolysis has not been proven to reduce mortality or the risk of recurrent PE. Thrombolytic therapy, however, should also be considered in patients with >50% obstruction of pulmonary perfusion on the lung scan. Recently published studies have suggested that it may be important from a therapeutic standpoint to divide patients in the hemodynamically stable group into those with and without evidence of right ventricular dysfunction. In the study by Goldhaber et al., in which patients randomized to receive heparin had a higher rate of recurrence than those treated with thrombolytic agents, PE recurred only in patients with baseline right ventricular hypokinesis. The authors suggested that the presence of right ventricular dysfunction might identify a subset of patients at risk for increased morbidity and mortality when treated with heparin alone. However, the role of thrombolytic therapy in patients who demonstrate acute right ventricular dilatation/failure is controversial.

Thrombolytic therapy is accompanied by a significantly greater risk of major hemorrhage than is treatment with heparin alone. There is also a small, but clinically important, risk of intracranial hemorrhage. Streptokinase tissue-type plasminogen activator (t-PA), and urokinase appear to be equally effective with a similar side-effect profile. The recommended dosages are listed in Table 13-3.

Vena Caval Interruption

No randomized controlled trial has been conducted that has compared heparin to vena caval interruption (alone) in the management of thromboembolic disease. However, the available evidence suggests that venal caval interruption is associated with a higher incidence of complications; particularly, recurrent DVT and postphlebitic syndrome. Because of presumed contraindications to heparin, vena caval filters have become commonplace for the primary and secondary prevention of PE. This is in spite of the lack of data on the relative safety and efficacy of vena caval interruption as compared with anticoagulant therapy. However, most of the presumed contraindications have never been subject to rigorous analysis to determine whether they are associated with a worse outcome than those treated with vena caval interruption. For example, intracranial neoplasms have been considered an absolute contraindication to anticoagulation. However, studies have suggested a high complication rate with Inferior Vena Caval (IVC) filters in these patients. Furthermore, in this patient population, anticoagulation is well tolerated, is associated with a low risk of intracerebral bleeding (if excessive anticoagulation is avoided), and results in a better quality of life than an IVC filter.

Absolute Contraindications for Anticoagulation With Heparin

- Recent intracerebral bleed (2 to 3 weeks).
- Recent gastrointestinal bleeding (2 weeks).
- Patients with heparin-associated thrombocytopenia; these patients can be treated with heparinoids, which do not cross-react with heparin.

■ SELECTED REFERENCES

1. Arcasoy SM, Kreit JW. Thrombolytic therapy of pulmonary embolism: a comprehensive review of current evidence. *Chest.* 1999;115:1695–1707.
2. Decousus H, Leizorovicz A, Parent F, et al. A clinical trial of vena caval filters in the prevention of pulmonary embolism in patients with proximal deep-vein thrombosis. Prevention du Risque d'Embolie Pulmonaire par Interruption Cave Study Group. *N Engl J Med.* 1998;338:409–415.
3. Goldhaber SZ, Haire WD, Feldstein ML, et al. Alteplase versus heparin in acute pulmonary embolism: randomised trial assessing right-ventricular function and pulmonary perfusion. *Lancet.* 1993;341:507–511.
4. Goldhaber SZ. Pulmonary embolism. *N Engl J Med.* 1998;339:93–104.
5. Gould MK, Dembitzer AD, Doyle RL, Hastie TJ, Garber AM. Low-molecular-weight heparins compared with unfractionated heparin for treatment of acute deep venous thrombosis. A meta-analysis of randomized, controlled trials. *Ann Intern Med.* 1999;130:800–809.
6. Joynt GM, Kew J, Gomersall CD, Leung VY, Liu EK. Deep venous thrombosis caused by femoral venous catheters in critically ill adult patients. *Chest.* 2000;117:178–183.
7. Konstantinides S, Geibel A, Olschewski M, et al. Association between thrombolytic treatment and the prognosis of hemodynamically stable patients with major pulmonary embolism: results of a multicenter registry. *Circulation.* 1997;96:882–888.
8. Levin JM, Schiff D, Loeffler JS, et al. Complications of therapy for venous thromboembolic disease in patients with brain tumors. *Neurology.* 1993;43:1111–1114.

9. Marik PE, Andrews L, Maini B. The incidence of deep venous thrombosis in ICU patients. *Chest*. 1997;111:661–664.
10. Meneveau N, Schiele F, Metz D, et al. Comparative efficacy of a two-hour regimen of streptokinase versus alteplase in acute massive pulmonary embolism: immediate clinical and hemodynamic outcome and one-year follow-up. *J Am Coll Cardiol*. 1998;31:1057–1063.
11. Meyer G, Gisselbrecht M, Diehl JL, Journois D, Sors H. Incidence and predictors of major hemorrhagic complications from thrombolytic therapy in patients with massive pulmonary embolism. *Am J Med*. 1998;105:472–477.
12. Prevention of pulmonary embolism and deep vein thrombosis with low dose aspirin: Pulmonary Embolism Prevention (PEP) trial. *Lancet*. 2000;355:1295–1302.
13. Quevedo JF, Buckner JC, Schmidt JL, Dinapoli RP, O'Fallon JR. Thromboembolism in patients with high-grade glioma. *Mayo Clin Proc*. 1994; 69:329–332.

14

Bronchoscopy in the Intensive Care Unit

Bronchoscopy is the endoscopic examination of the tracheobronchial tree. Flexible bronchoscopy has largely replaced rigid bronchoscopy as the procedure of choice for most endoscopic evaluations of the airway. Rigid bronchoscopy, however, is indicated for the removal of large foreign bodies, which may be difficult to remove with the flexible bronchoscope, and in the evaluation of patients with massive hemoptysis. Flexible bronchoscopy is easily performed, is associated with few complications, and allows greater visualization of the tracheobronchial tree than does rigid bronchoscopy. In intubated patients, the endotracheal tube provides easy access to the lower respiratory tract while still allowing ventilation. A size 8.0 mm or larger endotracheal tube is required to allow passage of the bronchoscope while allowing adequate ventilation (sometimes a size 7.5 tube may suffice). A number of diagnostic and therapeutic procedures can be performed with the fiberoptic bronchoscope including bronchoalveolar lavage (BAL), biopsy of intrabronchial lesions, protected microbiology specimen brush (PSB) and cytology sampling, as well as transbronchial biopsy. Many pulmonologists, however, are reluctant to perform transbronchial biopsy in ventilated ICU patients due to the high complication rate and low diagnostic yield in this setting.

BAL allows sampling of lower respiratory tract secretions and with the recent advances in molecular diagnostic methods is becoming an increasingly important diagnostic test. Furthermore, preliminary results from BAL sampling can usually be obtained within a few hours.

BAL is performed by infusing a sterile isotonic solution (usually normal saline) through the biopsy port of the bronchoscope. This fluid fills the intraluminal space of the conducting airways and the alveoli and is then recovered by aspiration. Because the fluid mixes with the intraluminal contents, the resulting lavage fluid effectively samples the intraluminal space of the lower respiratory tract. The procedure is performed by wedging the bronchoscope in a segmental or subsegmental bronchus. The wedged position allows the lavage fluid to be infused in a controlled manner into a single region of the lung. Usually at least 100 mL is infused, in aliquots varying in volume from 20 to 60 mL.

Because the lavage fluid effectively samples the peripheral intraluminal space, peripheral intraluminal infections can be diagnosed with a high degree of reliability. The diagnostic yield for *Pneumocystis carinii* is >95%. Viral infections can also be diagnosed reliably. For cytomegalovirus and herpes virus, pathognomic cytopathic changes can be recognized cytologically. The sensitivity for detecting viral material can be increased with the use of special techniques, including monoclonal antibodies, cDNA probes, and the polymerase chain reaction (PCR). PCR provides a very sensitive method for the detection of *Legionella*, mycoplasma, pneumocystis, *Chlamydia*, and mycobacterium and for an increasing number of viruses. Because aspergillus preferentially invades the vascular space, the intraluminal sampling technique of BAL may be diagnostic in only 50% of patients with invasive pulmonary aspergillosis. Furthermore, the presence of aspergillus in the BAL fluid is not necessarily diagnostic of invasive aspergillosis and may represent colonization. Similarly, the presence of *Candida* species and coagulase-negative staphylococci in BAL fluid almost always represents colonization rather than infection. Both routine and special cytological techniques can be used to diagnose pulmonary malignancies from fluid obtained from BAL.

As the upper airway (including the trachea, segmental and subsegmental bronchi) of intubated patients become colonized by gram-negative bacteria, staphylococci, and *Candida*, tracheal aspirates and/or BAL fluid culture cannot distinguish between colonization and infection. This problem can be overcome by performing quantitative culture on BAL fluid or by performing PSB sampling. A double-sheathed microbiology brush is used to perform PSB sampling. The PSB is contained within an inner and outer cannula, with its distal end protected by a wax plug. In PSB sampling, the bronchoscope is wedged in the subsegmental bronchus of the most involved bronchopulmonary segment. Once in place, the PSB catheter is advanced out of the bronchoscope into the desired subsegment, the distal plug ejected, and the brush advanced. The brush is then gently moved back and forth several times, and then retracted into the inner cannula and removed from the bronchoscope. The brush is advanced out of the PSB catheter and cut off from the wire into a sterile test tube containing 1 mL Ringer's lactate solution. This solution is then cultured using quantitative methods.

■ INDICATIONS

Bronchoscopy is best performed by a clinician well versed in this technique. The indications for bronchoscopy in the ICU include the following:

- *Diffuse parenchymal disease in patients testing positive for human immunodeficiency virus (HIV)*. BAL is the initial diagnostic procedure of choice in HIV-positive patients with a diffuse alveolar infiltrate. BAL has been shown to have a high sensitivity and specificity for the diagnosis of opportunistic pulmonary infections, especially *P. carinii* pneumonia. The role of BAL in isolating cytomegalovirus and its clinical significance in this population are controversial and much less well defined.
- *Diffuse parenchymal disease in non-HIV-immunocompromised patients (organ transplant, postchemotherapy neutropenia, immunosuppressive therapy, etc.)*. Immunocompromised patients are prone to develop various pulmonary complications, including cardiac failure, drug reactions, pulmonary emboli, and malignant spread; however, infections are the most common cause. These infections are caused by opportunistic as well as bacterial and viral pathogens. While the diagnostic yield of BAL is lower in this group of patients (diagnostic yield of approximately 40% to 70%) compared with HIV patients, it has a low complication rate, is easily performed, and should be considered the diagnostic test of first choice. Open lung biopsy has a diagnostic efficacy of about 65%, but because of attendant morbidity and mortality, this procedure should be performed in cases in which BAL has failed to yield a diagnosis and when clinical deterioration has occurred.
- *Atelectasis that has not improved despite aggressive physiotherapy*. The critically ill patient who is unable to move or cough effectively has multiple reasons to develop atelectasis and impaired mucociliary clearance. Lobar atelectasis in ICU patients may worsen oxygenation, predispose patients to pulmonary infection, and impair weaning attempts. Chest physiotherapy is considered the treatment of choice for atelectasis. Bronchoscopy is frequently performed when chest therapy fails to re-expand the lung. There are, however, no data to suggest that bronchoscopy is more efficacious than chest physiotherapy. It should be emphasized that the suction lumen of the bronchoscopic has a small diameter (1 to 2.6 mm), making the removal of thick tenacious secretions particularly difficult. The use of air insufflation through the bronchoscope has been reported for the treatment of persistent atelectasis.
- *Diagnosis of ventilator-associated pneumonia*. Bronchoscopy with PSB sampling or BAL together with quantitative culture is cur-

rently recommended as the procedure of choice for the diagnosis of ventilator-associated pneumonia. However, blind-PSB or mini-BAL with quantitative culture can be performed without bronchoscopy, has a sensitivity and specificity similar to bronchoscopic directed sampling, and is therefore a highly cost-effective alternative to the bronchoscopic sampling techniques.

- *Acute inhalational injury.* In patients exposed to smoke inhalation, fiberoptic laryngoscopy and bronchoscopy are indicated to identify the anatomic level and severity of injury.
- *The diagnosis of traumatic airway fracture.* After blunt trauma, patients who present with atelectasis, pneumomediastinum, and/or pneumothorax may have sustained a fractured airway.
- *Foreign bodies.* Forceps are available for use with the flexible bronchoscope, which may allow for the removal of foreign bodies.
- *Endotracheal intubation.* In difficult or failed intubations, the flexible bronchoscope may be used as an obturator for endotracheal intubation.

■ CONTRAINDICATIONS

- Refractory hypoxia. The Pao_2 will drop on average 20 mm Hg during the procedure.
- Poorly controlled asthmatics.
- Hemodynamically unstable patients.

■ PERFORMANCE OF BRONCHOSCOPY

- *Sedation and anesthesia:* Nonintubated patients should be lightly sedated with a short-acting benzodiazepine. It is important to ensure that patients are calm and yet cooperative during the procedure. Local anesthesia is used to limit the irritation caused by the bronchoscope. Intubated, mechanically ventilated patients should be well sedated, as coughing during the procedure increases airway pressure, interferes with ventilation, and hampers the procedure. As the endotracheal tube (or tracheostomy tube) bypasses the upper airways, local anesthesia is not required. Local anesthetic agents should not be used when performing PSB sampling.
- *Oxygenation:* It is essential that all patients be monitored with a pulse oximeter throughout the procedure and for several hours thereafter. If the patient desaturates during the procedure, the bronchoscope should be removed immediately. Intubated,

mechanically ventilated patients should be preoxygenated with 100% O_2. The Fio_2 should remain at 100% during the procedure and for some hours thereafter, because ventilation perfusing mismatching increases following bronchoscopy.

- *Insertion of the bronchoscope:* In the nonintubated patient, the two standard approaches to the lower airways are transnasal and transoral. The transnasal approach has the advantage of virtually bypassing the gag reflex. In the intubated patient, the bronchoscope is passed through the endotracheal tube. The endotracheal tube is fitted with an adapter, which allows for the simultaneous mechanical ventilation through one port and passage of the bronchoscope into the airway via the other. A size 8 (sometimes 7.5) or larger endotracheal tube is required to both ventilate the patient and to allow for the passage of the bronchoscope. In patients intubated with a smaller tube, a pediatric bronchoscope can be used, or the patient can be reintubated with a larger tube.

■ COMPLICATIONS

When performed by a trained specialist, flexible bronchoscopy is an extremely safe procedure. The complication rate increases significantly when transbronchial biopsy is performed. Complications include

- Complications associated with the use of sedation/anesthesia
- Hypoxemia
- Bleeding
- Pneumothorax
- Vasovagal reactions
- Pneumonia
- Bronchospasm
- Arrhythmias
- Acute myocardial infarction

15

Chest Physical Therapy in the Intensive Care Unit

Critically ill patients are nursed in the supine position for extended periods of time. In the supine patient, the abdominal contents push in a cephalad direction, decreasing the functional residual capacity and causing alveolar closure in the dependent lung zones. In addition, immobility results in accumulation of mucus in the dependent lung zones. Intubated, sedated, mechanically ventilated patients are unable to mobilize their respiratory secretions. As the endotracheal tube bypasses the glottic mechanism, coughing is ineffective in intubated patients. Furthermore, the endotracheal tube interferes with normal mucociliary transport. These patients are therefore at a high risk of developing segmental or lobar atelectasis. Thoracic and abdominal surgery further predispose patients to the development of atelectasis. The most common segment to develop atelectasis is the left lower lobe, possibly due to compression by the heart in the supine position and its poor drainage. Atelectasis impairs oxygenation, increases the risk of developing pneumonia, and delays attempts at weaning. Chest physical therapy is therefore a vital component in the management of all critically ill patients to prevent retention of secretions and atelectasis.

Chest therapy consists of postural drainage, percussion, vibration, coughing, suctioning, and patient mobilization. *None of these maneuvers have been studied vigorously in any type of clinical study.* While some form of chest therapy and endotracheal suctioning is essential in all mechanically ventilated patients, the most effective form of chest therapy has yet to be determined by controlled trials. Furthermore, while the role of routine chest therapy in postoperative patients is controversial, a number of studies have demonstrated that such therapy is effective in reducing postoperative pulmonary complications in patients who have undergone thoracic and abdominal surgery.

Mobilization and ambulation is the most effective method of chest therapy. Ambulation can be performed in intubated patients using a manual resuscitator bag. For obvious reasons, this technique cannot be performed in sedated patients; however, it is a highly effective method of facilitating weaning (liberation) in patients with chronic obstructive pulmonary disease (COPD). Percussion and vibration are the techniques most frequently recommended for patients who are intubated and mechanically ventilated and for patients with impaired cognition or poor coughing ability. Percussion and vibration are used to enhance mucociliary clearance from the central and peripheral airways. The exact mechanism of action of chest percussion is unknown.

Tracheal suctioning is an integral component of chest therapy for the intubated patient. Deep suctioning is usually necessary to mobilize secretions. Withholding suctioning may result in airway closure or even endotracheal tube occlusion. Because respiratory secretions are most prevalent after a change in patient position and following chest physical therapy, the suctioning procedure should be timed with these interventions.

The role of chest therapy in nonintubated ICU patients with respiratory disorders such as pneumonia, COPD, and asthma is unclear. Certainly, chest therapy is indicated if these patients develop atelectasis; however, in the absence of atelectasis, little data support such therapy.

16

Chest Radiography in the Intensive Care Unit Patient

Interpretation of a bedside film is fraught by numerous pitfalls. However, a number of studies have demonstrated that daily chest radiographs frequently demonstrate new, unexpected, or changing abnormalities, which result in changes in therapy. Daily portable chest examinations should therefore be performed in all but the most stable ICU patients.

The bedside chest radiograph is anteroposterior (AP) rather than posteroanterior (PA). On the AP view, the heart and mediastinum appear about 15% wider than on an upright PA chest radiograph. Most of this magnification occurs because portable radiography is performed with the x-ray tube closer to the patient than when done in the radiology department. Furthermore, magnification also occurs because of the increased distance of the heart from the film in the AP projection. Because of these factors, a false impression of cardiomegaly or a wide mediastinum may be obtained. In addition, portable chest radiographs may be difficult to interpret due to poor positioning with films taken in the supine position. Pleural effusion can easily be missed in the supine position; furthermore, the pulmonary vasculature is distorted on supine radiographs because blood no longer flows preferentially to the lower lobes. Thus, if the patient is imaged in the supine position, changes in lung blood flow, which are usually signs of congestive heart failure, can be mimicked. Every effort should therefore be made to position the patient upright. It should also be appreciated that, because lateral chest films cannot be obtained in the ICU, abnormalities in the posterior costophrenic angles, within the mediastinum and adjacent to the spine, can easily be missed. Notwithstanding these limitations, the routine portable chest radiograph provides vital information that is essential for the management of the critically ill ICU patient. In addition, chest radiographs should be obtained after the insertion of a subclavian or internal jugular central venous catheters to confirm correct placement of the catheter and to exclude a pneumothorax.

The chest radiograph should be studied systematically: First, the position of all the tubes and catheters should be evaluated, followed by an evaluation of the lung parenchyma, pleura, mediastinum, and diaphragm, followed by a search for signs of extra-alveolar air.

■ POSITION OF TUBES AND CATHETERS

- *Endotracheal tube.* With the head in a neutral position, the tip of the tube should be 7 ± 2 cm from the carina. It should be noted that, with movement of the head, from a flexed to an extended position, the tube can move by as much as 4 cm. A useful landmark for the tip of the endotracheal tube is the superior border of the aortic notch (Marik's sign) or the upper border of T4 (Figure 16-1).
- *Central venous catheters.* The tip of the catheter should be located beyond the venous valves of the subclavian or internal jugular vein but proximal to the right atrium (i.e., above the superior vena cava–right atrial junction). Placement in the right atrium may result in atrial perforation. Two useful radiographic landmarks for the position of the tip of the catheter follow (see Figure 16-1):
    The first costochondral junction
    A point 2 cm inferior to a line joining inferior margins of the clavicular heads
- *Pulmonary artery catheter.* The tip of the pulmonary artery catheter should be located in the proximal left or right branch of the pulmonary artery.
- *Other tubes and catheters.* The position of other tubes and catheters, such as the nasogastric tube, feeding tube, chest tubes, intra-aortic balloon catheter, and pacing wires should be noted.

■ LUNG PARENCHYMA, PLEURA, AND MEDIASTINUM

- *Pulmonary infiltrates.* The presence of pulmonary infiltrates should be noted. It should be noted whether the infiltrate is interstitial or alveolar (or both), unilateral or bilateral, and patchy or diffuse. An infiltrate may be caused by either water (cardiogenic

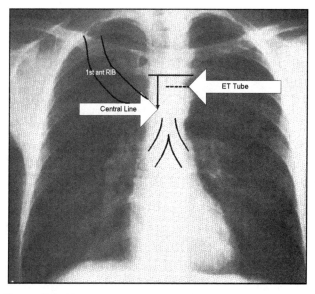

Figure 16-1. Idealized chest radiograph demonstrating the position of the central line and endotracheal tube.

or noncardiogenic pulmonary edema), cells (infection), and/or blood (pulmonary hematoma, intra-alveolar bleed). It should be appreciated that it may not be possible to distinguish between these entities by examination of the chest film alone. The following radiographic findings may help distinguish cardiac and noncardiac pulmonary edema:

Noncardiac pulmonary edema (acute lung injury)
Normal heart shape
Absence of septal lines
No peribronchial cuffing
Frequent air bronchograms
Patchy increased lung density
Peripheral increased lung density
Cardiogenic pulmonary edema
Base-to-apex blood flow inversion
Even distribution of increased lung density
Septal lines
Peribronchial cuffing

- *Pleural fluid.* In the supine position, fluid tracks posteriorly, resulting in a diffuse haziness of the lung fields. It is therefore very easy to miss a significant pleural collection. Fluid collections can be confirmed by lateral decubitus films or ultrasonography.
- *Mediastinum.* The width of the mediastinum should be noted (normal; <10 cm) as well as the presence of mediastinal nodes or masses.
- *Evidence of barotrauma.* The traditional apicolateral collection of air may not be present on portable supine films of patients with pneumothoraces. Free air will often be located in the anterior costophrenic sulcus, as this is the most superior portion of the pleural space in the supine patient. Other radiographic signs of a pneumothorax in the supine position include a relative hyperlucency over the upper abdominal quadrants and a deep costophrenic angle (the deep sulcus sign).

The portable chest radiograph is not ideal for evaluating the hilum and lung parenchyma. Conventional and high-resolution computed tomography (HRCT) may be useful for evaluating aortic dissection, pleural disease, lung parenchyma in immunocompromised patients with pulmonary infiltrates, characterization of diffuse infiltrative pulmonary disease, and suspected masses in the mediastinum or hilum. Routine CT evaluation of the chest can be done with or without intravenous administration of contrast media. Contrast is reserved for those cases in which mediastinal or hilar pathology is suspected.

HRCT differs from conventional CT not only in the use of a thinner x-ray beam (e.g., 1.5 mm vs. 1 cm) but also in the use of digitized x-ray construction, which allows for better spatial resolution and for more detailed images of the lung parenchyma. HRCT is therefore useful in the evaluation of patients with diffuse infiltrative lung diseases. Spiral CT differs from conventional CT primarily in that it allows continuous scanning of the patients. In spiral CT, the x-ray tube makes continuous 360-degree revolutions without interruption. The patient is moved through the circulating beam at a predetermined speed, and imaging information is then obtained as a solid cylinder, instead of one slice at a time. Spiral CT is most helpful in evaluating lesions at or near the diaphragm (less motion artifact), vascular structures (main pulmonary arteries in suspected pulmonary embolism), and small pulmonary nodules.

Part 2

The Cardiovascular System

17

Fluid and Pressor Resuscitation: The Management of Oliguria, Hypotension, and Prerenal States

The treatment of decreased intravascular volume (hypovolemia) is fluid resuscitation.

> . . . You need to fill the tank.

When the patient is not making urine, *do not* give Lasix (furosemide). It is a fundamental misunderstanding of human physiology to give a diuretic to a patient with acute oliguria. No scientific rationale or clinical evidence supports the use of loop diuretics in patients with acute oliguria; these agents should rarely if ever be used in this setting.

The intravascular volume of an average 70-kg man is approximately 5 L, of which 2 L are red cell volume and 3 L plasma volume. The intravascular extracellular fluid compartment equilibrates with the extracelluar extravascular fluid compartment ((ECF) 11 L), with a reduction in one compartment leading to a reduction of the other. A wide spectrum of medical conditions may reduce the total intravascular volume. The most common conditions include acute blood loss, gastrointestinal tract losses (diarrhea, vomiting, fistula), sepsis, hyperglycemia, decreased fluid intake due to acute medical conditions, and heat stroke.

A reduction in intravascular volume results in a fall in stroke volume, which is initially compensated for by an increase in heart rate, thereby maintaining cardiac output. However, with further volume depletion, cardiac output and then blood pressure fall. This is associated with a reduction in organ perfusion. At the organ level, local autoregulatory mechanisms come into play in an attempt to maintain tissue perfusion. A reduction in renal perfusion normally results in dilatation of the glomerular afferent arteriole and constriction of the glomerular efferent arteriole so that glomerular capillary hydrostatic pressure and glomerular filtration rate (GFR) remain constant. However, a decrease in *renal perfusion pressure* below the autoregulatory range (*mean arterial pressure* $< 80\,mmHg$) leads to an abrupt fall in GFR and urine output (oliguria). In the elderly and in patients with diseases affecting the integrity of the afferent arterioles, lesser degrees of hypotension may cause a decline in renal function and oliguria. While primary renal diseases and urinary tract obstruction may lead to oliguria, intravascular volume depletion with renal hypoperfusion is the most common cause of oliguria in clinical practice. The management of oliguria due to intravascular volume depletion is **aggressive fluid resuscitation.**

The effective circulating volume refers to that part of the intravascular volume that is in the arterial tree (normally about 700 mL in a 70-kg man) and is effectively perfusing the tissues.[1] Physiologically, the effective circulating volume is the *pressure perfusing the arterial baroreceptors* in the carotid sinus and glomerular afferent arterioles, since it is changes in pressure (or stretch) rather than volume or flow that is sensed. The effective circulating volume usually varies directly with the ECF volume. However, in some settings the effective circulating volume may be independent of the ECF volume, the plasma volume, or even cardiac output. In congestive heart failure, the effective circulating volume is reduced because a primary decrease in cardiac output lowers the pressure at the baroreceptors. This decline in pressure and flow induces compensatory fluid retention by the kidney, leading to expansion of the ECF. The net result is effective intravascular volume depletion in association with increases in both the plasma and total ECF volumes. The increase in volume in this setting is appropriate because the associated rise in intracardiac filling pressure can, by increasing cardiac stretch, improve cardiac contractility and raise cardiac output and systemic blood pressure toward normal (Frank-Starling mechanism). Sodium and water retention is therefore an appropriate compensation in that it restores tissue perfusion, even though it also augments the degree of edema. In patients with cirrhosis, the ECF volume is expanded, the plasma volume is increased, and the cardiac output is increased because of systemic vasodilation. Yet, in these patients the effective intravascular volume is reduced due to decreased systemic perfusion pressure and intense renal vasoconstriction.

Diuresis with loop diuretics in patients with normal or reduced effective intravascular volume is invariably associated with a fall in intravascular volume, a fall in plasma volume, a fall in GFR, and a rise in serum urea nitrogen (BUN). The fall in GFR has been correlated with the fall in intravascular volume. Contraction of the intravascular volume and fall in GFR may occur in the absence of a fall in cardiac output. Volume depletion is associated with a greater rise in the BUN than in the plasma creatinine due to increased passive reabsorption of urea that follows the hypovolemia-induced increase in sodium and water resorption in the kidney. An increasing BUN/creatinine ratio in a patient receiving a diuretic is a reliable sign of intravascular volume depletion and should prompt the immediate discontinuation of these agents.

Contrary to popular belief, the GFR falls (rather than rises) with loop diuretics. In the mammalian kidney, there is close coordination between the processes of glomerular filtration and tubular reabsorption. Coordination between the glomerulus and tubule is mediated by a system of tubuloglomerular feedback that operates within the juxtaglomerular apparatus of each nephron. Microperfusion experiments have demonstrated that an increase in flow rate of tubule fluid through the loop of Henle following the use of a loop diuretic is followed by a reduction in single-nephron GFR. This has been shown to be mediated via feedback control by the macula densa, which is the flow-dependent distal-sensing site. When the tubular glomerular feedback pathway is interrupted with a loop diuretic, there is an attenuation of the pressure-induced afferent arteriolar dilatation with impairment in blood flow autoregulation. In patients with extracellular volume depletion, this effect is exaggerated with a dramatic fall in GFR.

■ HYPOTENSION (OR OLIGURIA)

Treat patients with hypotension or oliguria with *fluid* (200- to 500-mL boluses).

In patients with respiratory failure and oliguria/hypotension, endotracheal intubation and or pressors should be considered before fluid challenges.

After 1500-mL resuscitation, *stop* and

- Reevaluate the patient (and diagnosis).
- Admit the patient to the ICU (if not in the ICU).
- Consider invasive hemodynamic monitoring.

■ ASSESSMENT OF INTRAVASCULAR VOLUME AND CARDIAC OUTPUT (SEE ALSO CHAPTER 18)

The clinical determination of the intravascular volume can be extremely difficult in critically ill ICU patients. A low urine output is a reliable indicator of intravascular volume depletion and/or a low cardiac output (in the absence of established renal failure). However, remember that hyperglycemia will result in a "good" urine output in dehydrated patients. Other clinical signs of inadequate intravascular volume/cardiac output include

- Postural hypotension and tachycardia (raise head of bed)
- Hypothermia
- Hypotension
- Altered sensorium
- Peripheral cyanosis
- Skin mottling
- Cold extremities
- Cold knees (Marik's sign); temperature gradient between thigh and knee
- Arterial systolic pressure variation during positive-pressure ventilation (fall in systolic blood pressure during inspiration)

The kidney (urine output) is an excellent barometer of intravascular volume/cardiac output. If the urine output does not increase with fluid challenges, invasive hemodynamic monitoring may be required (to exclude cardiac causes of diminished cardiac output).

Make sure the urinary catheter is not blocked.

The central venous pressure (CVP) is an extremely poor indicator of intravascular volume. Studies have demonstrated *no correlation* between the CVP and either the blood volume or the right ventricular end-diastolic volume. In fact, the CVP may fall with fluid resuscitation (due to decreased autonomic tone). Therapy guided by the CVP is likely to result in fluid overload and/or pulmonary edema. Many of the limitations to the use of the CVP apply to the pulmonary capillary wedge pressure (a poor indicator of intravascular volume and left ventricular end-diastolic volume). The REF catheter (right ventricular ejection fraction pulmonary artery catheter) allows for the computation of the right ventricular end-diastolic volume. A number of studies have shown this to be a useful determinant of intravascular volume and recruitable cardiac index (see Chapter 18).

■ THE TYPE OF FLUID (CRYSTALLOID VS. COLLOID)

The best type of resuscitation fluid in various clinical situations is a topic of much debate that is largely unresolved due to the lack of adequately powered, well-controlled clinical trials. Furthermore, the situation is complicated by the fact that certain patient groups may benefit from the combination of both crystalloids and a colloid. Furthermore, not all colloids are created equal. Two meta-analyses have provided some assistance in this area, namely,

- Colloids alone may be harmful in trauma patients.
- Albumin **should not** be used as a volume expander in critically ill patients (it increases mortality across subgroups of patients).

Crystalloids essentially resuscitate the *extravascular compartment*, whereas colloids resuscitate the *intravascular compartment*. It is important to assess the size of both compartments when deciding on the best fluid resuscitation protocol (Figure 17-1). Only about 20% to 25% of a crystalloid solution remains intravascular, whereas a colloidal solution will increase the intravascular volume in excess of the infused volume (>100%). Theoretically, colloids should not increase the interstitial compartment (extracellular extravascular compartment). However, recent studies indicate that albumin leaks into the interstitial compartment and significantly increases the size of this compartment (this effect may be more pronounced in septic patients). Hydroxyethyl starch (HES) solutions leak to some degree into the interstitial compartment. However, these solutions increase the plasma oncotic pressure more than the interstitial fluid oncotic pressure.

The type of resuscitation fluid will depend upon the patient's clinical diagnosis and the volume status of each compartment. Most patients who have lost intravascular volume have lost both colloid (plasma) and crystalloid (interstitial) fluid. Therefore, both fluid types, i.e., colloid and crystalloid, should be replaced. Replacing only colloid fluid may result in severe intracellular dehydration; replacing only crystalloid fluid may result in excessive tissue edema. As a general rule, patients should be resuscitated with a fluid similar to that lost (Tables 17-1 and 17-2); e.g., patients with diarrhea should receive 0.45 NaCl with supplemented potassium and bicarbonate. Remember that no body fluid is more hypertonic than plasma. Dehydrated patients (decreased intravascular volume) with either hypo- or hypernatremia should be volume resuscitated with either normal saline or Ringer's lactate until intravascular volume is restored; thereafter, the tonicity can be corrected. Five percent dextrose in water is not an intravascu-

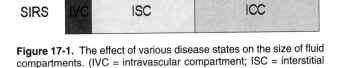

Figure 17-1. The effect of various disease states on the size of fluid compartments. (IVC = intravascular compartment; ISC = interstitial compartment; ICC = intracellular compartment; SIRS = systemic inflammatory response syndrome.)

lar volume expander and should **never** be used to volume resuscitate a patient.

Hemorrhage

In patients who have lost blood, fluid moves from the interstitial compartment to restore the blood volume (hence the hematocrit drops; it takes 72 hours for hematocrit to stabilize!). Therefore, both the intra- and extravascular compartments are decreased. Hemorrhage models in animals have demonstrated a higher mortality when animals are resuscitated with blood alone, as compared to blood and crystalloids. Patients who have lost blood should therefore be initially resuscitated with crystalloid and then with blood (and colloids).

Table 17-1. Electrolyte content of body fluids.

Type of Loss	Na+ mEq/L	K+ mEq/L	HCO₃⁻ mEq/L
Gastric	40–80	5–15	—
Pancreatic	140–150	0–10	80–100
Bile	140–150	0–10	40–50
Ileostomy	120–140	5–20	30–60
Diarrhea	40–140	20–50	30–50

Table 17-2. Constituents of common IV fluids.

	Na mEq/L	K mEq/L	Cl mEq/L	Lactate mEq/L	HCO₃ mEq/L	osm mOsm/L
5% glucose						278
NaCl 0.45%	77		77			154
NaCl 0.9%	154		154			308
Ringer's lactate	130	4	110	27		275
NaHCO₃ 4.2%	500				500	1000
NaHCO₃ 8.4%	1000				1000	2000
5% albumin	140		140			308
25% albumin	140		140			1500
6% hydroxyethyl starch	154		154			310

Dehydration

Patients who are dehydrated (from diarrhea, vomiting, diabetic osmotic diuresis, etc.) have lost both intravascular and extravascular volume. Volume replacement with crystalloids will resuscitate both compartments.

Sepsis and the Systemic Inflammatory Response Syndrome (Sepsis, Trauma, Pancreatitis, Postop)

As a consequence of leaky capillaries and third-space loss, these patients have a decreased effective intravascular compartment and tissue edema (enlarged interstitial compartment). Because <20% of infused crystalloids remains intravascular in these patients, the volume of crystalloids should be limited. Colloidal solutions such as HES have theoretical advantages in patients with sepsis and Systemic Inflammatory Response Syndrome (SIRS) (see Chapter 37).

Burns

Due to the thermal injury, these patients have a massive loss of interstitial fluid as well as a generalized capillary leak. Patients should be resuscitated with crystalloid during the first 24 hours.

Crystalloids

Isotonic crystalloid solutions are safe and effective for resuscitation of hypovolemic patients. Because isotonic fluids have the same osmolality as body fluids, there are no net osmotic forces tending to move water into or out of the intracellular compartment. Therefore, the electrolytes and water partition themselves in a manner similar to the body's extravascular water content: 75% extravascular and 25% intravascular. Three to four times the intravascular deficit therefore is required. The partitioning occurs within 30 minutes of infusion, and within 2 hours, <20% of the infused fluid remains within the intravascular space (may be significantly less in patients with leaky capillaries). When compared to colloids, fluid challenges with crystalloids are associated with only a small increase in cardiac output and oxygen delivery. Excessive administration of crystalloid is associated with pulmonary and generalized tissue edema.

- *0.9% NaCl.* This is the only crystalloid that can be mixed with blood. Patients may develop a hyperchloremic metabolic acidosis and/or hypernatremia.
- *Ringer's lactate.* This has a more physiologic electrolyte composition. The added lactate is converted to bicarbonate in the liver, which occurs readily except in patients with profound liver dysfunction and shocked liver. Ringer's lactate does not cause acidosis in these circumstances, because the lactate is in the form of the base.

Colloids

Colloids are solutions that rely on high-molecular-weight species for their osmotic effect. Because the barrier between the intravascular space is only partly permeable to the passage of these molecules, colloids tend to remain in the intravascular space for longer periods than do crystalloids. Smaller quantities of colloids are therefore required to restore intravascular volume. Because of their oncotic pressure, colloids tend to draw fluid from the extravascular compartment into the intravascular space.

Albumin

Albumin is available as a 5% solution. The serum half-life of exogenous albumin is <8 hours, though <10% leaves the vascular space within 2 hours of administration. After 2 days, only 25% of the administered dose remains within the intravascular compartment. In patients with the leaky capillary syndrome, these molecules may leak from the intravascular space, lowering the colloid osmotic pressure of the plasma, and drawing more fluid into an already compromised interstitium.

Hetastarch (Hespan)

Hetastarch is a synthetic hydroxyethyl starch that is available as a 6% solution dissolved in normal saline. It is a polydispersed solution with molecular weights ranging from 10,000 to 2,000,000. The average molecular weight is approximately 450,000, or nearly seven times larger than albumin. About half the administered dose is excreted by the kidneys within 2 days and about 65% within 8 days. The large-molecular-weight moieties are taken up by the reticuloendothelial system and can be detected for as long as 42 days. Hetastarch may cause a thrombocytopenia and prolongation of the partial thromboplastin time due to an interaction of the large-molecular-weight moieties with platelets and factor VIII. Both small- and large-molecular-weight species filter into the interstitial fluid; however, the plasma oncotic pressure increases to a greater extent than that of the interstitial fluid oncotic pressure. Contrary to popular belief, HES is safe in patients with renal failure and is, in fact, the volume expander of choice in patients who become hypotensive during hemodialysis.

■ TREATMENT OF HYPOALBUMINEMIA

Hypoalbuminemia is a common finding in critically ill patients. It has been well documented that hypoalbuminemic patients have a higher morbidity and mortality when compared to patients with a normal serum albumin. Consequently, hypoalbuminemic patients are commonly treated with exogenous albumin in the hope of improving their outcome. A review of the prospective, randomized studies that have been reported to date does not support this practice. The administration of albumin for the purpose of raising reduced serum levels has been described as the *"ultimate metabolic misunderstanding."*

One of the major motivations for the use of albumin in the critically ill patient has been to prevent pulmonary and tissue edema by enhancing the plasma colloid osmotic pressure (COP). However, in the critically ill patient there is a very poor relationship between the serum albumin and COP. Furthermore, endothelial injury with leaky capillaries (reduced σ in the Starling equation) is common in critically ill patients, reducing the importance of the COP in influencing fluid flux. Albumin supplementation has only a transitory effect on the serum albumin concentration, due to the redistribution of albumin from the intravascular to the extravascular space.

A recent meta-analysis of the use of albumin in critically ill patients has suggested that albumin administration increases mortality. The pooled relative risk of death with albumin administration was 1.68 (1.26 to 2.23). For every 17 critically ill patients treated with albumin, there was one additional death. There is therefore no evidence that albumin administration reduces mortality in critically ill patients with hypovolemia, burns, or hypalbuminemia, and there is a strong suggestion that it may increase mortality. These data suggest that use of human albumin should not be used outside the context of rigorously conducted, randomized controlled trials.

The only circumstances in which the treatment of hypoalbuminemia with exogenous albumin has been proven to be of benefit are when combined with a loop diuretic in cirrhotic patients with refractory ascites, large-volume paracentesis, and in nephrotic patients with anasarca.

■ PRESSOR AGENTS IN THE CRITICALLY ILL

The available pressor agents and their receptor occupation are listed in Table 17-3. Patients who remain hypotensive despite "adequate" fluid resuscitation may benefit from the addition of a vasopressor agent. Pulmonary artery catheterization is not a prerequisite for the use of vasopressor agents. Norepinephrine, dobutamine, and dopamine are the vasoactive agents most commonly used in the ICU setting. No randomized, controlled studies have been performed demonstrating the superiority of one these agents over the other in various hemodynamic settings. The agent(s) of choice should be based on the drug's hemodynamic profile and its effect on blood flow redistribution.

While there are no strong data to demonstrate the benefit of either norepinephrine, dobutamine, or dopamine in the critically ill, a number of studies have demonstrated that epinephrine and phenylephrine may have deleterious effects. Epinephrine has been shown to cause a significant increase in the serum lactate concentration with an associated fall in the serum pH. This increase in lactate has been associated with an increase in the lactate/pyruvate ratio, a marker of anaerobic metabolism. This rise in lactate has not been demonstrated

Table 17-3. Pressor agents: Receptor occupation and hemodynamic effects.

	Epinephrine	Norepinephrine	Dopamine	Dobutamine	Phenylephrine
α_1	+++	+++	++ (3rd)	+	+++
α_2	+++	+++	++	+	0
β_1	++++	+++	+++ (2nd)	++++	0
β_2	++	0	+	++	0
DA 1&2 dopamine receptors	0	0	+++ (1st)	0	0
Cardiac index	+++	+	+++	+++	—
Heart rate	+++	+	+++	++	+/−
Systemic vascular resistance	+/−	+++	+/−	—	+++
Left cardiac work index	+++	++	+++	++	++
O_2 consumption	++	0 / +	++	+	0
Blood glucose	+++	0 / +	+	+	0

with the use of the other commonly used inotropic agents. Epinephrine increases glycogenolysis, increases free fatty acid levels, and impairs insulin-mediated glucose uptake. These metabolic effects are undesirable in the critically ill. Phenylephrine has no beta-receptor activity and will decrease cardiac output: there is no medical condition that benefits from a reduction of cardiac output.

Dobutamine should be used with extreme caution in hypotensive patients (particularly volume-depleted patients), as it may exacerbate the hypotension. Dobutamine is the drug of choice to increase myocardial contractility. Norepinephrine is the drug of choice to increase systemic vascular resistance. Dobutamine and norepinephrine may be a useful combination in patients with depressed myocardial contractility and a low systemic vascular resistance, i.e., patients with underlying heart disease who develop sepsis or patients with severe myocardial depression due to sepsis (see Chapter 42). Dopamine increases cardiac output more than norepinephrine; however, its use may be limited by tachycardia. Low-dose dopamine has no proven role in oliguric states (see Chapter 32). Contrary to popular opinion, norepinephrine has been demonstrated to increase both splanchnic and renal blood flow in sepsis, with an improvement of gastric intramucosal pH (or Pco_2) and creatine clearance. Vasopressin causes profound splanchnic ischemia and appears to have a limited role as a pressor agent.

■ SELECTED REFERENCES

1. Bessey PQ, Brooks DC, Black PR, Aoki TT, Wilmore DW. Epinephrine acutely mediates skeletal muscle insulin resistance. *Surgery*. 1983;94:172–179.
2. Desjars P, Pinaud M, Bugnon D, Tassea F. Norepinephrine therapy has no deleterious renal effects in human septic shock. *Crit Care Med*. 1989;17:-426–429.
3. Ernest D, Belzberg AS, Dodek PM. Distribution of normal saline and 5% albumin infusions in septic patients. *Crit Care Med*. 1999;27:46–50.
4. Human albumin administration in critically ill patients: systematic review of randomised controlled trials. Cochrane Injuries Group Albumin Reviewers. *BMJ*. 1998;317:235–240.
5. Korent VA, Conhaim RL, McGrath AM, DeAngeles DA, Harms BA. Molecular distribution of hetastarch in plasma and lung lymph of unanesthetized sheep. *Am J Respir Crit Care Med*. 1997;155:1302–1308.
6. Levy B, Bollaert PE, Charpentier C, et al. Comparison of norepinephrine and dobutamine to epinephrine for hemodynamics, lactate metabolism, and gastric tonometric variables in septic shock: a prospective, randomized, study. *Intensive Care Med*. 1997;23:282–287.
7. Practice parameters for hemodynamic support of sepsis in adult patients in sepsis. *Crit Care Med*. 1999;27:639–660.

8. Schrier RW. An odyssey into the milieu interieur: pondering the enigmas. *J Am Soc Nephrol.* 1992;2:1549–1559.
9. van der Sande FM, Luik AJ, Kooman JP, Verstappen V, Leunissen KML. Effect of intravenous fluids on blood pressure course during hemodialysis in hypotensive-prone patients. *J Am Soc Nephrol.* 2000;11:550–554.

18

Hemodynamic Monitoring: Pulmonary Artery and Arterial Catheterization

No conclusive data demonstrates an improvement in patient outcome with the use of the pulmonary artery catheter (PAC). The merits of the PAC must therefore be carefully evaluated in each patient.

The bedside assessment of cardiac performance and ventricular preload is perhaps one of the most difficult and yet vitally important problems in critical care medicine. The traditional clinical signs of cardiac function such as blood pressure, jugular venous distension, skin perfusion, and skin turgor are unreliable in the ICU setting. According to the Frank-Starling principle, the vigor of cardiac contraction relates directly to muscle fiber length at end-diastole. This presystolic fiber stretch, or preload, is proportionate to end-diastolic volume. Left ventricular end-diastolic volume (preload) is therefore a major factor determining cardiac output. To make rational management decisions in terms of fluid and vasoactive drug therapy, the intensivist needs to correctly assess the patient's preload.

■ THE PULMONARY ARTERY CATHETER

It is clear that the inappropriate use and poor understanding of the PAC leads to excessive mortality. It is also evident that the PAC is a very useful diagnostic tool that aids in the management of critically ill patients. PACs should therefore be used only by physicians who have extensive experience in their use. Furthermore, the data must be interpreted in the context of the clinical scenario. Too often, the attending physician reviews the patient's "numbers" without ever setting eyes on the patient.

PAC may be useful in the evaluation and optimization of intravascular volume status in

- Refractory shock
- Acute respiratory distress syndrome and acute lung injury
- Acute myocardial infarction complicated by acute cardiac failure
- High-risk surgical patients (perioperative management)

Insertion of a PAC

Central venous access is obtained as outlined in Chapter 56. It is easier to "float" a PAC from either the left subclavian or right internal jugular vein. Before inserting the PAC through the introducer, gently shake (jiggle) the tip and look at the waveform on the monitor; an undamped "sinusoidal" wave should appear. It is absolutely essential to ensure that an adequate waveform can be obtained before inserting the catheter. Also check the patency of the balloon. The catheter is advanced through the introducer. Once the introducer is cleared (approximately 20 cm), the balloon should be inflated with 1.5 mL of air. The catheter is then advanced until the right ventricular tracing is obtained (approximately 30 cm from subclavian or internal jugular access). If the right ventricular tracing is not encountered, the balloon should be deflated and the catheter withdrawn into the central venous system. The catheter is then readvanced, and the procedure repeated until a right ventricular tracing is obtained. Once the catheter is placed in the right ventricle, the catheter should be advanced into the pulmonary artery (an additional 10 to 15 cm) until a wedge tracing is obtained.

Complications Associated With PAC

Both minor and major life-threatening complications may follow PAC. These include

- Complications associated with central venous access
- Arrhythmias during insertion
- Catheter-associated sepsis
- Balloon rupture
- Intracardiac knotting of catheter
- Pulmonary infarction

- Pulmonary artery perforation
- Tricuspid and pulmonary valve damage and/or endocarditis
- Cardiac perforation (with pacing electrode)
- Heparin-associated thrombocytopenia (from heparin bonding)
- Thrombotic and embolic complications

Thermodilution Cardiac Output

There is no true reference technique for the clinical determination of cardiac output. The reproducibility and accuracy of the thermodilution method of cardiac output determination have been compared with both the Fick and dye-dilution methods. An analysis of these data reveals that the three methods are of equal merit and can be used as independent references. However, an assessment of the reproducibility of the thermodilution technique demonstrates that there must be a difference of at least *15% between the mean of three cardiac output determinations* to be clinically significant.

Determination of the Pulmonary Artery Occlusion Pressure and Pulmonary Capillary Wedge Pressure

Data suggest that as many as *50% of all pulmonary artery occlusion pressure (PAOP) readings are incorrectly determined and/or interpreted, resulting in incorrect therapeutic maneuvers.* It is likely that this single factor is the major reason leading to the "increased mortality" that has been reported in patients who are treated with a PAC. It is therefore important that all the following steps be diligently followed to minimize errors:

- The transducer must be zeroed to atmospheric pressure and fixed to a point that is level with the patient's fourth intercostal space in the midaxillary line (do not guess; use a builder's level, and *mark the chest position for consistency*).
- The patient ***must lie supine*** when the transducer is leveled and the PAOP is measured.
- The dynamic compliance of the system should be checked (Figure 18-1). This is most easily done by using the rapid flush feature of the continuous irrigation device to provide a pressure signal that terminates abruptly. Observe the waveform on the screen. This procedure should produce a square waveform with an oscillating wave at the end of the waveform.
  An overdamped system may be produced by
    Air bubbles
    Kinking of the PAC or tubing
    Too many stopcocks

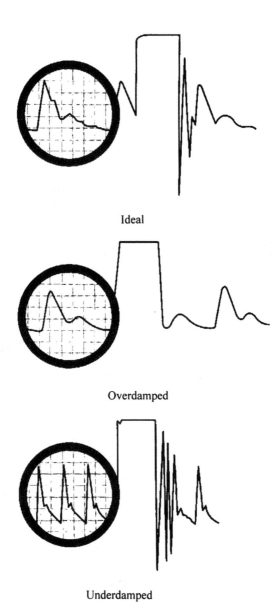

Ideal

Overdamped

Underdamped

Figure 18-1. Assessment of dynamic compliance.

Highly compliant tubing
Blood clots in the tubing
Tubing that is too long
An underdamped system may be produced by
Tubing that is too short
Tubing that is too stiff
- The PAOP tracing should have the following characteristics:
  The PAOP cannot be greater than the pulmonary artery diastolic pressure.
  The phasic PAOP recording must be consistent with an atrial pressure waveform.
  The PAOP waveform should fluctuate with changes in intrapleural pressure. A catheter wedged outside zone 3 of the lung will show marked respiratory variation, a smooth waveform, and misleadingly high pressures (PAOP > PA diastolic).

As the balloon of the PAC is gradually inflated, the catheter "floats" into and obstructs a branch of the pulmonary artery. Once balloon obstruction occurs and forward flow ceases, a static column of blood is created between the inflated balloon and the left atrium, allowing the indirect determination of the left ventricular end-diastolic filling pressure (LVEDP). With balloon occlusion, the pulmonary artery pressure tracing changes to an atrial pressure tracing. The transition from the pulsatile pulmonary artery pressure to the nonpulsatile PAOP shows an initial rapid phase, followed by a more gradual pressure change. The initial rapid phase may represent the pressure across the pulmonary arteries, whereas the slower phase represents the pressure drop across the pulmonary veins. To measure the PAOP accurately, the balloon must totally occlude the branch of the pulmonary artery, and sufficient time must be allowed to elapse so that the pressures fully equilibrate across the vascular tree. The PAOP must then be measured at *end-expiration and end-diastole* (Figures 18-2 and 18-3). It is critical that the PAOP is recorded at a point in the respiratory cycle when pleural pressure has returned as close as possible to baseline value. It is critically important to identify end-expiration on the PCWP tracing; *the waveform looks different after a spontaneous and a ventilator breath.*

Several investigators have recommended that the average of three or more end-expiratory values should be recorded to minimize interpolation error and the respiratory cycle-to-cycle variation, particularly when the patient makes forceful efforts to breathe. In patients having large fluctuation in intrathoracic pressure (due to both patient and ventilator), it may be impossible to determine end-expiration and accurately measure the PAOP. In this situation, I recommend transiently changing the ventilator mode to CPAP (leaving the positive end-expiratory pressure [PEEP] and fraction of inspired oxygen [Fio$_2$]

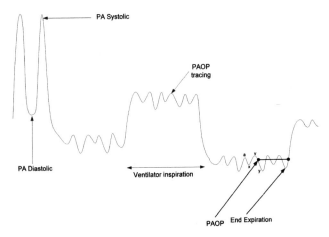

Figure 18-2. Idealized pulmonary artery and PAOP/PCWP tracing.

unchanged) and then determining the PAOP (at patient end-expiration). *It is essential that the PAOP be accurately determined if therapeutic decisions are to be based on this measurement.*

Isovolumetric ventricular contraction begins after the A wave at the onset of the C wave on the left atrial tracing. The AC wave junction (X' descent) may be difficult to see on the PAOP tracing. Consequently, the mean PAOP (midpoint between top of A wave and X descent) can be used to estimate the LVEDP (see Figure 18-2). When measuring the PAOP, it is important that the same reference point be used with each subsequent measurement to achieve consistency.

Although convenient, the digital displays on the oscilloscope are inaccurate, uninterpretable, and totally misleading for determining the pulmonary artery pressures and the PAOP because of the unselective nature of the time-based electrical sampling and averaging. The oscilloscope is designed to calculate and display systemic arterial pressures, which (normally) do not fluctuate significantly throughout the respiratory cycle. However, the oscilloscope cannot tell inspiration from expiration, and it averages the peaks (during ventilator inspiration) and the troughs (during patient inspiration or ventilator expiration) over a few cycles and then displays these as the pulmonary artery systolic and diastolic pressures (these are obviously bogus numbers;

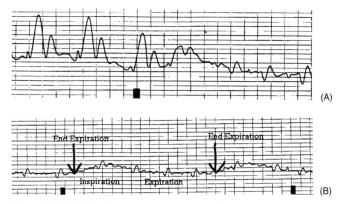

Figure 18-3. (A) Pulmonary artery occlusion. (B) Measurement of PAOP at end-expiration once tracing is stabilized (third breath).

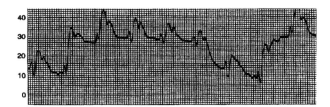

Figure 18-4. Effect of respiratory cycles on pulmonary artery pressure (PAP) tracing. Monitor displayed 42/7 mm Hg. "Real" PAP is 34/27 mm Hg.

see Figure 18-4). The pulmonary artery pressures and the PAOP should therefore be determined from the waveform of a calibrated oscilloscope or hard copy "strip." When measuring the PAOP, it is essential to ensure that the balloon is fully inflated, the PAOP tracing has fully equilibrated, and at least three respiratory cycles have transpired (Figure 18-3).

PAOP and Preload

Since its introduction into clinical medicine almost 30 years ago, the PAC has been assumed to be a reliable and valid indicator of left ventricular preload. Indeed, perhaps the most common reason for inserting a PAC in the ICU is to measure the PAOP to assess a patient's volume status. However, it was not long after the introduction of the PAC that studies began to appear demonstrating that the PAOP was a poor reflection of preload. Despite the fact that this observation has been confirmed in a multitude of studies, *many physicians still erroneously believe that the PAOP provides an accurate assessment of a patient's intravascular volume. This factor, together with the incorrect interpretation of the PAOP, may largely explain the excess mortality associated with the use of the PAC.*

It must be emphasized that the PAOP is a measure of left ventricular end-diastolic *pressure* (LVEDP) and *not* left ventricular end-diastolic *volume* (LVEDV) or left ventricular preload. The use of the PAOP to measure left ventricular preload in absolute or relative terms assumes a direct relationship between the LVEDP and LVEDV. This pressure–volume curve, which describes left ventricular compliance, is normally curvilinear. Furthermore, alterations in left ventricular compliance shifts the pressure–volume curve. Factors that alter left ventricular compliance include left ventricular preload, left ventricular afterload, left ventricular mass, and ventricular fiber stiffness. Myocardial ischemia, sepsis, diabetes, obesity, aging, sustained tachycardia, dialysis, cardioplegia, as well as other factors alter myocardial fiber stiffness. In addition, the left ventricular pressure–volume curve is affected by the degree of right ventricular filling. Since the two ventricles are physically coupled by the interventricular septum and by the constraining effects of the pericardium, the end-diastolic pressure–volume curve of either ventricle is dependent upon the diastolic volume of the other. Indeed, in patients with pulmonary hypertension and an elevated PAOP, volume unloading with a reduction of the PAOP may paradoxically increase the LVEDV. The increase in LVEDV occurring in association with a decrease in RVEDV is referred to as *diastolic ventricular interaction*. In critically ill patients, many of the factors that determine left ventricular compliance are in a state of dynamic flux, making it exceedingly difficult to estimate the LVEDV from the LVEDP. This alteration in the left ventricular pressure–volume curve is the major factor accounting for the poor relationship between the PAOP and LVEDV.

The distending pressure resulting in left ventricular diastolic filling is the difference between the simultaneous intracavity pressure and the juxtacardiac pressure. A noncompliant ventricle or one surrounded by increased intrathoracic pressure requires a higher than normal intracavitary pressure to achieve any specified presystolic volume. Increased intrathoracic pressure associated with positive-pressure ventilation and PEEP has a significant effect on juxtacardiac pressure. PEEP >8 to 10 cm H_2O increases juxtacardiac pressure, and therefore the pressure gradient between the left atrium and atmospheric pressure, but not the transmural distending pressure. This artifactually increases the PAOP. Formulas that subtract a percentage of the PEEP from the PAOP are of little practical value, as the fraction of the PEEP, which is transmitted to the heart, is difficult to estimate.

Pitfalls in the Interpretation of the PAOP

- PEEP (> 5 to 8 cm H_2O) increases intrapleural pressure (and intracardiac pressure) and therefore the pressure gradient between the left atrium (ventricle) and atmospheric pressure. This artifactually increases the PAOP. The "true" PAOP can only be determined if the intrapericardial pressure can be measured or estimated. Esophageal manometry may be useful in this instance.
- Pericardial tamponade and tension pneumothorax will increase the PAOP while decreasing LVEDV.
- Changes in myocardial compliance will alter the PCWP. Myocardial ischemia decreases myocardial compliance, giving a higher PAOP for any given end-diastolic volume.
- The PAOP will not reflect LVEDV in patients with mitral stenosis and pulmonary–veno-occlusive disease.
- Patients with mitral incompetence will have a large CV wave, making interpretation of the PAOP difficult.

From the available data, the PAOP must be regarded as an unreliable index of the LVEDV both in large patient groups as well as in individual patients assessed over time. The change in PAOP in response to fluid loading reflects left ventricle compliance rather than the adequacy of left ventricular filling. The change in cardiac output in response to fluid loading, however, provides an indication of the position of the ventricle on the Frank-Starling curve.

Oximetric Pulmonary Artery Catheters

Pulmonary artery catheters with fiberoptic capabilities, which provide continuous mixed venous O_2 saturation (Svo_2) measurements, have been developed and are widely utilized. Svo_2 monitoring, however, is fraught with numerous pitfalls (see Chapter 53).

The Volumetric Pulmonary Artery Catheter

The use of a PAC with a rapid-response thermistor and an electro-cardiographic electrode allows recognition along the rewarming phase of the thermodilution curve of a series of plateaus, which are due to the pulsatile ejection of blood from the right ventricle. The temperature drop between two successive beats allows computation of the right ventricular ejection fraction (RVEF). Once the RVEF is known, the right ventricular end-systolic and end-diastolic volumes can be calculated from the stroke volume. Several groups of investigators have validated the RVEF measurements obtained by the thermodilution technique by comparison with radionuclide imaging, echocardiography, and biplane angiography.

It has been suggested that the right ventricular end-diastolic volume index (RVEDVI) is a better indicator of preload in a critically ill patient than the PAOP. Several groups of investigators have reported an excellent correlation between the RVEDVI and cardiac index and have found the RVEDVI to be superior to the PAOP in determining the preload status of patients.

The value of the RVEDVI is the ability to predict the change in cardiac output in response to a fluid challenge. The optimal RVEDVI will depend upon right ventricular function (i.e., RVEF), and it is likely that this value will change during the course of a patient's illness. The optimal RVEDVI has been reported to range from 90 to $140 \, mL/m^2$. When a volumetric PAC is used, the "optimal" RVEDVI should be determined by plotting RVEDVI against the cardiac index (see Figure 18-5). The volumetric PAC is particularly useful in determining the preload in patients who are being ventilated with PEEP, a setting in which the PAOP reading becomes uninterpretable.

Derived Hemodynamic and Oxygen Transport Variables

The simultaneous measurement of cardiac output, cardiac pressures, as well as arterial and mixed venous blood gas analysis will allow for the generation of an impressive number of derived physiological variables. The formulas and normal values of these variables are listed in Table 18-1, and the hemodynamic profiles in common clinical disorders listed in Table 18-2. It is important, however, not to fall into the "trap" of treating numbers and forgetting to treat the patient.

■ ARTERIAL PRESSURE MONITORING

The arterial blood pressure has traditionally been measured with a mercury sphygmomanometer and stethoscope. This time-honored

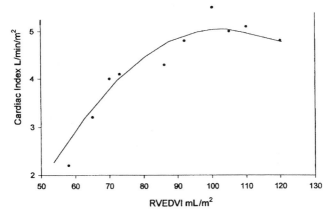

Figure 18-5. Right ventricular function curve (derived from RV PAC).

method is reliable, reproducible, simple, and cheap and not associated with any major complications. The disadvantages of this method include operator variability, absence of Korotkoff sounds when the arterial pressure is low, and poor correlation with directly measured intra-arterial pressure at the extremes of pressure. Automated manometer cuffs have been developed, which correlate well with the standard mercury sphygmomanometer.

Despite the proven reliability of the sphygmomanometer, over half of all patients admitted to an ICU have an arterial line inserted. With technological improvements and a better understanding of the complications associated with intra-arterial catheterization, the complication rates have been reduced. However, the complications associated with intra-arterial catheterization are not minor and cannot be ignored, and include

- Pain and swelling
- Arterial thrombosis
- Embolization
- Limb (digit) ischemia
- Catheter-related infection
- Hemorrhage
- Pseudoaneurysm
- Arteriovenous fistula
- Nerve damage
- *Excessive* diagnostic studies and blood loss

Table 18-1. Measured and derived hemodynamic and oxygenation parameters.

Parameter	Equation	Normal range
Mean arterial pressure	From oscilloscope	70–105 mm Hg
Mean pulmonary artery pressure (MPAP)	From oscilloscope/printout	10–20 mm Hg
Pulmonary artery occlusion pressure (PAOP)	From oscilloscope/printout	6–12 mm Hg
Central venous pressure (CVP)	From oscilloscope/printout	0–6 mm Hg
Cardiac output (CO)	Thermodilution computer	4.0–8.0 L/min
Cardiac index (CI)	CO/body surface area (BSA)	2.6–4.0 L/min
Stroke volume (SV)	CO/HR	60–100 mL
Stroke index (SI)	SV/BSA	40–50 mL/M^2
Right ventricular ejection fraction (RVEF)	Thermodilution computer	40%–60%
Right ventricular end-diastolic volume index (RVEDVI)	Thermodilution computer	60–100 mL/M^2
Left ventricular stroke work index (LVSWI)	$0.0136 \times SI \times (MAP - PAOP)$	50–62 g.M/M^2
Right ventricular stroke work index (RVSWI)	$0.0136 \times SI \times (PAP - CVP)$	5–10 g.M/M^2
Systemic vascular resistance (SVR)	$(MAP - CVP) \times 80/CO$	800–1200 dynes.sec/cm^5
Systemic vascular resistance index (SVRI)	$SVR \times BSA$	2000–2400 dynes.sec/cm^5/M^2
Pulmonary vascular resistance (PVR)	$(MPAP - PAOP) \times 80/CO$	100–250 dynes.sec/cm^5
Pulmonary vascular resistance index (PVRI)	$PVR \times BSA$	255–300 dynes.sec/cm^5/M^2
Arterial O$_2$ content (CaO$_2$)	$(Hb \times 1.34 \times Sat) + (0.031 \times PaO_2)$	17–20 mL/dL
Mixed venous O$_2$ content (CvO$_2$)	$(Hb \times 1.34 \times Sat) + (0.031 \times PvO_2)$	12–15 mL/dL
Arteriovenous O$_2$ difference (avDO$_2$)	$CaO_2 - CvO_2$	4–6 mL/dL
Oxygen extraction ratio (O$_2$ER)	$avDO_2/CaO_2$	20%–30%
Venous admixture ratio (Qs/Qt)	$(Ccapo_2 - CaO_2)/(Ccapo_2 - CvO_2)$	3%–5%
Oxygen delivery (DO$_2$)	$(CO \times CaO_2)/10$	950–1150 mL/min
Oxygen delivery index (DO$_2$I)	DO_2/BSA	500–600 mL/min/M^2
Oxygen consumption (VO$_2$)	$(CO \times avDO_2) / 10$	200–250 mL/min
Oxygen consumption index (VO$_2$I)	VO_2/BSA	120–160 mL/min/M^2

Table 18-2. Typical hemodynamic profiles obtained in various disorders.

Diagnosis	CI	MAP	CVP	PCWP	SVRI	PVRI
Cardiogenic shock	↓	↓	↑	↑	↑	N – ↑
Severe LV failure	↓	N – ↓	N – ↑	↑	↑	N
RV infarction	↓	↓	↑	N – ↓	↑	N
Cardiac tamponade (PA diastolic = CVP = PCWP)	↓	↓	↑	↑	↑	N – ↑
Severe mitral stenosis	↓	N – ↓	↑	↑	↑	↑
Cor pulmonale	↓	N – ↓	↑	N	↑	↑
Septic shock	↓ – ↑	↓	↓ – ↑	↓ – ↑	↓	↑
Hemorrhagic shock	↓	↓	↓	↓	↑	N – ↑
End-stage liver disease	↑	↓	↓ – ↑	↓ – ↑	↓	N – ↑
Massive pulmonary embolism	↓	↓	↑	N – ↓	↑	↑

(CI = cardiac index; CVP = central venous pressure; MAP = mean arterial pressure; PCWP = pulmonary capillary wedge pressure; PVRI = pulmonary vascular resistance index; SVRI = systemic vascular resistance index.)

Indwelling arterial catheters result in excessive blood volume being taken for diagnostic tests and an excessive number of samples for blood gas analyses. Data suggest that the number of blood gas analyses performed on patients is related to the presence or absence of an arterial catheter rather than the clinical indications for such sampling.

Before the placement of an intra-arterial radial catheter, an Allen test should be performed to confirm the patency of the ulnar artery. The risk of complications is reported to be similar with femoral and radial sites. I prefer the femoral site due to the ease of placement and stability of the catheter.

Indications for Intra-arterial Catheterization

- Shocked hemodynamically unstable patients being treated with vasoactive agents, i.e., patients with a mean arterial pressure (MAP) < 60 mm Hg
- Hypertensive emergencies
- Major vascular, thoracic, and abdominal surgeries

Contraindications for Intra-arterial Catheterization

- Local vascular insufficiency
- Post-thrombolytic therapy
- Local infection

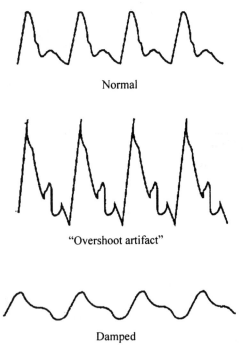

Normal

"Overshoot artifact"

Damped

Figure 18-6. Quality of arterial pressure tracing.

Waveform Analysis

When setting up the arterial pressure monitoring system, the same precautions should be taken as when setting up the PAC (i.e., determination of the dynamic compliance and zeroing). See Figures 18-1 and 18-6.

The arterial waveform has two major peaks (Figure 18-7): (1) the anacrotic notch (or inotropic spike), which is the initial steep upstroke and is related to the rate of acceleration of blood (contractility), and (2) the volume displacement curve produced by the continued ejection of the stroke volume from the left ventricle. The height of the volume displacement curve is essentially related to the stroke volume. The dicrotic notch is on the descending limb of the waveform and is

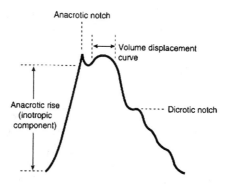

Figure 18-7. Idealized arterial pressure tracing.

caused by aortic valve closure. Normally, the amplitude of the inotropic spike and the volume displacement curve are the same. However, under various hemodynamic conditions, either peak may be taller and determine the peak systolic pressure. Hemodynamic monitors interpret and digitally display the taller peak as the systolic pressure.

Causes of Increased Inotropic Component

- Overshoot artifact (see below)
- Increased contractility/rate of pressure generation
- Hypertension
- Increased systemic vascular resistance (vasoconstriction)

Causes of Decreased Inotropic Component

- Decreased contractility
- Hypotension (inotropic spike may disappear)
- Hypovolemia
- Decreased SVR (vasodilation)

The interpretation of the blood pressure when there is dominance of one peak over the other is simple: Record the *MAP*. The MAP remains unaffected because the inotropic spike contributes little to the area under the arterial waveform.

The arterial waveform changes as one moves from the aorta to the periphery so that the lower extremity systolic pressure is considerably higher than the systolic pressure of an upper extremity (even with the patient supine). However, the *MEAN* arterial pressure (MAP) is essentially the same at all points within the arterial circulation, and it is this value that should be monitored. Furthermore, it is the MAP that determines renal and cerebral blood flow.

Overshoot Artifact

Systolic overshoot is a common artifact. Overshoot of the systolic pressure due to catheter/transducer underdamping or inadequate frequency response relative to that of the pressure signal may produce a falsely high systolic pressure (inotropic spike). The possibility of this artifact must be investigated by dynamic response (snap, square root) testing and ruled out before beginning possibly inappropriate antihypertensive therapy. The overshoot artifact may occur transiently because the patient's pressure pulse signal contains high-frequency components that equal those of the monitoring system. This occurs in patients who develop hyperdynamic circulations and/or rapid heart rates. *Note again: Antihypertensive treatment should be based on the MAP and not the systolic overshoot.*

■ SELECTED REFERENCES

Pulmonary Artery Catheterization

1. Calvin JE, Driedger AA, Sibbald WJ. Does the pulmonary capillary wedge pressure predict left ventricular preload in critically ill patients. *Crit Care Med.* 1981;9:437–443.
2. Connors AF, Speroff T, Dawson NV, et al. The effectiveness of right heart catheterization in the initial care of critically ill patients. *JAMA.* 1996;276:889–897.
3. Diebel L, Wilson RF, Heins J, et al. End-diastolic volume versus pulmonary artery wedge pressure in evaluating cardiac preload in trauma patients. *J Trauma.* 1994;37:950–955.
4. Diebel L, Wilson R, Tagett MG, Line RA. End diastolic volume; a better indicator of preload in the critically ill. *Arch Surg.* 1992;127:817–822.
5. Morris AH, Chapman RH, Gardner RM. Frequency of technical problems encountered in the measurement of pulmonary artery wedge pressure. *Crit Care Med.* 1984;12:164–170.
6. Pinsky M, Vincent JL, De Smet JM. Estimating left ventricular filling pressure during positive end-expiratory pressure in humans. *Am Rev Respir Dis.* 1991;143:25–31.
7. Trottier SJ, Taylor RW. Physicians' attitudes toward and knowledge of the pulmonary artery catheter: Society of Critical Care Medicine Membership Survey. *New Horiz.* 1997;5:201–206.

Arterial Catheterization

1. Clark VL, Kruse JA. Arterial catheterization. *Crit Care Clin.* 1992;8:687–697.
2. Frezza EE, Mezghebe H. Indications and complications of arterial catheter use in surgical or medical intensive care units: analysis of 4932 patients. *Am Surg.* 1998;64:127–131.
3. Thomas F, Burke JP, Parker J, et al. The risk of infection related to radial vs femoral sites for arterial catheterization. *Crit Care Med.* 1983;11:807–812.

19

Supraventricular and Ventricular Arrhythmias

■ ACUTE ATRIAL FIBRILLATION/FLUTTER

Atrial tachyarrhythmias are the most common arrhythmias occurring in ICU patients, with a reported prevalence of 28%. Atrial fibrillation (AF) is the most common atrial arrhythmia (52%) followed by atrial flutter (27%) and multifocal atrial tachycardia (MAT). Since the etiology and management strategies of atrial fibrillation and atrial flutter overlap, for the purposes of this discussion, they will be considered one entity, AF. Patients who develop AF have a worse prognosis than those who remain in sinus rhythm (SR); however, the attributable mortality of AF is unclear. Loss of atrioventricular synchrony will compromise stroke volume and cardiac output to a variable degree, depending upon ventricular compliance, venous filling pressure, ventricular rate, and other hemodynamic factors.

AF is particularly common in ICU patients with cardiovascular disorders, respiratory failure, and sepsis. The etiology is largely multifactorial, with hypoxia, electrolyte disturbance, myocardial ischemia, increased sympathetic tone, and atrial distention being implicated. Pulmonary hypertension with right atrial distention may be an important precipitant in patients with respiratory failure and sepsis. Despite the high prevalence of AF in ICU patients, only two prospective studies and one retrospective study (total of 83 patients) have reported on the management of AF in critically ill ICU patients (Table 19-1).

The components of the acute management of AF include (1) assessment of the need for urgent cardioversion, (2) correction of treatable precipitating factors, (3) control of the ventricular response rate, (4) conversion to SR, and (5) prophylaxis against thromboembolic events in those patients who remain in AF. Conversion to SR may be par-

Table 19-1. Trials of acute atrial fibrillation in ICU patients.

Author	Year	No patients	P/R	Drugs Studied	Conversion Success Rate
Chapman	1993	24	P	procainamide vs. amiodarone	71% vs. 70%
Moran	1995	21	P	magnesium vs. amiodarone	78% vs. 50%
Clemo	1998	38	R	amiodarone	48%

(P = prospective; R = retrospective).

ticularly important in critically ill patients, as AF may be associated with a significant fall in cardiac output and rendering vulnerable tissue beds hypoxic. Furthermore, prompt termination may obviate the need for anticoagulation.

Urgent Cardioversion

Electrical cardioversion is a time-honored, highly effective method for converting AF to SR. It is probably underutilized in ICU patients. Urgent cardioversion is indicated when the ventricular response is > 130 beats/min in association with

- Angina/myocardial ischemia on electrocardiogram (ECG)
- Acute cardiac failure
- Hypotension (mean arterial pressure [MAP] < 70 mm Hg or fall in MAP > 15 mm Hg)
- Indices of inadequate tissue perfusion

Patients should be well sedated and given an analgesic before cardioversion. The combination of midazolam (2 to 10 mg) and fentanyl (50 to 150 μg) may be used in nonintubated patients. Ketamine (a neuroleptic anesthetic agent with potent analgesic properties) is an alternative in nonintubated patients in whom respiratory depression (e.g., chronic obstructive pulmonary disease [COPD]) needs to be avoided.

The aim of electrical therapy is to provide a current through the myocardium to change enough myocardial cells to the same electrical state, for sufficient time to break the re-entrant circuits or produce electrical homogeneity. This allows a stable rhythm to be re-established from the sinus node. Animal experiments have shown that the period of homogeneity needs to be 4 to 12 ms. More organized arrhythmias such as AF require less energy to break the circuit (5 to 10 J internal, 20 to 100 J external) compared to disorganized rhythms (e.g., ventricular fibrillation, 10 to 13J internal, 200 to 300J external). The current delivered to the heart is determined by both the energy chosen (J) and the transthoracic impedance. The use of bare paddles without a couplant (gel/cream) results in very high transthoracic impedance. The paddles/pads should be placed in a position that will maximize current flow through the myocardium. The most commonly employed placement is apex-anterior. The anterior electrode should be placed on the right of the upper sternum below the clavicle; the apex electrode should be placed to the left of the nipple, with the center of the electrode in the midaxillary line. In women, placement of paddles on the breast should be avoided, since in this position, transthoracic impedance is high. Placement of the apex electrode adjacent to or under the breast is preferable. Synchronization of shocks is extremely important. Properly synchronized shocks rarely, if ever, induce ventricular fibrillation; failure to synchronize shocks on the R wave may lead to inadvertent delivery of a shock in the vulnerable period and is likely to produce ventricular fibrillation. Because some defibrillators default to an unsynchronized mode after each shock, the operator must remember to reenable the synchronizer before each subsequent shock. Shocks to convert atrial fibrillation should begin at energy levels of 100J with the energy for subsequent shocks increased in increments of 50 to 100J. Atrial flutter is an easier rhythm to convert, and shocks should begin at 50J.

For those patients who fail cardioversion, pace termination of AF may be effective. Recently, Oral and colleagues have demonstrated that pretreatment of patients with ibutilide increased the efficacy and decreased the mean energy required for successful transthoracic cardioversion. The role of this approach in ICU patients remains to be determined. In the ICU setting, it is highly likely that the AF will recur soon after successful cardioversion, as the precipitating conditions still exist. Consequently, antiarrhythmic drugs such as procainamide or amiodarone, administered before or soon after the cardioversion, may be useful for prevention of recurrence. Due to the risk of torsades de pointes, all antiarrhythmics should be avoided for at least 4 to 6 hours in patients who have received ibutilide.

Rate Control

Rate control can improve hemodynamics even if the patient remains in AF. Digoxin is commonly used in the treatment of AF in ICU patients. Yet, in the critically ill ICU patient, digoxin is probably the *most ineffective drug* in controlling the ventricular response in AF. Digoxin decreases ventricular response in AF by vagotonic mechanisms. In critically ill patients, AF occurs in the setting of high sympathetic tone and frequently with the use of vasopressors and inotropic agents, a situation in which digoxin is likely to be ineffec-

Table 19-2. Parenteral agents used for rate control in atrial fibrillation.

Agent	Loading Dose	Maintenance Dose
Digoxin	10–15 µg/kg LBW (8–10 µg/kg)*	0.125–0.25 mg daily
Esmolol	0.5 mg/kg over 1 min	0.05–0.2 mg/kg/min
Metoprolol	5 mg over 2–4 min May repeat every 5 min to 15 mg	5–10 mg q6h
Diltiazem	0.25–0.35 mg/kg over 2 min	5–15 mg/h

*Patients age > 70 years and renal failure.

tive. In addition, this drug has a very narrow therapeutic index and should be avoided except in patients with poor left ventricular function.

Diltiazem appears to be an effective alternative to digoxin for rate control. Studies have demonstrated a response rate of between 93% and 97%. Esmolol, an ultrashort-acting cardioselective beta-blocker, has been demonstrated to be effective in controlling the ventricular response in AF. However, beta-blockers may cause hypotension in ICU patients. Magnesium has also been shown to reduce the ventricular response in AF, with a greater effect when combined with digoxin.

Magnesium may act by increasing the atrio-His interval and atrioventricular nodal refractoriness. The dosages of drugs used for rate control are listed in Table 19-2.

Digoxin and calcium channel blockers should not be given to patients who have AF with an anterograde conducting accessory pathway, because blocking atrioventricular nodal conduction may provoke conduction down the accessory pathway, leading to an increase rather than decrease in the ventricular rate and hemodynamic collapse. The emergent treatment for such patients is intravenous procainamide.

Pharmacological Cardioversion

A number of randomized, controlled clinical trials (RCTs) have evaluated procainamide, amiodarone, flecainide, sotalol, propafenone, and ibutilide in patients presenting to hospital with acute atrial fibrillation (non-ICU setting). In general, these studies have found the rate of conversion with the antiarrhythmic drug to be similar to that with placebo, with approximately 60% of patients spontaneously converting to SR within 24 hours. The natural history of AF in acutely ill ICU patients has not been studied. However, it is likely that the untreated arrhythmia will persist until the underlying medical condition that precipitated the arrhythmia has improved or resolved. Procainamide and amiodarone are generally considered to be the antiarrhythmic agents of choice in acutely ill ICU patients. However, the efficacy of these agents in critically ill ICU patients has never been tested in an RCT. The choice between amiodarone and procainamide is determined largely by the drug's side-effect profile and cost, with amiodarone being recommended in patients with severe left ventricular dysfunction. Hypotension and bradycardia, the most common adverse events reported with intravenous amiodarone, usually occur during the loading infusion. Acute hepatotoxicity with liver function test abnormalities have been reported in 9% to 17% of patients. Amiodarone has also been associated with acute pulmonary toxicity presenting as acute respiratory distress syndrome (ARDS). High inspired oxygen concentration and preexisting ARDS may be risk factors for acute amiodarone pulmonary toxicity. Procainamide is negatively inotropic and may cause severe hypotension during intravenous loading. A close relationship has been found between the plasma concentration and the therapeutic effects of procainamide, with a suggested therapeutic range varying from 4 to 8 μg/mL. QT prolongation and polymorphic ventricular tachycardias (torsades de pointes) may occur with this drug, necessitating daily monitoring of both drug levels and the QTc interval on a 12-lead ECG.

Based on the foregoing information, the following approach is recommended in critically ill patients with AF. Hemodynamically unstable patients should be electrically cardioverted followed by an infusion of procainamide or amiodarone. A loading dose of procainamide, amiodarone, or ibutilide followed by repeated attempts at direct-current cardioversion should be considered after three failed attempts at cardioversion. In "hemodynamically stable" patients with AF, all correctable factors such as hypokalemia (K < 4 mmol/L), anemia, and hypoxemia should be corrected. Magnesium supplementation (2 g magnesium sulphate in 10 mL dextrose in water over 5 minutes) should be considered except in hypermagnesemic patients (serum magnesium > 2.5 mg/dL). Drugs such as aminophylline and dopamine should be stopped. Pain and anxiety, which increase sympathetic activity, should be treated. Rate control with diltiazem is suggested (5-mg boluses every 5 minutes until rate control is achieved or a maximal dose of 15 mg is administered, followed by an infusion of up to 15 mg/h). Procainamide or amiodarone should be considered in patients who remain in AF. In patients who remain in AF despite 12 to 24 hours of antiarrhythmic therapy, direct-current electrical cardioversion should be attempted. This algorithm is outlined in Figure 19-1. The dosages of the agents used for cardioversion of AF are listed

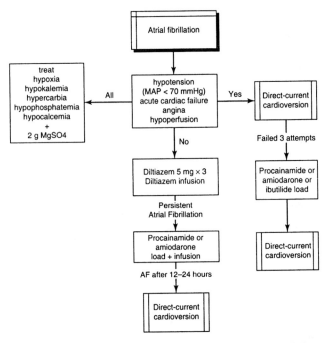

Figure 19-1. Approach to the management of atrial fibrillation. *Source*: Marik PE, Zaloga GP. The management of atrial fibrillation/flutter in the ICU. *J Intensive Care Med.* 2000;15:181–190.

in Table 19-3. There are no data on the optimal duration of antiarrhythmic therapy. However, as AF is likely to recur if the drug is terminated prematurely, I suggest continuation of the drug (intravenously or orally) until the precipitating factors have either improved or resolved.

Anticoagulation

According to the most recent guidelines on antithrombotic therapy from the American College of Chest Physicians, anticoagulation is not required for AF of <48 hours. This recommendation is supported by the study of Weigner and colleagues, who

Table 19-3. Agents used for cardioversion in atrial fibrillation.

Agent	Loading Dose	Maintenance Dose	$t_{1/2}$ (hours)	Steady State (hours)
Procainamide	5–15 mg/kg over 15 min max 1000 mg	2–4 mg/min	3–4	12
Amiodarone	150 mg over 20–30 min	1 mg/min 6 h then 0.5 mg/min	3–21 (acute)	NA
Ibutilide	1 mg over 30 min May be repeated once	None	6	NA
Flecainide	PO: 50–150 mg q8h	50–100 mg q12h	16–20	48–72
Propafenone	PO: 130–300 mg q8h	PO: 130–300 mg q8h	2–10	24–36

demonstrated three thromboembolic events in 357 patients (1%) with new-onset AF who converted to SR. However, in patients in whom the arrhythmia lasts >48 hours or in whom its duration is uncertain, full anticoagulation is required. In patients planned for pharmacological cardioversion in whom the arrhythmia has been present for >48 hours, transesophageal echocardiography is required to exclude the presence of an atrial thrombus before attempts at cardioversion.

■ MULTIFOCAL ATRIAL TACHYCARDIA

MAT has been defined as a rhythm with an atrial rate > 100 beats/min, at least three morphologically distinct P waves, irregular P-P intervals, and an isoelectric baseline between P waves. An exacerbation of COPD is the most common setting in which MAT arises. The treatment of COPD may promote the arrhythmia. A weak relationship exists between MAT and pulmonary embolism. This arrhythmia is typically an epiphenomenon of an underlying disorder and should usually not be treated. MAT is commonly transient and will often resolve after precipitating causes are reversed. MAT should be treated only if it causes hypotension, congestive heart failure, or myocardial ischemia. Calcium channel blockers, beta-blockers (avoid in acute exacerbation of COPD), and magnesium have demonstrated some utility in treating this arrhythmia. Magnesium may be particularly effective and should probably be the first line of treatment (a loading dose of 2 g in 10 mL dextrose in water over 5 minutes, followed by 10 g in 500 mL dextrose in water over 5 hours).

■ PAROXYSMAL SUPRAVENTRICULAR TACHYCARDIA

Atrioventricular nodal reentrant tachycardia is usually not associated with underlying heart disease and may be precipitated by the same factors as atrial fibrillation/atrial flutter. This arrhythmia is characterized by a sudden onset and sudden termination. The rate may range from 150 to 200 beats/min but most often is 180–200 beats/min. In the common atrioventricular nodal reentrant tachycardia, there is antegrade conduction over the slow atrioventricular nodal pathway and retrograde conduction over the fast pathway. As there is almost simultaneous excitation of both the atria and ventricles, the P wave occurs at the time of the QRS complex and is difficult to appreciate on the ECG. In 10% of patients, the reentrant pathway is reversed. This tachycardia, referred to as the *uncommon atrioventricular nodal reentrant tachycardia*, is characterized by clearly visible P waves that are inverted in leads II, III, and aVF.

Management

- Vagal maneuvers are the initial treatment of choice:
  Valsalva's maneuver.
  Müller's maneuver: deep inspiration against a closed glottis.
  Carotid sinus massage: Check that the patient has no carotid bruit or history of transient ischemic attack.
- Electrical cardioversion if the patient is hemodynamically unstable; 100 to 200 J.
- Adenosine is the pharmacologic agent of choice in patients who have failed vagal maneuvers. The usual dose is 6 to 12 mg by slow intravenous push. After termination of the tachycardia, brief periods of asystole are common.
- Diltiazem or verapamil are also effective in terminating a paroxysmal supraventricular tachycardia.
- Due to denervation hypersensitivity, adenosine should not be given to heart transplant recipients.

■ SUPRAVENTRICULAR TACHYCARDIA MEDIATED BY ACCESSORY PATHWAYS

Accessory pathways are anomalous bands of conducting tissue that form a connection between the atrium and ventricle. When there is antegrade accessory-pathway conduction during SR, ventricular preexcitation occurs. This results in the combination of a short PR interval and a delta wave, the electrocardiographic features of the Wolff-Parkinson-White (WPW) syndrome. Nearly 25% of accessory pathways are capable of only retrograde conduction (concealed bypass tracts).

The most common supraventricular tachycardia (SVT) in patients with WPW is the orthodromic atrioventricular reentrant tachycardia; the impulse travels anterograde over the atrioventricular (AV) node and then retrograde through the accessory pathway. In about 10% of patients with WPW, the reentrant circuit travels in the opposite direction (antidromic). This tachycardia is characterized by a wide QRS configuration (exaggeration of the delta wave).

Atrial fibrillation and atrial flutter are frequently seen in patients with the WPW syndrome because most accessory pathways have rapid conduction. These patients may achieve ventricular rates that approach 300 beats/min; ventricular fibrillation may occur under such circumstances.

A number of acute therapies are available for an orthodromic reciprocating tachycardia:

- Electrical cardioversion if the patient is hemodynamically unstable.
- Adenosine is the pharmacologic agent of choice (6 to 12 mg intravenously).
- Procainamide may be safely used in WPW syndrome.
- *Digoxin, Verapamil* and *Diltiazem should not be administered,* as these drugs can shorten the refractory period of the bypass tract.
- Adenosine, digoxin, and calcium channel blockers should *not* be given to patients who have atrial fibrillation with an accessory pathway, because blocking AV nodal conduction may provoke conduction down the accessory pathway, leading to an increase in the ventricular rate and hemodynamic collapse. The treatment of choice in these patients is procainamide.

■ SINUS BRADYCARDIA

Sinus bradycardia is not uncommon in ICU patients. This may occur due to myocardial ischemia, digoxin toxicity, sick sinus syndrome, and beta-blockers and calcium channel blockers. The patient should be treated *only* if symptomatic and/or hypotensive.

- Atropine, 0.5 mg repeated up to total of 3 mg
- Isoproterenol, 1–2 µg/min up to 20 µg/min
- A dopamine infusion, especially in hypotensive patients
- Pacing
    Transvenous temporary pacemaker
    External pacemaker (transcutaneous)

■ SICK SINUS SYNDROME

Sick sinus syndrome is also known as the tachycardia-bradycardia syndrome. As the name implies, these patients have episodes of both tachycardia and bradycardia. The critically ill patient with this syndrome often requires temporary pacing in order to achieve hemodynamic stability.

■ ACCELERATED IDIOVENTRICULAR RHYTHM

Accelerated idioventricular rhythm is characterized by a wide QRS complex and a regular ventricular rate, usually 60 to 110 beats/min. This is a benign rhythm that is usually asymptomatic and should just be observed.

■ VENTRICULAR PREMATURE COMPLEXES AND BIGEMINY

Ventricular premature complexes (VPCs) and bigeminy are recognized by wide QRS complexes (>120 ms) with a bizarre configuration. Identify and treat possible precipitating factors, such as hypoxia and electrolyte disturbances. Ensure that the $K^+ > 4 \, mEq/L$ and that the $Mg^{++} > 2 \, mg/dL$. Treat the underlying cause and *not* the VPCs. Frequent VPCs (>6/min), multifocal VPCs, couplets, and "R on T" VPCs occurring within the first 6 hours of an acute myocardial infarction are often treated with lidocaine. These VPCs increase the risk of ventricular fibrillation. There are, however, no convincing data that suppression of these "complex" VPCs reduces the incidence of ventricular fibrillation or impacts on patient outcome. Complex VPCs occurring later in the course of an acute myocardial infarction are of prognostic import; however, there is no evidence that antiarrhythmic therapy, other than beta-blocking agents, alters patient outcome. The Cardiac Arrhythmia Suppression Trial (CAST) demonstrated an increase in mortality among post-AMI patients with VPCs who were treated with flecainide and encainide. These patients should be treated with a beta-blocking agent such as metoprolol (if no contraindications exist to the use of this class of drugs).

■ NONSUSTAINED VENTRICULAR TACHYCARDIA

Nonsustained ventricular tachycardia is defined as from three consecutive PVCs up to 30 seconds at a rate of >100 beats/min. This arrhythmia is usually associated with underlying heart disease and is associated with an increased mortality. In the ICU setting, precipitating factors should be diagnosed and treated. In the setting of acute myocardial ischemia, progressively longer runs of this arrhythmia may herald the onset of ventricular fibrillation and should therefore be suppressed. In most other situations, unless the patient is symptomatic, this arrhythmia should just be observed.

■ SUSTAINED VENTRICULAR TACHYCARDIA

A wide QRS complex tachycardia: How to distinguish between ectopy or aberration.

Factors Favoring Ectopy

- AV dissociation
- R or qR in V1 with taller *left* rabbit ear
- QS or RS in V6
- Bizarre frontal plane axis
- Concordant V leads
- Left bundle branch block pattern with wide R in V1

Factors Favoring Supraventricular Tachycardia (SVT) with Aberration

- Preceding P wave
- Right bundle branch block pattern

- Triphasic contour in V1 and V6
- Initial vector identical with that of flanking conducted beats
- qRs in V6

If there is any question of doubt, the arrhythmia should be considered to be ventricular rather than supraventricular. Adenosine may be used to differentiate between these two arrhythmias. The treatment of a ventricular tachycardia with a calcium channel blocker can result in a fatal outcome.

Sustained ventricular tachycardias usually occur in patients with severe underlying heart disease, usually ischemic heart disease. The prognosis depends largely on that of the underlying heart disease. The treatment of patients with ventricular tachycardia (VT) is dependent on the hemodynamic consequences. Cardioversion is the treatment of choice in hemodynamically compromised patients. If the patient is asymptomatic or only mildly symptomatic, a number of therapeutic options can be pursued (alone and in combination), including

- Elective synchronized cardioversion.
- Procainamide is considered the drug of choice. A loading dose of 15 mg/kg at a rate of 25 to 50 mg/min is followed by an infusion at 1 to 4 mg/min. Monitor levels and ECG as described above.
- Amiodarone.
- Implantable antitachycardia device.

■ SUSTAINED VENTRICULAR TACHYCARDIA IN THE SETTING OF ACUTE ISCHEMIA

- Treat the underlying ischemia.
- Lidocaine: 1 mg/kg loading dose, followed by 0.5 mg/kg in 20 minutes, infusion of 1 to 4 mg/min.
- Beta-blocking agent.
- Bretylium: 5 to 10 mg/kg loading dose, followed by infusion, 0.5 to 4 mg/min.
- Amiodarone.

■ POLYMORPHIC VENTRICULAR TACHYCARDIA (TORSADES DE POINTES)

The hallmark of polymorphic ventricular tachycardia (PVT) is a QRS morphology that changes constantly. Torsades de pointes translated means "twisting of the points." Multiple leads may be required to demonstrate this phenomenon. This arrhythmia is classified as being associated with either (1) a normal QT interval or (2) a prolonged QT interval.

Normal QT Interval

- Acute myocardial ischemia
- Hypertrophic cardiomyopathy
- Dilated cardiomyopathy

Prolonged QT Interval

- Congenital long-QT syndrome
- Acute myocardial ischemia
- Anti-arrhythmic drugs especially class 1 agents; rarely sotalol (hypokalemia) and amiodarone
- Other drugs, including phenothiazines, tricyclic antidepressants, erythromycin, ampicillin, pentamidine
- Electrolyte disturbances
  Hypokalemia
  Hypomagnesemia
  Hypocalcemia
- Acute intracranial pathology, such as subarachnoid hemorrhage and intracerebral bleeding

Management

- Electrolyte abnormalities must be aggressively corrected, particularly potassium and magnesium deficiency.
- Magnesium sulphate (1 to 2 g) is usually highly successful, even in the absence of magnesium deficiency: 2 g (10 mL of 20% solution) is given intravenously over 10 minutes, followed by 4 g over 4 to 8 hours as an infusion.
- Accelerating the heart rate is a simple and quick method of shortening the QT interval. Transvenous pacing is a safe and effective method of controlling this arrhythmia. As an immediate measure, transcutaneous pacing may be used while preparations are being made for electrode placement.
- An infusion of isoproterenol (2 to 8 μg/min) titrated to increase the heart rate above 120/min is sometimes used if pacing is not available. Isoproterenol is contraindicated in patients with an acute myocardial infarction, active ischemia, and severe hypertension.
- If the arrhythmia occurs during therapy with a type 1A agent, amiodarone may terminate the arrhythmia.

- PVT occurring in the setting of myocardial ischemia does not usually respond to antiarrhythmic therapy. These patients usually require coronary revascularization. If the QT interval is prolonged, standard class I antiarrhythmic agents should not be used.
- Patients with the congenital long-QT syndrome are usually treated with beta-blockers or phenytoin.

■ SELECTED REFERENCES

1. American Heart Association's standard and guidelines for cardiopulmonary resuscitation (CPR) and emergency care. *JAMA*. 1992;268:2184–2241.
2. Intravenous digoxin in acute atrial fibrillation. Results of a randomized, placebo-controlled multicentre trial in 239 patients. The Digitalis in Acute Atrial Fibrillation (DAAF) Trial Group. *Eur Heart J*. 1997;18:649–654.
3. Klein AL, Grimm RA, Black IW, et al. Cardioversion guided by transesophageal echocardiography: the ACUTE Pilot Study. A randomized, controlled trial. Assessment of Cardioversion Using Transesophageal Echocardiography. *Ann Intern Med*. 1997;126:200–209.
4. Kowey PR, Marinchak RA, Rials SJ, Filart RA. Acute treatment of atrial fibrillation. *Am J Cardiol*. 1998;81:16C–22C.
5. Marik PE, Zaloga GP. The management of atrial fibrillation/flutter in the ICU. *J Intensive Care Med*. 2000;15:181–190.
6. Moran JL, Gallagher J, Peake SL, Cunningham DN, Salagaras M, Leppard P. Parenteral magnesium sulphate versus amiodarone in the therapy of atrial tachyarrhythmia: a prospective, randomized study. *Crit Care Med*. 1995;23:1816–1824.
7. Oral H, Souza JJ, Michaud GF, et al. Facilitating transthoracic cardioversion of atrial fibrillation with ibutilide pretreatment. *N Engl J Med*. 1999;340:-1849–1854.
8. Preliminary report: effect of encainide and flecainide on mortality in a randomized trial of arrhythmia suppression after myocardial infarction. The Cardiac Arrhythmia Suppression Trial (CAST) Investigators. *N Engl J Med*. 1989;321:406–412.
9. Weigner MJ, Caulfield TA, Danias PG, Silverman DI, Manning WJ. Risk for clinical thromboembolism associated with conversion to sinus rhythm in patients with atrial fibrillation lasting less than 48 hours. *Ann Intern Med*. 1997;126:615–620.

20

Hypertensive Emergencies

Accelerated hypertension is among the most misunderstood and mismanaged of "acute" medical problems. Most physicians have an urgent need to rapidly lower an elevated blood pressure without considering the pathophysiological principles involved. It should be appreciated that most patients who present to the hospital with an elevated blood pressure are chronically hypertensive with a rightward shift of the pressure/flow cerebral (and renal) autoregulation curve (Figure 20-1). Furthermore, most patients with severe hypertension (diastolic pressure ≥120 mm Hg) have no acute, end-organ damage. Rapid antihypertensive therapy in this setting may be associated with significant morbidity. There are, however, true hypertensive emergencies in which the rapid (controlled) lowering of blood pressure is indicated.

The clinical differentiation of hypertensive emergencies from hypertensive urgencies depends on the presence of target organ damage, rather than the level of blood pressure. Hypertensive crisis is classified into *hypertensive emergencies*, characterized by the presence of end-organ damage, as opposed to *hypertensive urgency*, characterized by the absence of end-organ damage. Patients with hypertensive emergencies require immediate control of the blood pressure to terminate ongoing end-organ damage *but not* to return blood pressure to normal levels. In patients with hypertensive urgencies, blood pressure is lowered gradually over a period of 24 to 48 hours, usually with oral medication.

Indications for the Emergent Lowering of Severe Hypertension

- Hypertensive encephalopathy and/or papilledema
- Dissecting aortic aneurysm (diastolic >110 mm Hg)

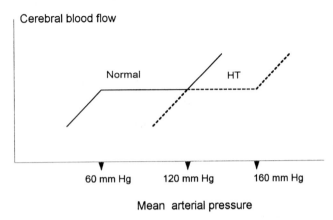

Figure 20-1. Cerebral autoregulation in normal and hypertensive patients. *Source*: Varon J, Marik PE. The diagnosis and management of hypertensive crises. *Chest*. 2000;118:214–227.

- Acute pulmonary edema with respiratory failure
- Acute myocardial infarction/unstable angina (diastolic >110 mm Hg)
- Eclampsia (diastolic >110 mm Hg)
- Acute renal failure
- Microangiopathic hemolytic anemia

These are the *only* indications for the immediate and rapid reduction of a markedly elevated blood pressure. In patients who have suffered a major cerebrovascular event, the blood pressure *should not* be immediately lowered (may cause further cerebral ischemia; see Chapter 31). In all other patients, the blood pressure can be lowered slowly using oral agents.

■ MANAGEMENT OF HYPERTENSIVE EMERGENCIES

The elevated blood pressure in patients with hypertensive emergencies should be treated in a controlled fashion in an ICU. The patient should be admitted to an ICU as an emergency, and the blood pressure should be reduced in a controlled fashion. The rapid and uncontrolled reduction of blood pressure will result in cerebral and renal ischemia/infarction. Intra-arterial blood pressure monitoring is recommended in these patients.

The immediate goal of intravenous therapy is to reduce the diastolic blood pressure by 10% to 15% or to about 110 mm Hg. In patients with a dissecting aneurysm, this goal should be achieved within 5 to 10 minutes. In the other patients, this end point should be achieved within 30 to 60 minutes. Once the end points of therapy have been reached, the patient can be started on oral maintenance therapy. In pregnancy-related hypertension, intravenous drug therapy is reserved for those patients with persistent systolic blood pressures >180 mm Hg or persistent diastolic blood pressures >110 mm Hg (105 mm Hg in some institutions). Before delivery, it is desirable to maintain the diastolic blood pressure >90 mm Hg. This pressure allows for adequate uteroplacental perfusion.

The antihypertensive agents used in the management of hypertensive crisis are listed in Table 20-1. The antihypertensive agents of choice for specific hypertensive crises are listed in Table 20-2. Contrary to popular belief, nitroglycerin is not an effective vasodilator. Nitroglycerin is a potent venodilator and only at high doses affects arterial tone. Nitroglycerin reduces blood pressure by reducing preload and cardiac output—undesirable effects in patients with compromised cerebral and renal perfusion. Hydralazine has a long half-life and is poorly titratable. This drug should therefore be avoided in the management of hypertensive emergencies. The use of sublingual nifedipine must be strongly condemned; this agent may result in a precipitous and uncontrolled fall in blood pressure. Given the seriousness of the reported adverse events and the lack of any clinical documentation attesting to a benefit, the use of nifedipine capsules for hypertensive emergencies and pseudo-emergencies should be abandoned.

Sodium Nitroprusside and Nitroprusside-Related Cyanide Poisoning

Sodium nitroprusside is an arterial and venous vasodilator that decreases both afterload and preload. Nitroprusside is a very potent agent. The onset of action of this drug is within seconds, with a duration of action of 1 to 2 minutes and a plasma half-life of 3 to 4 minutes. If the infusion is stopped abruptly, the blood pressure begins to rise immediately and returns to the pretreatment level within 1 to 10 minutes. In patients with coronary artery disease, a significant reduction in regional blood flow (coronary steal) can occur. In a large randomized, placebo-controlled trial, nitroprusside was shown to increase mortality when infused in the early hours after acute myocardial infarction (mortality at 13 weeks, 24.2% vs. 12.7%). This agent

Table 20-1. Intravenous antihypertensive medications used in hypertensive crises.

Drug	Characteristics and Dosage
Labetalol	Labetalol is a combined blocker of alpha- and beta-adrenergic receptors (the alpha- to beta-blocking ratio is 1:7). The elimination half-life after IV administration is 4.9 h. Labetalol's hypotensive effect begins within 2–5 min after an IV dose, reaches its peak at 5–15 min, and persists for about 2–4 h.
	Initial bolus 5–20 mg, followed by boluses of 5–80 mg or an infusion starting at 2 mg/min. Although the recommended maximum cumulative daily dose is 300 mg, patients may tolerate doses of up to 600 mg or more daily. Labetalol should be titrated to effect.
Esmolol	Esmolol is a cardioselective, beta-adrenergic blocking agent that has an extremely short duration of action. The drug has an elimination half-life of 9 min with a duration of action of 10–20 min.
	Loading dose of 250 to 500 μg/kg over 1 min, followed by an infusion at 25–50 μg/kg/min, which may be increased by 25 μg/kg/min every 10–20 min until desired response to a maximum of 300 μg/kg/min.
Nicardipine	Nicardipine is a dihydropyridine derivative calcium channel blocker.
	Dose: 5 mg/h, titrate to effect by increasing 2.5 mg/h every 5 min to a maximum of 15 mg/h.
Enalaprilat	Intravenous angiotensin-converting enzyme inhibitor.
	Intravenous injection of 1.25 mg over 5 min q6h, titrated by increments of 1.25 mg at 12- to 24-h intervals to a maximum of 5 mg q6h.
Fenoldopam	Fenoldopam is a dopamine agonist (DA1 agonist) that is short acting and has the advantages of increasing renal blood flow and sodium excretion.
	An initial dose of 0.1 μg/kg/min, titrated by increments of 0.05–0.1 μg/kg/min to a maximum of 1.6 μg/kg/min.
Nitroprusside	0.5 μg/kg/min, titrate as tolerated to maximum of 2 μg/kg/min.
Phentolamine	1- to 5-mg boluses. Maximum dose 15 mg.
Trimethaphan	0.5–1 mg/min, titrate by increasing by 0.5 mg/min as tolerated. Maximum dose 15 mg/min.

Table 20-2. Treatment of specific hypertensive emergencies.

Condition	Preferred Treatment
Acute pulmonary edema	Nitroprusside or fenoldopam in combination with nitroglycerin (up to 200 μg/min) and a loop diuretic.
Acute myocardial ischemia	Labetalol or esmolol in combination with nitroglycerin (up to 200 μg/min). Nicardipine or fenoldopam may be added if pressure is controlled poorly with labetalol/esmolol alone.
Hypertensive encephalopathy	Labetalol, nicardipine, or fenoldopam.
Acute aortic dissection	Labetalol or combination of nitroprusside and esmolol.
Eclampsia	Hydralazine (traditional). In the ICU, labetalol or nicardipine are preferred.
Acute renal failure/ microangiopathic anemia	Fenoldopam or nicardipine.
Sympathetic crisis	Nicardipine, verapamil, or fenoldopam.

Source: Varon J, Marik PE. The diagnosis and management of hypertensive crises. *Chest.* 2000, 118:214–227.

may cause cerebral blood flow to decrease in a dose-dependent manner. Furthermore, both clinical and experimental studies demonstrate that nitroprusside *increases intracranial pressure.* Sodium nitroprusside has been demonstrated to cause cytotoxicity through the release of nitric oxide, with hydroxyl radical and peroxynitrite generation leading to lipid peroxidation. Nitroprusside may also cause cytotoxicity due to the release of cyanide with interference of cellular respiration.

Nitroprusside contains 44% cyanide by weight. Cyanide is released nonenzymatically from nitroprusside, the amount generated being dependent on the dose of nitroprusside administered. Cyanide is metabolized in the liver to thiocyanate. Thiosulfate is required for this reaction. Thiocyanate is 100 times less toxic than cyanide. The thiocyanate generated is excreted largely through the kidneys. Cyanide removal therefore requires adequate liver function, adequate renal function, and adequate bioavailability of thiosulfate.

Cyanide toxicity has been documented to result in unexplained cardiac arrest, coma, encephalopathy, convulsions, and irreversible focal neurological abnormalities. The current methods of monitoring for cyanide toxicity are insensitive. Metabolic acidosis is usually a preterminal event. A rise in serum thiocyanate levels is a late event and not directly related to cyanide toxicity. Obtaining red blood cell cyanide concentrations (although not widely available) may be a more reliable method of monitoring for cyanide toxicity. A red blood cell cyanide concentration >40 nmol/mL results in detectable metabolic changes. Levels >200 nmol/L are associated with severe clinical symptoms, and levels >400 nmol/mL are considered lethal. Data suggest that nitroprusside infusion rates in >4 µg/kg/min, for as little as 2 to 3 hours, may lead to cyanide levels in the toxic range. The "standard" recommended doses of nitroprusside of up to 10 µg/kg/min result in cyanide formation at a far greater rate than human beings can detoxify.

Considering the severe toxicity of nitroprusside, this drug should be used only in exceptional circumstances (i.e., acute pulmonary edema when other drugs are not available) and then only in patients with normal renal and hepatic function. The duration of treatment should be as short as possible, and the infusion rate should not exceed 2 µg/kg/min. An infusion of thiosulfate should be used in patients receiving higher dosages (4 to 10 µg/kg/min) of nitroprusside. It has been demonstrated that hydroxocobalamin (vitamin 12a) is safe and effective in preventing and treating cyanide toxicity associated with the use of nitroprusside. This may be given as a continuous infusion at a rate of 25 mg/h. Hydroxocobalamin is unstable and should be stored dry and protected from light. Cyanocobalamin (B12), however, is ineffective as an antidote and is not capable of preventing cyanide toxicity.

■ HYPERTENSIVE URGENCIES AND SYMPATHETIC CRISIS

Abrupt discontinuation of a short-acting sympathetic blocker (such as clonidine or propranolol) can lead to severe hypertension. Control of blood pressure can be achieved in this setting by readministration of the discontinued drug. If evidence of pulmonary edema or coronary ischemia is present, the patient should be treated as outlined above.

In addition to drug withdrawal, increased adrenergic activity can lead to severe hypertension in a variety of other clinical settings. These include (1) the use of sympathomimetic drugs such as cocaine, amphetamines, phencyclidine, or the combination of a monoamine oxidase inhibitor and the ingestion of tyramine-containing foods, and (2) pheochromocytoma and autonomic dysfunction as in Guillain-Barré syndrome.

Beta-blockers (including labetalol) should be avoided in these patients, since inhibition of beta-receptor-induced vasodilation results in unopposed alpha-adrenergic vasoconstriction and a further rise in blood pressure. Control of blood pressure in these patients is best achieved with nicardipine, fenoldopam, or verapamil. Phentolamine and nitroprusside are alternative agents.

■ SELECTED REFERENCES

1. Cohn JN, Franciosa JA, Francis GS, et al. Effect of short-term infusion of sodium nitroprusside on mortality rate in acute myocardial infarction complicated by left ventricular failure: results of a Veterans Administration cooperative study. *N Engl J Med.* 1982;306:1129–1135.
2. Gray RJ. Managing critically ill patients with esmolol. An ultra short-acting beta-adrenergic blocker. *Chest.* 1988;93:398–403.
3. Grossman E, Messerli FH, Grodzicki T, Kowey P. Should a moratorium be placed on sublingual nifedipine capsules given for hypertensive emergencies and pseudoemergencies? *JAMA.* 1996;276:1328–1331.
4. Izumi Y, Benz AM, Clifford DB, Zorumski CF. Neurotoxic effects of sodium nitroprusside in rat hippocampal slices. *Exp Neurol.* 1993;121:14–23.
5. Varon J, Marik PE. The diagnosis and management of hypertensive crises. *Chest.* 2000;118:214–227.
6. Pasch T, Schulz V, Hoppenshauser G. Nitroprusside-induced formation of cyanide and its detoxication with thiosulphate during deliberate hypotension. *J Cardiovasc Pharmacol.* 1983;5:77–85.

21

Management of the Patient with Unstable Angina/Non-Q-Wave Myocardial Infarction

Unstable angina most often results from disruption of an atherosclerotic plaque and a subsequent cascade of pathologic processes that decrease coronary blood flow. Most patients who die during unstable angina do so because of sudden death or an intervening myocardial infarction (MI).

Canadian Cardiovascular Classification of Angina

- Class 1: Pain is precipitated only by severe and unusually prolonged exertion.
- Class 2: Pain on moderate effort. There is slight limitation of ordinary activity.
- Class 3: Marked limitation of ordinary activity; pain occurs on mild exertion, usually restricting daily chores. The patient is unable to walk two blocks on a level at a comfortable temperature and at a normal pace.
- Class 4: Chest discomfort on almost any physical activity.

Definition of Unstable Angina

- Symptoms of angina at rest (usually prolonged >20 minutes)
- New onset (≤2 months) exertional angina
- Recent (≤2 months) acceleration of angina
- Variant angina
- Post-MI (>24 hours) angina

Differential Diagnosis

- Acute myocardial infarction (AMI)
- Aortic dissection
- Esophagitis
- Pleurisy
- Leaking or ruptured thoracic aneurysm
- Acute pericarditis
- Pulmonary embolism
- Pneumothorax
- Esophageal rupture

■ DIAGNOSIS OF ANGINA/AMI

The distinction between an AMI and unstable angina can sometimes be difficult at presentation. Patients with ≥1 mm ST elevation in two or more contiguous leads, or ST depression in V1–V3 or left bundle branch block with a consistent history should be managed as if they have an AMI.

Clinical Features Associated With a Higher Probability of AMI

- History of angina or prior MI
- Pain duration ≥1 hour
- Pain worse than prior angina or equivalent to prior MI
- Radiation of pain to the neck, left shoulder, or left arm

■ RISK STRATIFICATION

It is important to assess the likelihood that the patient has an unstable coronary syndrome, as this largely determines the management strategy. Risk stratification depends on the patient's clinical symptoms and initial electrocardiogram(s) (ECGs):

High Risk

- ST-segment elevation or depression ≥1 mm
- Deep symmetrical T-wave inversion in multiple precordial leads
- ECG change occurring during pain
- Ongoing "anginal"-type pain despite aspirin and sublingual nitroglycerin

Intermediate Risk

- ST-segment elevation or depression of ≥0.5 mm but <1 mm
- T-wave inversion ≥1 mm in leads with dominant R waves
- Nonspecific ST- and T-wave changes

Low Risk

- Normal ECG. A completely normal ECG in the emergency department does not exclude the possibility of acute ischemic heart disease, since 1% to 6% of such patients will eventually prove to have had an acute MI, and 4% or more will be found to have unstable angina.

■ PROGNOSIS

Risk of death or ischemic complications in patients with unstable angina is lower than with AMI but higher than with stable angina. The prognosis of patients presenting with symptoms suggestive of unstable angina is determined by the likelihood of coronary artery disease (CAD), the tempo of the recent clinical course, and factors that affect the likelihood that a patient will survive an acute ischemic event. Prospective studies have found that 12% of patients hospitalized with unstable angina progress to MI within 2 weeks of diagnosis. One-year mortality of patients with unstable angina ranges from 5% to 14%, with approximately half of these deaths occurring within 4 weeks of diagnosis.

■ MEDICAL MANAGEMENT

Initial Management in the Emergency Room/Physician's Office

The patient should undergo a focused history and physical examination to exclude other likely causes of chest pain. Baseline ECG and cardiac enzymes should be performed. Treatment at this stage should include acetylsalicylic acid (ASA) and sublingual nitroglycerine (NTG). The patients should then be triaged.

Triage of Patients

- High-risk patients should be admitted initially to an ICU.
- Intermediate-risk patients should be admitted to an ICU or monitored cardiac bed.

- Low-risk patients can be evaluated in an unmonitored hospital setting or be evaluated as an outpatient.

General Management

The goals of this phase of care are to relieve pain and ischemia and to prevent the progression of the underlying disease process to AMI or death.

- All patients should have serial cardiac enzymes and ECGs to exclude the possibility of acute AMI.
- Patients with obvious cyanosis, respiratory distress, or high-risk features should receive supplemental oxygen. A finger pulse oximetry or arterial blood gas determination should be used to confirm adequate arterial oxygen saturation and continued need for supplemental oxygen. No evidence is available to support the common medical practice of administering oxygen to all patients with acute chest pain syndromes in the absence of signs of respiratory distress.
- Continuous ECG monitoring for ischemia and arrhythmia detection.
- Patients should remain at bed rest for the first 24 hours.

Pharmacologic Management

The aggressiveness of drug dosage will depend on the severity of symptoms and, for many drugs, will require modification throughout the subsequent hospital course.

Aspirin

Aspirin (ASA), 160 to 324mg, should be given immediately on presentation and daily thereafter unless contraindicated.

Intravenous Heparin/LMWH

The efficacy of heparin (without ASA) in reducing cardiac events has been well established. The efficacy of ASA and heparin in combination is suggested, but this benefit has not been unequivocally demonstrated. Nevertheless, heparin is generally recommended in high-risk patients. A recent meta-analysis found a 33% reduction in risk of MI or death in patients with unstable angina treated with ASA plus heparin compared to those treated with aspirin alone. Heparin infusion should be continued for 2 to 5 days or until revascularization is performed. Most of the trials evaluating the use of heparin in unstable angina have continued therapy for ≥5 days. Initial heparin dosage is 80 U/kg bolus and intravenous infusion of 18 U/kg/h. The partial thromboplastin time should be monitored and kept between 46 and 70 seconds or 1.5 to 2.5 times control. Antithrombotic therapy with low-molecular-weight heparin plus aspirin has been shown to be more effective than unfractionated heparin plus aspirin in reducing the incidence of ischemic events in patients with unstable angina or non-Q-wave MI. In patients with unstable angina or non-Q-wave MI, the recommended dose of Lovenox injection is 1 mg/kg (up to 80 mg) administered subcutaneously every 12 hours in conjunction with oral aspirin therapy (100 to 325 mg once daily).

Glycoprotein IIb/IIIa Receptor Antagonists

Aggregation of platelets is the pathophysiologic basis of the acute coronary syndromes. The IIb/IIIa receptor is the final common pathway for platelet aggregation. A monoclonal antibody, as well as a number of peptide and nonpeptide high-affinity inhibitors of the platelet glycoprotein IIb/IIIa receptor have been developed. These receptor antagonists have been demonstrated to have a small incremental benefit beyond that of heparin and ASA in reducing the frequency of adverse outcomes in patients with unstable angina/non-Q-wave infarction. It appears, however, that the benefit of GIIb/IIIa-receptor antagonists is limited to those patients who have an early revascularization procedure. The role of these drugs in patients who are not selected for revascularization remains to be determined.

Nitroglycerin

All patients with ongoing chest pain should receive sublingual nitroglycerin (NTG). Pooled analysis of studies of NTG in patients with AMI from the prethrombolytic era suggest a 35% reduction in mortality. However, the ISIS-4 and GISSI-3 trials in AMI patients receiving thrombolytic therapy failed to confirm this benefit. Despite these findings, intravenous (IV) NTG is recommended in patients whose symptoms are not fully relieved with three or more doses of sublingual NTG, as well as high-risk patients. Intravenous NTG should be used cautiously in hypotensive patients. Furthermore, IV NTG should not be abruptly stopped, as this has been associated with exacerbation of ischemic changes on ECG.

Intravenous NTG should be started at a dose of 10 μg/min by continuous infusion and titrated up by 10 μg/min every 5 to 10 minutes until relief of symptoms or until limiting side effects occur (headache or hypotension with systolic blood pressure <90 mm Hg or >30% below starting mean arterial pressure). Patients on IV NTG should be switched to oral or topical nitrate therapy once they have been symptom-free for 24 hours. Tolerance to nitrates is dose- and duration-dependent and typically becomes significant only after 24 hours of continuous therapy.

Beta-Blockers

Beta-blockers, IV (for high-risk patients) or oral (for intermediate- and low-risk patients), should be started in the absence of contraindications (see Tables 21-1 and 21-2). Meta-analysis of the available trials indicates a 13% reduction in risk of progression to AMI.

Patients with marked first-degree atrioventricular (AV) block (i.e., ECG PR segment [PR] >0.24 seconds), any form of second- or third-degree AV block, a history of asthma, or severe left ventricular (LV) dysfunction with congestive heart failure (CHF) or cardiogenic shock should not receive beta-blockers. Patients with significant sinus bradycardia (heart rate ≤60 beats/min) or hypotension (systolic blood pressure ≤90 mm Hg) generally should not receive beta-blockers until these conditions have resolved. Patients with significant chronic obstructive pulmonary disease (COPD) that may have a component of reactive airway disease should be given beta-blockers cautiously; initially, low doses of a beta-selective agent should be used.

Choice of the specific agent is not as important as ensuring that appropriate candidates receive this therapy. If there are concerns about patient intolerance due to existing pulmonary disease—especially asthma, LV dysfunction, or risk of hypotension or severe

Table 21-1. Beta-blockers in unstable angina.

Metoprolol:
  Metoprolol 5 mg IV (over 1–2 min) repeated every 5 min for a total dose of 15 mg; followed in 1–2 h by 25–50 mg po every 6 h

Metoprolol (conservative protocol):
  1–2 mg repeated every 5 min for 3 doses; followed in 1–2 h by 25 mg po every 6 h

Propranolol:
  Propranolol 0.5–1.0 mg, followed in 1–2 h by 40–80 mg po every 6–8 h

Esmolol:
  Esmolol is given as a starting maintenance dose of 0.1 mg/kg/min with titration in increments of 0.05 mg/kg/min every 10–15 min as tolerated by blood pressure until the desired therapeutic response has been obtained, limiting symptoms develop, or a dose of 0.20 mg/kg/min is reached. An optional loading dose of 0.5 mg/kg may be given by slow IV administration (2–5 min) for more rapid onset of action.

Atenolol:
  In patients suitable for a longer acting agent, IV atenolol can be initiated with a 5-mg IV dose followed 5 min later by a second 5-mg IV dose and then 50–100 mg orally per day initiated 1–2 h after the IV dose.

Table 21-2. Beta-blockers in clinical use.

Drug	Intrinsic Sympathomimetic Activity	β_1-Selective	Lipid Sol.	$t_{1/2}$ (hours)	Starting Daily Dose (mg)	Usual Total Daily Dose (mg)
Acebutolol	+	+	Low	3–4	200–400	400–800
Atenolol	–	+	Low	6–9	25–50 (5 IV)	50–100
Labetalol	?	–	Low	3–4	100–400 (5–20 IV)	500–1000 (bd/tid)
Metoprolol	–	+	Inter	3–4	25–100 (5 IV)	50–200 (bd/qd)
Nadolol	–	–	Low	14–24	40–80	40–160
Pindolol	++	–	Inter	3–4	5–15	10–15 (bd/qd)
Propranolol	–	–	High	3–4	10–80 (1 IV)	160 (q6/qd)
Sotalol	–	–	Low	8–10	80	160 (bd/qd)
Timolol	–	–	Low	5–10	5–10	10–20 (bd/qd)

bradycardia—initial selection should favor a short-acting agent, such as propranolol, or metoprolol, or the ultra-short-acting agent esmolol. Mild wheezing or a history of COPD should prompt a trial of a short-acting agent at a reduced dose (e.g., 2.5 mg IV metoprolol, 12.5 mg oral metoprolol, or 25 µg/kg/min esmolol as initial doses) rather than complete avoidance of beta-blocker therapy.

Monitoring during IV beta-blocker therapy should include frequent checks of heart rate and blood pressure and continuous ECG monitoring, as well as auscultation for rales or bronchospasm. After the initial IV load, patients without limiting side effects may be converted to an oral regimen. The target heart rate for beta blockade is 50 to 60 beat/min.

Morphine Sulphate

Morphine sulphate may be necessary if pain is not resolved with initial therapy. Morphine sulphate at an IV dose of 2 to 5 mg is recommended for any patient whose symptoms are not relieved after three serial sublingual NTG tablets or whose symptoms recur with adequate anti-ischemic therapy unless contraindicated by hypotension or intolerance.

Anxiolytic Therapy

Anxiety and fear are almost universal findings in patients with an unstable coronary syndrome. The increased sympathetic stimulation causes tachycardia and may increase the risk of arrhythmias. Therefore, almost all patients should receive an anxiolytic. Lorazepam 1 to 2 mg given every 4 to 8 hours is usually effective.

Calcium Channel Blockers

The dihydropyridine calcium channel blockers have not been shown to improve the outcome of patients with unstable angina; in fact, these agents may be harmful. However, a recent study demonstrated that IV diltiazem was more effective in reducing ischemic events in patients with unstable angina than IV NTG. Diltiazem, however, should not be used as first-line therapy but, rather, should be used in patients who have "failed" medical therapy or in patients in whom a beta-blocker is contraindicated. Diltiazem should be used very cautiously in patients receiving a beta-blocker.

ACE Inhibitors

Angiotensin-converting enzyme (ACE) inhibitors should not be used as initial therapy in patients with unstable angina. These agents, however, have an important role in the management of patients with LV dysfunction.

Thrombolytic Therapy

A number of studies (including the TIMI IIIB) have been unable to demonstrate a benefit of thrombolytic therapy in patients with unstable angina (including the high-risk group).

Cardiac Catheterization: An Early Invasive or Conservative Approach

Two randomized trials compared medical and surgical therapy in unstable angina. Both studies included patients with progressive or rest angina accompanied by ST- and T-wave changes. Follow-up for up to 2 years failed to show any differences in survival between the therapies. Routine early angiography and percutaneous transluminal coronary angioplasty (PTCA) appear to have a limited role in the management of patients with unstable angina. The TIMI IIIB study failed to demonstrate an advantage from early cardiac catheterization and angioplasty (when feasible). Similarly, the VANQWISH trial failed to demonstrate a benefit from routine early invasive management of patients with non-Q-wave MI as compared to a conservative "ischemia-guided" approach, consisting of medical therapy and noninvasive testing, with subsequent invasive management if indicated by the development of spontaneous or inducible ischemia.

Failure of Medical Therapy

If chest discomfort with objective evidence of ischemia persists for ≥ 1 hour after aggressive medical therapy, emergency cardiac catheterization should be strongly considered. Cardiac catheterization should also be considered in patients with recurrent ischemic episodes despite appropriate medical therapy.

Indications for Cardiac Catheterization

- Failure to stabilize with adequate medical therapy.
- Recurrent unstable angina.
- High-risk result of noninvasive test.
- Patients who present with intermediate- or high-risk unstable angina and a history of a prior PTCA or prior coronary artery bypass graft surgery represent a group for whom a strategy of early coronary angiography is generally indicated. In this group

of patients, stenting has been shown to result in a lower incidence of restenosis compared to PTCA alone.

- Diagnosis or exclusion of significant CAD.
- Patients with CAD and known or suspected poor LV function have sufficient probability of benefit from revascularization procedures to merit direct coronary angiography without preceding functional testing.

Management of the Stable Patient

The large majority of unstable angina patients will stabilize and become pain free with appropriate intensive medical therapy. Transfer from intensive to nonintensive medical management is undertaken when the patient is hemodynamically stable (including no uncompensated CHF) and when ischemia has been successfully suppressed for ≥24 hours. Heparin should continue for 3 to 5 days. ASA and beta-blockers should continue without interruption.

All patients hospitalized for unstable angina should undergo non-invasive testing after stabilization has been achieved and before discharge or as soon as possible thereafter. In patients who have had evidence of ischemia, previous infarction, or conduction abnormalities on their resting ECG or who have cardiomegaly by physical examination or chest radiograph, resting LV function should be assessed using either a radionuclide ventriculogram or a two-dimensional echocardiogram. The resting ejection fraction (EF) is one of the most potent prognostic factors in CAD. Patients with low EFs (≤0.50) should receive careful consideration for revascularization therapy because of the risk with medical therapy that increases as a function of decrease in EF. Patients with low EFs are also candidates for therapy with ACE inhibitors.

■ SELECTED REFERENCES

1. A comparison of aspirin plus tirofiban with aspirin plus heparin for unstable angina. Platelet Receptor Inhibition in Ischemic Syndrome Management (PRISM) Study investigators. *N Engl J Med.* 1998;338:1498–1505.
2. Anderson HV, Cannon CP, Stone PH, et al. One year results of the Thrombolysis in Myocardial Infarction (TIMI) IIIB clinical trial. A randomized comparison of tissue-type plasminogen activator versus placebo and early invasive versus early conservative strategies in unstable angina and non-Q wave myocardial infarction. *J Am Coll Cardiol.* 1995;26:1643–1650.
3. Bar FW, Verheugt FW, Col J, et al. Thrombolysis in patients with unstable angina improves the angiographic but not the clinical outcome. Results of UNASEM, a multicenter, randomized, placebo-controlled, clinical trial with anistreplase. *Circulation.* 1992;6:131–137.

4. Boden WE, O'Rourke RA, Crawford MH, et al. Outcomes in patients with acute non-Q-wave myocardial infarction randomly assigned to an invasive as compared with a conservative management strategy. Veterans Affairs Non-Q-Wave Infarction Strategies in Hospital (VANQWISH) Trial Investigators. *N Engl J Med.* 1998;338:1785–1792.

5. Cohen M, Demers C, Gurfinkel EP, et al. A comparison of low-molecular-weight heparin with unfractionated heparin for unstable coronary artery disease. Efficacy and Safety of Subcutaneous Enoxaparin in Non-Q-Wave Coronary Events Study Group. *N Engl J Med.* 1997;337:447–452.

6. Distante A, Maseri A, Severi S, et al. Management of vasospastic angina at rest with continuous infusion of isosorbide dinitrate. A double crossover study in a coronary care unit. *Am J Cardiol.* 1979;44:33–39.

7. Figueras J, Lidon R, Cortadellas J. Rebound myocardial ischaemia following abrupt interruption of intravenous nitroglycerin infusion in patients with unstable angina at rest. *Eur Heart J.* 1991;12:5–11.

8. Gurfinkel EP, Manos EJ, Mejail RI, et al. Low molecular weight heparin versus regular heparin or aspirin in the treatment of unstable angina and silent ischemia. *J Am Coll Cardiol.* 1995;26:313–318.

9. Inhibition of platelet glycoprotein IIb/IIIa with eptifibatide in patients with acute coronary syndromes. The PURSUIT Trial investigators. Platelet Glycoprotein IIb/IIIa in Unstable Angina: Receptor Suppression Using Integrilin Therapy. *N Engl J Med.* 1998;339:436–443.

10. Oler A, Whooley MA, Oler J, Grady D. Adding heparin to aspirin reduces the incidence of myocardial infarction and death in patients with unstable angina. A meta-analysis. *JAMA.* 1996;276:811–815.

11. Parisi AF, Khuri S, Deupree RH, et al. Medical compared with surgical management of unstable angina. 5-year mortality and morbidity in the Veterans Administration Study. *Circulation.* 1989;80:1176–1189.

12. White HD, French JK, Norris RM, et al. Effects of streptokinase in patients presenting within 6 hours of prolonged chest pain with ST segment depression. *Br Heart J.* 1995;73(6):500–505.

13. Yeghiazarians Y, Braunstein JB, Askari A, Stone PH. Unstable angina pectoris. *N Engl J Med.* 2000;342:101–114.

22

Management of Acute Myocardial Infarction

■ DIAGNOSIS OF ACUTE MYOCARDIAL INFARCTION AND STRATIFICATION OF PATIENTS WITH CHEST PAIN

According to the World Health Organization definition, the diagnosis of acute myocardial infarction (AMI) is based on the presence of at least two of the following three criteria:

- A clinical history of ischemic-type chest discomfort
- Changes on serially obtained electrocardiographic tracings
- A rise and fall in serum cardiac markers

Approximately 70% to 80% of patients with AMI present with ischemic-type chest discomfort. Conversely, <25% of patients admitted to the hospital with ischemic-type chest discomfort are subsequently diagnosed as having had an acute AMI. Although ST-segment elevation and/or Q waves on the electrocardiogram (ECG) are highly indicative of AMI, about 50% of patients with AMI do not exhibit ST elevation but display other or nondiagnostic ECG changes. In patients with ischemic-type chest discomfort, ST-segment elevation on the ECG has a specificity of 91% and a sensitivity of 46% for diagnosing AMI. In patients with chest pain at rest who do not exhibit ST elevation of the ECG, laboratory tests including (creatine phosphokinase MB isoenzyme (CPK-MB) and troponin T/I) are required to differentiate AMI from unstable angina. In the management of patients presenting with acute chest pain, it is useful to divide these patients into two groups; namely, those showing ST elevation (in two or more contiguous leads) and those without ST elevation. Only patients with ST elevation have been demonstrated to benefit from thrombolytic

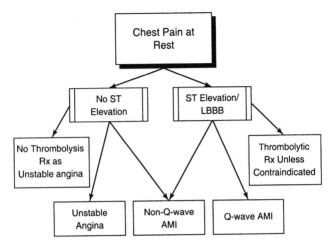

Figure 22-1. Approach to patients with chest pain.

therapy or primary percutaneous transluminal coronary angioplasty (PTCA); thrombolytic therapy is associated with a worse outcome in patients without ST elevation. It should be noted that mortality increases with the number of ECG leads showing ST elevation and the degree of ST elevation. Symptoms consistent with AMI and left bundle branch block (LBBB) should be managed like ST-segment elevation (Figures 22-1 and 22-2).

■ MANAGEMENT OF PATIENTS IN THE EMERGENCY DEPARTMENT

When the patient with suspected AMI reaches the emergency department (ED), evaluation and initial management should take place promptly. The initial evaluation of the patient ideally should be accomplished within 10 minutes of his or her arrival in the ED. On arrival in the ED, the patient with suspected AMI should immediately receive

- Oxygen by nasal prongs
- Sublingual nitroglycerin (unless systolic blood pressure <90 mm Hg or heart rate <50 or >100 beats/min)

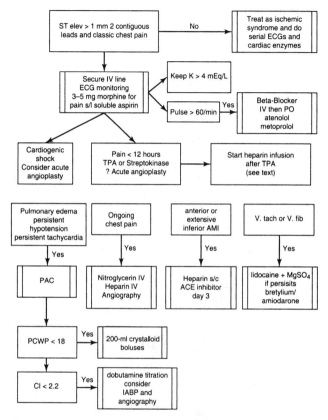

Figure 22-2. Summary of the management of acute myocardial infraction. (ACE = angiotension-converting enzyme; ECG = electrocardiogram; IABP = intraaortic balloon pump; PAC = pulmonary artery catheter; PCWP = pulmonary capillary wedge pressure; PO = orally; s/l = sublingual; TPA = tissue plasminogen activator).

- Adequate analgesia with morphine sulphate
- Aspirin, 160 to 325 mg orally

Effective analgesia should be administered promptly at the time of diagnosis and should not be delayed on the premise that it will mask symptoms of ongoing ischemia. Long-acting oral nitrates should be

Table 22-1. Streptokinase vs. t-PA: Additional cost per year gained ($).

Age	<41	41–60	61–75	>75
Inferior AMI	203,000	74,000	27,000	16,000
Anterior AMI	123,000	49,000	20,000	13,000

Data from Mark et al.

avoided. Continuous ECG and pulse oximetry should be initiated. Patients with an arterial saturation of <90% should be treated with a venturi or continuous positive airway pressure mask.

The 12-lead ECG in the ED is at the center of the decision pathway because of the strong evidence that ST-segment elevation identifies patients who benefit from reperfusion therapy. Patients with ST-segment elevation ($\geq 1\,mV$) in contiguous leads are candidates for immediate reperfusion therapy, either by fibrinolysis or primary PTCA. In contrast, patients without ST-segment elevation should not receive thrombolytic therapy. The benefit of primary PTCA in these patients remains uncertain. The TIMI-IIIB trial compared primary PTCA versus conservative therapy in patients with unstable angina/AMI with nondiagnostic ECG changes. This study showed no difference in the primary outcome measures.

■ THROMBOLYTIC THERAPY

Unless contraindicated, all patients presenting with chest pain and ST elevation (>0.1 mv in two or more contiguous leads)/LBBB within 12 hours after the onset of chest pain should receive thrombolytic therapy. Primary PTCA is an alternative to thrombolytic therapy only if performed in a timely fashion by individuals skilled in the procedure and supported by personnel in high-volume centers. Primary PTCA should be considered in patients who present in cardiogenic shock.

A review of the major thrombolytic trials for AMI demonstrates an 18% proportional reduction in 35-day mortality when compared with placebo. In the GUSTO study, the combined clinical outcomes of death and nonfatal disabling stroke were 7.7% for streptokinase and 6.9% for front-loaded t-PA. Mark and co-workers performed an analysis to determine those patients in whom tissue-type plasminogen activator (t-PA) is cost-effective (Table 22-1). These authors used a threshold of $50,000 per life year gained, as has been suggested by health economists. The dosages of thrombolytics approved for treatment of AMI, are listed in Table 22-2.

Table 22-2. Dosages of thrombolytic agents.

Agent	Dosage
t-PA—conventional	100 mg or 1 mg/kg for those <65 kg over 3 h with 10% of the dose given as an initial bolus
t-PA—front loaded	100 mg over 1.5 h with 15-mg initial bolus
Streptokinase	1,500,000 U over 1 h

Contraindications and Cautions for the Use of Thrombolytic Therapy in Myocardial Infarction

Contraindications

- Active peptic ulcer, recent bleeding
- Suspected aortic aneurysm
- Recent head injury or cerebral neoplasm
- Cerebrovascular accident (CVA) within 2 months
- Previous hemorrhagic stroke at any time
- Trauma or major surgery within 6 weeks
- Recent prolonged or traumatic cardiopulmonary resuscitation
- Diabetic retinopathy or other ophthalmic hemorrhagic lesions
- Acute pancreatitis

Relative Contraindications

- Severe uncontrolled hypertension on presentation (blood pressure >180/110 mm Hg)
- History of prior (CVA) or known intracerebral pathology not covered in contraindications
- Current use of anticoagulants in therapeutic doses (international normalized ratio 2 to 3);
- Known bleeding diathesis
- Noncompressible vascular punctures
- Recent (within 2 to 4 weeks) internal bleeding
- For streptokinase/anistreplase: prior exposure (especially within 5 days to 2 years) or prior allergic reaction
- Pregnancy
- Active peptic ulcer
- History of chronic severe hypertension

Primary Angioplasty

The GUSTO IIB and more recent studies have demonstrated that angioplasty provides a small-to-moderate, short-term clinical advantage over thrombolytic therapy with t-PA in patients with AMI. Primary angioplasty, when it can be accomplished promptly at experienced centers, should be considered an alternative method for myocardial reperfusion. In addition, primary stenting of the infarct-related artery, compared with optimal primary angioplasty, results in a lower rate of major adverse events related to recurrent ischemia and a lower rate of angiographically detected restenosis or reocclusion of the infarct-related artery (IRA).

■ MANAGEMENT DURING THE FIRST 24 HOURS

- Admission to an ICU or telemetry (low-risk patients)
- ECG monitoring
- Aspirin, 160 to 325 mg
- Heparin, in patients who have received t-PA or primary PTCA
- 7500 U subcutaneous heparin in patients without a contraindication who are not receiving intravenous (IV) heparin
- IV nitroglycerin, unless contraindicated
- An IV beta-blocker followed by an oral beta-blocker, unless contraindicated
- An oral angiotensin-converting enzyme (ACE) inhibitor in patients with ST elevation or LBBB

The patient should be monitored closely for adverse electrical or mechanical events because reinfarction and death occur most frequently within the first 24 hours. The patient's physical activities should be limited for at least 12 hours, and pain and/or anxiety should be minimized with appropriate analgesics. Although the use of prophylactic antiarrhythmic agents in the first 24 hours of hospitalization is not recommended, atropine, lidocaine, transcutaneous pacing patches or a transvenous pacemaker, a defibrillator, and epinephrine should be immediately available. Supplemental oxygen can be discontinued in patients whose oxygen >90% on room air.

Considering the superior performance of accelerated r-tPA plus IV heparin in the GUSTO trial, it seems judicious to give heparin intravenously for at least 48 hours after alteplase is given. The TIMI 9 and GUSTO IIa studies have shown that unless the partial thromboplastin time (PTT) is closely monitored and the upper limit of the PTT reduced, there is an excessive incidence of intracranial bleeding. Hence, when using heparin- and fibrin-specific activators, the PTT must be closely monitored and kept in the range of 55 to 80 seconds. A weight-based dosing protocol has been recommended with a

70-U/kg bolus followed by 15-μ/kg/h and adjusted as required. *Nitro-glycerin has been reported to increase the dosage requirements of heparin.* This is of particular importance when the infusion of nitro-glycerin is stopped, as the activated PTT (aPTT) may become exces-sively prolonged with an increased risk of bleeding. When primary PTCA is performed, high-dose IV heparin is recommended. Aspirin, 160 to 325 mg daily, initially given in the ED, should be continued indefinitely.

Despite the absence of definitive outcome data, it is reasonable to treat the patient with AMI and without hypotension, bradycardia, or excessive tachycardia with IV nitroglycerin for 24 to 48 hours after hospitalization. Concern exists about oral nitrate preparations in the patient with AMI because of inability to titrate the dose to effect in an acutely evolving hemodynamic situation, whereas IV infusion of nitroglycerin can be titrated successfully with frequent measurement of heart rate and cuff blood pressure. Nitroglycerin should not be used as a substitute for narcotic analgesics, which are often required in the patient with AMI.

The patient with evolving AMI should receive early IV beta-adrenergic blocker therapy, followed by oral therapy, provided that there is no contraindication. Beta-adrenoceptor blocker therapy should be initiated regardless of whether reperfusion therapy was given, because several studies in the prethrombolytic as well as the thrombolytic era showed that beta-adrenoceptor blockers diminish morbidity and mortality. The recommended dosages of beta-blockers are listed in Table 22-3. Calcium channel blockers have not been shown to reduce mortality in patients with AMI, and in certain patients, they appear to be harmful. In the patient without ST-segment elevation or LBBB in whom pulmonary congestion is absent, dilti-azem may reduce the incidence of recurrent ischemic events, but its benefit beyond that of beta-adrenoceptor blockers and aspirin is unclear. Immediate-release dihydropyridines (e.g., nifedipine) are contraindicated in the patient with AMI.

Table 22-3. Dosages of beta-blockers in AMI.

Agent	IV	Oral 1st 7 days	1 week to 2 years
Atenolol	5 mg over 5 min, repeated 10 min later	10 min after last IV-dose, 50 mg	50 mg
Metoprolol	5 mg over 5 min, repeated 5 min later and again 5 min later	8 h after IV dose, 25 to 50 mg q12h	50–100 mg q12h

In the patient with evolving AMI with ST-segment elevation or LBBB, an ACE inhibitor should be initiated within hours of hospitalization, provided that the patient does not have hypotension or a contraindication. Subsequently, the ACE inhibitor should be continued indefinitely in the patient with impaired left ventricular (LV) systolic function (ejection fraction <40%) or clinical congestive heart failure (CHF). In patients without complications and no evidence of symptomatic or asymptomatic LV dysfunction by 6 weeks, ACE inhibitors can be stopped. On admission to the hospital, a lipid profile and serum electrolyte concentration (including magnesium) should be measured in all patients.

■ AFTER THE FIRST 24 HOURS

Patients who have had an uncomplicated course in the coronary care unit during the first 24 hours are unlikely to develop a complication and can be discharged to a step-down unit/telemetry unit after 24 hours of observation. Further management should include the following:

- Aspirin, 160 to 325 mg/day continued indefinitely.
- Beta-adrenergic blocker continued indefinitely.
- Subcutaneous heparin continued until the patient is fully ambulatory.
- ACE inhibitor continued for at least 6 weeks. ACE inhibitor continued indefinitely in patients with an ejection fraction <40% or evidence of congestive heart failure (CHF).
- Nitroglycerin should be infused intravenously for 24 to 48 hours.
- For the patient receiving alteplase, it is current practice to give intravenous heparin for an additional 48 hours.
- Unless contraindicated, a low-level stress test should be performed before discharge from the hospital.
- Patients at an increased risk of systemic emboli should receive therapeutic doses of heparin followed by warfarin (INR 2.5 to 3.5) for up to 3 months, and then long-term aspirin (warfarin and aspirin should not be given concurrently except in situations of very high embolic risk). These patients include those with
    Large anterior Q-wave infarction
    Severe LV dysfunction
    CHF
    History of systemic or pulmonary emboli
    Two-dimensional echocardiographic evidence of mural thrombus
    Atrial fibrillation (indefinite therapy)

■ COMPLICATIONS

Recurrent Chest Pain Post-AMI

The two most common causes of recurrent chest pain are acute pericarditis and ischemia. An ECG taken during the recurrent chest pain and compared with the previous ECGs is helpful in distinguishing between these two conditions. Cardiac rupture may also result in recurrent chest pain.

Pericarditis

Pericarditis has been reported to occur in 20% of patients following AMI and occurs with extension of myocardial necrosis throughout the wall to the epicardium. The pain associated with pericarditis is pleuritic in nature and positional. The ECG features of pericarditis include J-point elevation, concave-up ST-segment elevation, and PR-segment depression. It is not associated with re-elevation of the creatine phosphokinase MB isoenzyme (CPK-MB). Aspirin is the treatment of choice, but high doses (650 mg every 4 to 6 hours) may be required.

Ischemia

Reinfarction during the first 10 days postinfarction has been reported to occur in about 10% of patients who have not received thrombolytic therapy compared to approximately 3% of patients who have been thrombolysed. Coronary angiography is indicated in patients with suspected ischemic-type chest pain. Prompt reperfusion using PTCA or an additional thrombolytic may be feasible.

Left Ventricular Failure and Low Output States

Patients can be grouped according to hemodynamic status by the Forrester Classification (see Table 22-4).

Table 22-4. Forrester Classification of acute myocardial infarction.

Class	Pulmonary Capillary Wedge Pressure (mmHg)	Cardiac Index L/min
I	<18	>2.2
II	>18	>2.2
III	<18	<2.2
IV	>18	<2.2

Adequate Output, Pulmonary Congestion (Forrester Class II)

In the early hours of acute infarction, ischemia often contributes substantially to LV dysfunction. The elevated pulmonary capillary wedge pressure is largely due to the poorly compliant ischemic left ventricle. In patients with a systolic blood pressure >100 mm Hg with adequate tissue perfusion and features of pulmonary congestion, gentle diuresis with furosemide in combination with pre- and afterload reduction with IV nitroglycerin may improve LV function. Nitroglycerin may also relieve ischemia by dilating epicardial coronary arteries. Nitroprusside has been demonstrated to cause coronary steal and should be avoided.

Poor Output, Clear Chest (Forrester Class III)

Due to a combination of factors including poor oral intake, sweating, nausea and vomiting, as well as nitrates, LV preload may be reduced. These patients should be treated with repeated fluid challenges (200-mL boluses of Ringer's lactate or normal saline). Right ventricular infarction (see below) should also be considered.

Poor Output, Pulmonary Congestion (Forrester Class IV)

Patients with a systolic blood pressure <90 mm Hg and/or who have signs of inadequate tissue perfusion together with pulmonary congestion have significant LV dysfunction with elevated left-sided filling pressures. Intravenous norepinephrine should be administered and titrated to increase the mean arterial pressure >65 to 70 mm Hg. Dobutamine, 5 to 20 µg/kg/min should be added to improve cardiac function. Pulmonary artery catheterization should be considered in these patients to optimize preload and allow the more rational use of vasoactive agents. In addition, consideration should be given to initiating intra-aortic counterpulsation. Reperfusion by PTCA or coronary artery by pass grafting may improve the outcome of these patients.

Right Ventricular Infarction

Diagnosis

- *Clinical*: A raised jugular venous pressure (JVP), hypotension, and clear chest in a patient with an acute inferior myocardial infarction is characteristic of right ventricular (RV) infarction. Kussmaul's sign may be positive.
- *Hemodynamic criteria*: Right atrial (RA) pressure >10 mm Hg or a pulmonary artery/pulmonary capillary wedge pressure >0.8 in patient with no features of cor pulmonale.

- *ECG criteria*: ST-segment elevation in V4R. ST elevation in V1 with ST depression in V2 is said to be characteristic of RV infarction.
- *Radionuclide techniques*: These are the most sensitive diagnostic methods. Multiple gated (MUGA) or pyrophosphate scan.

Management of RV Infarction

- Fluid administration (despite a raised JVP) is the cornerstone of therapy. The optimal central venous pressure is between 10 and 14 mm Hg.
- Stop/avoid use of nitrates.
- Patients who have not responded to fluid challenges should have a therapeutic trial of dobutamine. Pulmonary artery catheter (PAC) may be useful in these patients.
- High-degree heart block is common in these patients. Atrioventricular (AV) sequential pacing improves right ventricular filling and increase in cardiac output (even in patients who have not improved with ventricular pacing alone).

Atrial Fibrillation

Atrial fibrillation (AF) associated with AMI most often occurs within the first 24 hours and is usually transient but may recur. The incidence of AF in acute AMI ranges from 10% to 16%. In the patient with AMI, the appearance of AF is often a manifestation of extensive LV systolic dysfunction.

- If the occurrence of AF causes hemodynamic compromise or ongoing ischemia, direct-current cardioversion should be performed.
- In the absence of CHF, bronchospastic disease, or AV block, the most effective means of slowing the ventricular rate in AF is the use of IV beta-adrenoceptor-blocking agents such as atenolol or metoprolol.
- Rapid digitalization will control the ventricular rate and improve LV function. This method provides a slower response than intravenous beta-adrenoceptor-blocking agents. Acute digitalization, however, may cause coronary and splanchnic vasoconstriction.
- Rate slowing may also be achieved with IV diltiazem. However, because of their negative inotropic effect and concerns regarding the use of calcium channel blockers in AMI, these agents are not recommended as first-line agents.
- The role of Class I and Class III antiarrhythmic agents and electric shock for converting persistent AF are unclear, as is the role

of antiarrhythmic agents for the prevention of further episodes of AF in patients who convert to sinus rhythm.
- Anticoagulation with heparin is indicated in patients who remain in AF for more than 24 hours or who have recurrent episodes of AF.

Ventricular Tachycardia/Ventricular Fibrillation

- Episodes of ventricular fibrillation and sustained ventricular tachycardia (more than 30 seconds or causing hemodynamic compromise) should be treated with immediate direct-current countershock; the same is true for episodes of monomorphic ventricular tachycardia associated with angina, pulmonary congestion, or hypotension.
- Monomorphic ventricular tachycardia not accompanied by chest pain, pulmonary congestion, or hypotension should be treated with IV lidocaine, procainamide, or amiodarone.
- Infusions of antiarrhythmic drugs may be used after an episode of ventricular tachycardia/ventricular fibrillation, but these drugs should be discontinued after 6 to 24 hours; the need for further arrhythmia management should then be assessed.
- Electrolyte and acid–base disturbances should be corrected to prevent recurrent episodes once the initial episode has been treated.

Bradyarrhythmias and Heart Block

Sinus bradycardia occurs in up to 40% of patients with an AMI, especially within the first hour of an inferior AMI and with reperfusion of the right coronary artery. Heart block develops in about 6% to 14% of patients with AMI. The increased mortality associated with heart block and intraventricular conduction delay is related more to extensive myocardial damage than to heart block as such. Indeed, pacing has not been shown to reduce mortality in these patients. Atropine is indicated in patients with symptomatic bradycardia (generally heart rate <50 beats/min associated with hypotension, ischemia, or ventricular escape rhythm and symptomatic AV block.

Transcutaneous Pacing

The newly available transcutaneous pacemaker systems are suitable for providing standby pacing in AMI, especially for those not requiring immediate pacing and at only moderate progression to AV block.

Indications for Temporary Transvenous Pacing

- Sinus bradycardia unresponsive to drug therapy
- Mobitz type II second-degree AV block
- Third-degree heart block
- Bilateral bundle branch block (BBBB) (alternating left bundle branch block and right bundle branch block (RBBB) or RBBB with alternating left anterior fasicular block (LAFB)/left posterior fascicular block (LPFB))
- Bifascicular block in conjunction with first-degree AV block.

■ SELECTED REFERENCES

1. A clinical trial comparing primary coronary angioplasty with tissue plasminogen activator for acute myocardial infarction. The Global Use of Strategies to Open Occluded Coronary Arteries in Acute Coronary Syndromes (GUSTO IIb) Angioplasty Substudy investigators. *N Engl J Med.* 1997;336: 1621–1628.
2. An international randomized trial comparing four thrombolytic strategies for acute myocardial infarction. The GUSTO investigators. *N Engl J Med.* 1993;329:673–682.
3. Antoniucci D, Santoro GM, Bolognese L, Valenti R, Trapani M, Fazzini PF. A clinical trial comparing primary stenting of the infarct-related artery with optimal primary angioplasty for acute myocardial infarction: results from the Florence Randomized Elective Stenting in Acute Coronary Occlusions (FRESCO) trial. *J Am Coll Cardiol.* 1998;31:1234–1239.
4. Every NR, Parsons LS, Hlatky M, Martin JS, Weaver WD. A comparison of thrombolytic therapy with primary coronary angioplasty for acute myocardial infarction. Myocardial Infarction Triage and Intervention investigators. *N Engl J Med.* 1996;335:1253–1260.
5. Gersh BJ. Current issues in reperfusion therapy. *Am J Cardiol.* 1998;82: 3P–11P.
6. Mark DB, Hlatky MA, Califf RM, et al. Cost effectiveness of thrombolytic therapy with tissue plasminogen activator as compared with streptokinase for acute myocardial infarction. *N Engl J Med.* 1995;332:1418–1424.
7. Suryapranata H, van't Hof AW, Hoorntje JC, de Boer MJ, Zijlstra F. Randomized comparison of coronary stenting with balloon angioplasty in selected patients with acute myocardial infarction. *Circulation.* 1998;97: 2502–2505.
8. Zijlstra F, Beukema WP, van't Hof AW, et al. Randomized comparison of primary coronary angioplasty with thrombolytic therapy in low risk patients with acute myocardial infarction. *J Am Coll Cardiol.* 1997;29:908–912.

23

Management of Cardiac Failure in the Intensive Care Unit

■ INDICATIONS FOR ADMISSION TO THE ICU

Heart failure is a serious condition affecting an estimated 2 million Americans and is a common reason for hospitalization. Patients presenting with an acute deterioration of cardiac function are often admitted to the ICU. These patients are likely to benefit from treatment in an ICU. However, patients with end-stage cardiac failure whose condition has progressed slowly and inexorably despite maximal medical therapy are poor candidates for admission to the ICU, unless they are candidates for cardiac transplantation or have suffered from an acute medical complication. The following patients with cardiac failure may benefit from admission to an ICU:

- Worsening pulmonary edema with acute respiratory failure
- Acute myocardial ischemia
- Acute hemodynamic compromise due to arrhythmias
- Severe complicating disease, e.g., pneumonia

■ CONFIRM THE DIAGNOSIS OF CARDIAC FAILURE

Many other diseases may cause symptoms that mimic cardiac failure. Dyspnea can be caused by a wide range of conditions. It may be difficult to distinguish dyspnea caused by cardiac failure as opposed to that caused by chronic obstructive pulmonary disease; this distinction is critically important in the management of patients with a history of cardiac failure who become dyspneic. Patients with peripheral edema may be inappropriately labeled as having heart failure when there is another cause for the edema. Physical examination is not sensitive for diagnosing heart failure. Many patients with severely impaired left ventricular function have no signs of heart failure. Marantz et al. reported that 20% of patients with an ejection fraction (EF) <40% had no clinical features of heart failure; and only 42% of patients with left ventricular EFs of <30% had dyspnea on exertion.

■ EVALUATION OF THE PATIENT WITH CARDIAC FAILURE

It is important to determine the precipitating factor(s) that have led to a deterioration of cardiac function. The most important include

- Myocardial ischemia
- Poorly controlled hypertension
- Arrhythmias, particularly atrial arrhythmias
- Poor compliance with medication
- Drug reactions/side effects
- Fluid overload due to deterioration of renal function
- Anemia
- Intercurrent illness, particularly infections

Assessment of left ventricular function is a critical step in the evaluation and management of patients with heart failure. All patients should undergo echocardiography, unless this investigation or angiography has been performed recently (within the last year). An EF of <45%, with or without symptoms of heart failure, is accepted as evidence of left ventricular systolic dysfunction. Between 8% and 18% of patients will have technically inadequate echocardiograms, in which case radionuclide ventriculography should be performed. A substantial proportion (up to 40% in some studies) of patients with signs and symptoms of heart failure have preserved systolic function (EFs >45%). The cause of heart failure in these patients is valvular disease or diastolic dysfunction. In many patients it may be difficult to determine clinically whether the patient has predominantly systolic or diastolic left ventricular dysfunction. This distinction is critically important, as the management of these patients differs considerably. Digoxin, angiotensin-converting enzyme (ACE) inhibitors, and nitrates may be potentially harmful in patients without left ventricular systolic dysfunction. Furthermore, quantitative assessment of left ventricular function provides important prognostic information, as the

EF is the most important predictor of the 5-year survival rate. The findings from echocardiography or radionuclide ventriculography, however, do not always provide information for determining the cause of the patient's heart failure.

■ MANAGEMENT OF ACUTE PULMONARY EDEMA

Intravenous furosemide in a dose of 40 to 80 mg should be given. Sublingual nitroglycerin will acutely reduce preload, providing symptomatic relief until the diuretic effect of the loop diuretic is maximal. Small doses of morphine sulphate (1 to 2 mg) are useful in alleviating anxiety (they also decrease preload). Large doses of morphine may suppress the respiratory drive, resulting in worsening hypoxemia. Patients in pulmonary edema may benefit from positive-pressure ventilation with positive end-expiratory pressure (PEEP) or nasal continuous positive airway pressure/bilevel positive airway pressure (CPAP/BiPAP). Positive-pressure ventilation (plus PEEP) is good for the left ventricle; it reduces the work of breathing, reduces preload, and reduces left ventricular (LV) afterload.

■ PHARMACOLOGIC MANAGEMENT OF SYSTOLIC DYSFUNCTION

Diuretics

Diuretics should be used in patients with signs of *intravascular volume overload*. Diuretics have no place in the management of heart failure in the absence of symptoms or signs of pulmonary congestion. It is widely (although incorrectly) believed that diuresis improves cardiac function in patients with congestive cardiac failure. It has been postulated that diuretic-induced changes in preload increase ventricular performance by two mechanisms: either by shifting the ventricle to a more optimal position on the descending limb on the Starling's curve or by reducing LV size and thereby reducing systolic wall stress (afterload) by the Laplace effect. However, it has been clearly demonstrated that in the physiological range there is *no* descending limb of the LV stroke volume–pressure curve (Starling's curve) in the mammalian heart (this includes humans). Furthermore, currently no evidence supports the contention that diuresis increases stroke volume or cardiac output in patients with congestive cardiac failure. Braunwald and colleagues demonstrated an average fall in cardiac output of 20% following diuresis in patients with impaired cardiac function both at rest and during exercise. A single, randomized, placebo-controlled study has been reported that has evaluated the efficacy of diuretics in patients with LV dysfunction. In this study, furosemide was no better than placebo in preserving LV function.

Diuretics are appropriate therapy in patients with *symptomatic* cardiogenic pulmonary edema. However, it is important to realize that patients with failing hearts (chronic) are able to tolerate high pulmonary venous pressures without developing pulmonary edema. Patients with severe chronic left heart failure frequently lack pulmonary rales on examination or alveolar edema on chest x-ray, despite high pulmonary venous pressure (and features of pulmonary venous hypertension on chest x-ray). These patients may have pulmonary venous pressures >30 mm Hg. This observation is explained by reduced pulmonary microvascular permeability as well as increased lymphatic flow in these patients.

Overdiuresis should be avoided, as this may excessively reduce LV preload, with decreased stroke volume and cardiac output, leading to further neurohormonal activation and further impairment of LV function. It is important to avoid excessive diuresis before starting ACE inhibitors; this may lead to profound hypotension and/or renal insufficiency/failure. The serum urea nitrogen (BUN) should be closely followed in patients with cardiac failure who are receiving diuretics. Diuretics should be *stopped* in the face of a rising BUN and/or oliguria; do not wait until uremic frost develops before stopping the diuretic. In addition, it is extremely dangerous to use "crackles" as the end point of diuretic therapy: "*all the crackles is not failure.*"

Recently, the aldosterone-receptor antagonist spironolactone (12.5 mg up to 50 mg daily), when used in conjunction with an ACE inhibitor, has been demonstrated to reduce the risk of death from progressive heart failure and sudden death from cardiac causes in patients with severe heart failure. The drug is well tolerated with few side effects. It has been suggested that the beneficial effect of spironolactone may be mediated by preventing myocardial and vascular fibrosis associated with increased circulating levels of aldosterone. Spironolactone should therefore be added to the regimen of an ACE inhibitor in patients with severe heart failure due to LV systolic dysfunction. The serum potassium level should be closely monitored and the dose reduced (or stopped) if hyperkalemia develops.

ACE Inhibitors

All patients with heart failure due to LV systolic dysfunction should be given a trial of ACE inhibitors unless specific contraindications exist. ACE inhibitors have been shown to improve functional status and reduce the mortality in patients with moderate and severe heart failure. ACE inhibitors have been demonstrated to be more effective in reducing morbidity and mortality than the combination of isosorbide dinitrate and hydralazine. ACE inhibitors may be considered as sole therapy in the subset of heart failure patients who present with fatigue or mild dyspnea on exertion and who do not have any signs or symptoms of volume overload. A diuretic (spironolactone) should be added if symptoms persist (monitor serum potassium levels). ACE inhibitors have been demonstrated to be useful in patients with moderate-to-severe aortic incompetence and in patients with mitral incompetence.

ACE inhibitors are contraindicated in patients with moderate-to-severe aortic stenosis, bilateral renal artery stenosis, hypertrophic obstructive cardiomyopathy, and pericardial tamponade. ACE inhibitors should not be started (or discontinued) in patients with a serum potassium >5.5 mEq/L. In addition, ACE inhibitors should be avoided in patients whose renal function has acutely declined. ACE inhibitors should be used very cautiously in patients with poorly controlled angina, as ACE inhibitors may cause an increase in angina in these patients.

Low doses of an ACE inhibitor (captopril 6.25 mg or intravenous enalapril 1.25 mg) should be used in patients with a systolic blood pressure <100 mm Hg, patients with a serum sodium of <135 mEq/L, patients who have a serum creatinine >2.0 mg/dL (or an estimated creatinine clearance of <40 mL/min) and in patients with severe LV dysfunction. The renal function of these patients should be closely monitored and the drug discontinued if renal function deteriorates. Potassium-sparing diuretics should be stopped in all patients who are being started on ACE inhibitors regardless of the serum potassium.

Isosorbide Dinitrate and Hydralazine

Isosorbide dinitrate and hydralazine are appropriate alternatives in patients with contraindications or intolerance to ACE inhibitors. Isosorbide is initiated at a dose of 10 mg tid and increased slowly to 40 mg tid as tolerated. Hydralazine should be initiated at a dose of 10 to 25 mg tid and increased slowly up to 75 mg tid (over a few weeks).

Digoxin

Digoxin is clearly indicated in patients with LV systolic dysfunction and chronic atrial fibrillation. The role of digoxin in patients with heart failure who remain in sinus rhythm has been much debated. Digoxin can prevent clinical deterioration in patients with heart failure due to LV systolic dysfunction. The recently completed Digitalis Investigation Group (DIG) Study did not demonstrate a benefit of digoxin on mortality but did demonstrate a reduction in the hospitalization rate in the digoxin group as compared with placebo. Similarly, the RADIANCE study demonstrated that the withdrawal of digoxin from patients with chronic heart failure resulted in worsening heart failure and a higher rate of hospitalization compared to patients who continued to receive this drug. Digoxin should therefore be used in patients with severe heart failure and should be added to the medical regimen of patients with mild or moderate heart failure who remain symptomatic after optimal management with ACE inhibitors and diuretics. Digoxin should be used with caution after an acute myocardial infarction (AMI). A number of studies have suggested that digoxin increases mortality in patients with acute ischemic syndromes.

Digoxin has a very narrow therapeutic index, and unless the patient is dosed precisely and the serum levels monitored, the patient is likely to suffer significant toxicity. Recent data suggest that a serum *>1.2 ng/mL* offers very little therapeutic advantage but increases the risk of toxicity. The patient's age, weight, and renal function must be taken into account when dosing (loading and maintenance) (Table 23-1). An intravenous loading dose may be appropriate in the ICU setting. However, a loading dose should be used very cautiously in patients currently receiving digoxin. Furthermore, the volume of distribution of digoxin is reduced by up to 50% in renal failure, and therefore the loading dose must be reduced by up to 50% in these patients. The prescriber should also be cognizant of the many drugs that alter digoxin pharmacokinetics (Table 23-2).

Beta-Blockers

Beta-blockers have been shown to be of benefit in "stable" patients with cardiac failure. These agents improve New York Heart Association functional class and left ventricular ejection fraction (LVEF) in patients with idiopathic or ischemic cardiomyopathy. They should not be used, however, in patients who have acutely decompensated unless the patients have diastolic dysfunction. The progressive increase in the dose of the beta-blocking agent appears to be an important factor allowing hemodynamic and functional benefit in patients with heart failure (correction of neurohormonal milieu). Studies have shown that improvement in EF takes several months to develop. In contrast, the nonprogressive administration of antihypertensive doses of beta-blockade often leads to hemodynamic as well as functional status deterioration. These data suggest that beta-blockers **should not** be used in patients with acute decompensated cardiac failure but rather should be used in stable patients already receiving maximal medical therapy. Beta-blockers have been shown to reverse the remodeling that occurs in the failing heart—and thereby interrupt the destructive cycle of neurohormonal signaling, abnormal growth, mechanical

Table 23-1. Digoxin dosing guidelines.

Loading Doses:	IV 10–15 µg/kg LBW (8–10 µg/kg)*
	po 15–20 µg/kg LBW (15 µg/kg)*
	*Patients over age 70 and renal failure

Maintenance Dosing:

CrCL (mL/min)	<60 kg <132 lb	60–70 kg 132–154 lb	70–80 kg 154–176 lb	>80 kg >176 lb	Weeks to SS
<10	0.125 mg qod	0.125 mg qod	0.125 mg qd	0.125 mg qd	3–4
10–30	0.125 mg qod	0.125 mg qod	0.125–0.25 mg qd	0.25 mg qd	2.5–3
30–50	0.125 mg qd	0.25 mg qd	0.25 mg qd	0.25 mg qd	2
>50	0.25 mg qd	0.25 mg qd	0.25 mg qd	0.25–0.375 mg qd	1–2

LBW: Males = 50 + (2.3 × inches over 5 feet)
Females = 45.5 + (2.3 × inches over 5 feet)

Estimated CrCl (mL/min)
Males = [114 – (0.8 × age)] / Scr
Females = above × 0.9

Use LBW if weight greater than 1.5 × LBW.
(LBW = Lean Body Weight; qd = daily; qod = every other day)

Table 23-2. Digoxin interactions.

Drug interactions that increase serum digoxin levels:
  Amiodarone
  Cyclosporine
  Diltiazem
  Propafenone
  Quinidine
  Triamterene
  Verapamil
  Macrolide antibiotics
  Ibuprofen
  Itraconazole

Drug interaction that decrease serum digoxin levels:
  Hydantoins

Electrolyte disturbances that potentiate digoxin toxicity:
  Hypokalemia/hyperkalemia
  Hypomagnesemia
  Hypercalcemia

deterioration, and myocyte destruction that is set in motion when the ventricle fails. After 3 months of therapy, LV performance is markedly improved in the vast majority of patients. After 3 to 6 months of therapy with beta-blockers, reductions are seen in both systolic and diastolic volumes. After 18 months of therapy, regression in LV mass is seen and the ventricle becomes more elliptical or normal in shape.

Metoprolol, bucindolol, carvedilol, bisoprolol, and nebivolol have been demonstrated to improve the outcome of patients with cardiac failure. Carvedilol, however, appears to have a greater effect on mortality reduction than the other beta-blockers. In the U.S. Carvedilol Heart Failure Study Group, carvedilol was associated with a 65% mortality reduction. Carvedilol has unique characteristics that distinguish it from other beta-blockers, including alpha-blockade and antioxidant properties. Whether these features account for the benefits reported cannot be determined from current data.

Calcium Channel-Blocking Drugs

First-generation calcium channel-blocking drugs such as verapamil, diltiazem, and nifedipine should be avoided in patients with LV systolic dysfunction, as these agents have been demonstrated to increase morbidity and mortality. The PRAISE study demonstrated that amlodipine does not adversely affect the natural history of chronic heart failure. This drug should be considered second-line therapy for the management of hypertension or angina in patients with LV dysfunction.

Dobutamine

Dobutamine may have a role in patients with acute LV failure due to myocardial ischemia. In this setting, dobutamine may recruit hibernating myocardium and improve cardiac function. The role of dobutamine in patients with chronic heart failure is unclear. Chronic heart failure is characterized by sympathetic hyperactivation and beta-receptor downregulation. Short-term infusions or continuous beta-stimulant therapies have not been demonstrated to be beneficial in these patients. This therapy is associated with an increased frequency of ventricular arrhythmias, which may increase mortality. However, intermittent pulsed (<1 hour) stimulation with dobutamine has been demonstrated to produce beneficial changes analogous to the effects of physical training. This effect is not seen when dobutamine is given for >4 hours.

■ ANTICOAGULATION

Routine anticoagulation is not recommended. Patients with a history of systemic or pulmonary embolism, recent atrial fibrillation, or mobile LV thrombi should be anticoagulated to a prothrombin time ratio of 1.2 to 1.8 times control (international normalized ratio, 2.0 to 3.0).

■ MANAGEMENT OF ATRIAL FIBRILLATION

Atrial fibrillation (AF) may occur in up to 50% of patients with severe heart failure. If AF causes sudden severe worsening of heart failure, immediate cardioversion may be necessary. However, most patients can be stabilized by using digoxin to control heart rate. Approximately 60% of patients with acute AF (<1 week) will spontaneously revert back to sinus rhythm. A recent randomized, placebo-controlled study demonstrated that the rate of conversion of acute AF to sinus rhythm was similar in the group of patients treated with amiodarone compared to the group receiving placebo. Patients with recent-onset AF who do not spontaneously convert back to sinus rhythm, and patients with a history of AF of <1 year (and with a left atrial diameter of <50 mm) should be considered for elective cardioversion.

■ PERSISTENT HYPERTENSION DESPITE ACE INHIBITORS AND DIURETICS

Reduction of blood pressure may in itself have a beneficial effect on the signs and symptoms of heart failure. Hypertension is a relative concept in patients with heart failure. Although a blood pressure of 135/85 mm Hg may be acceptable for a patient with a normal EF, that same blood pressure may be harmful for a patient with LV systolic dysfunction. Patients' symptoms may improve with blood pressure reduction due to an increase in cardiac output. Hydralazine is a useful drug in these patients. Alpha-1-adrenergic blocking drugs or centrally acting alpha-blockers are alternatives. Calcium channel blockers should be avoided in patients with systolic dysfunction. Amlodipine is a newer generation calcium channel blocker that may have a role in these patients (see "Calcium Channel-Blocking Drugs," above).

■ ANTIARRHYTHMIC DRUGS AND IMPLANTABLE DEFIBRILLATORS

Ventricular arrhythmias in patients with congestive heart failure are associated with increased rates of overall mortality and sudden death. However, attempts at suppressing ventricular arrhythmias with antiarrhythmic agents have not been demonstrated to improve survival. The CAST study has shown that the suppression of arrhythmias with encainide or flecainide increased mortality among patients postmyocardial infarction. In a recent study, amiodarone failed to reduce the incidence of sudden death or prolong survival among patients with heart failure. Antiarrhythmic drugs are not currently recommended to suppress ventricular arrhythmias except in patients with life-threatening arrhythmias who have undergone careful evaluation, with electrophysiologic testing demonstrating the effectiveness and safety of the chosen drug. Implantable defibrillators appear to have a role in patients with cardiac failure and ventricular arrhythmias. The MADIT study demonstrated that, in patients with prior myocardial infarction who have an EF <35%, a documented episode of asymptomatic ventricular tachycardia (VT) and inducible, nonsuppressible VT during Electrophysiological Study (EPS), prophylactic therapy with an implantable defibrillator led to improved survival as compared to conventional therapy. The AVID study demonstrated that an implantable cardioverter–defibrillator resulted in lower mortality than antiarrhythmic drug therapy among patients resuscitated from ventricular fibrillation or symptomatic, sustained VT with hemodynamic compromise.

■ EVALUATION OF PATIENTS FOR REVASCULARIZATION

Coronary artery disease is currently the most common cause of heart failure in the United States, and some heart failure patients may benefit from revascularization. Patients with a history of angina or AMI should undergo physiologic testing for ischemia, followed by coronary artery angiography if ischmic regions are detected. Patients with heart failure who have significant angina (exercise limiting, occurring at rest, recurrent episodes of pulmonary edema) should undergo coronary arteriography as the initial test for operable coronary lesions.

■ CONSIDERATION FOR HEART TRANSPLANTATION

Consideration should be given to cardiac transplantation in patients with severe limitation or repeated hospitalizations because of heart failure despite aggressive medical therapy in whom revascularization is not likely to convey benefit.

■ MANAGEMENT OF PATIENTS WITH DIASTOLIC DYSFUNCTION

As many as 40% of patients with a clinical diagnosis of heart failure have preserved LV systolic function and no evidence of valvular heart disease. Most of these individuals have LV diastolic dysfunction. In diastolic heart failure, the LV has increased diastolic stiffness (reduced compliance and is unable to fill adequately at normal diastolic pressures). This condition results in reduced end-diastolic volume and elevated end-diastolic pressures. The reduced LV filling leads to decreased stroke volume and symptoms of low cardiac output, whereas the increased filling pressure leads to symptoms of pulmonary congestion.

Hypertension is the most common cause of diastolic dysfunction, which can develop even in the absence of LV hypertrophy. Left ventricular compliance decreases with aging; this syndrome is therefore not uncommon in the elderly hypertensive patient. Coronary artery disease is also an important cause of LV diastolic dysfunction. The optimal treatment of diastolic dysfunction is not well defined. Beta-blocking drugs, calcium channel blockers, and diuretics are the treatments of choice. Excessive diuresis may reduce stroke volume and cardiac output. Digitalis may further decrease LV compliance. Vasodilators (hydralazine) may cause severe uncompensated hypotension. The role of ACE inhibitors is not clear.

■ SELECTED REFERENCES

1. A comparison of antiarrhythmic-drug therapy with implantable defibrillators in patients resuscitated from near-fatal ventricular arrhythmias. The Antiarrhythmics versus Implantable Defibrillators (AVID) investigators. *N Engl J Med.* 1997;337:1576–1583.
2. CAST investigators. Preliminary report: effect of encainide and flecainide on mortality in a randomized trial of arrhythmia suppression after myocardial infarction. *N Engl J Med.* 1989;321:406–412.
3. CIBIS investigators. A randomized trial of beta-blockade in heart failure: The cardiac insufficiency bisoprolol study. *Circulation.* 1994;90:1765–1773.
4. CONSENSUS Trial Study Group. Effects of enalapril on mortality in severe congestive heart failure. *Engl J Med.* 1987;316:1429–1435.
5. Davies SW, Bailey J, Keegan J, et al. Reduced pulmonary microvascular permeability in severe chronic left heart failure. *Am Heart J.* 1992;124:137–142.
6. Dries F, Krell MJ, Whitloe, et al. Intermittent dobutamine in ambulatory patients with chronic heart failure. *Circulation.* 1986;74(suppl II):II-38.
7. The effect of digoxin on mortality and morbidity in patients with heart failure. The Digitalis Investigation Group. *N Engl J Med.* 1997;336 (8):525–533.
8. Eichhorn EJ. Restoring function in failing hearts: the effects of beta blockers. *Am J Med.* 1998;104:163–169.
9. Galve E, Rius T, Ballester, et al. Intravenous amiodarone in treatment of recent-onset atrial fibrillation: results of a randomized, controlled study. *J Am Coll Cardiol.* 1996;27:1079–1082.
10. Marantz PR, Tobin JN, Wassertheil-Smoller S, Steingart RM, Wexler JP, Budner N, Lense L, Wachspress J. The relationship between left ventricular systolic function and congestive heart failure diagnosed by clinical criteria. *Circulation.* 1988;77(3):607–612.
11. Moss AJ, Hall WJ, Cannon DS, et al. Improved survival with an implanted defibrillator in patients with coronary disease at high risk for ventricular arrhythmias. *N Engl J Med.* 1996;335:1933–1940.
12. O'Connor CM, Carson PE, et al. Effect of amlodipine on mode of death among patients with advanced heart failure in the PRAISE trial. Prospec-

tive Randomized Amlodipine Survival Evaluation. *Am J Cardiol.* 1998;82(7):881–887.

13. Packer M, Bristow MR, et al. The effect of carvedilol on morbidity and mortality in patients with chronic heart failure. U.S. Carvedilol Heart Failure Study Group. *N Engl J Med.* 1996;334(21):1349–1355.

14. Packer M, Gheorghiade M, Young JB, et al. Withdrawl of digoxin from patients with chronic heart failure treated with angiotensin-converting-enzyme inhibitors. *N Engl J Med.* 1993;329:1–7.

15. Pitt B, Zannad F, Remme WJ, et al. The effect of spironolactone on morbidity and mortality in patients with severe heart failure. Randomized Aldactone Evaluation Study Investigators. *N Engl J Med.* 1999;341:709–717.

16. Sharpe N, Murphy J, Smith H, Hannan S. Treatment of patients with symptomless left ventricular dysfunction after myocardial infarction. *Lancet.* 1988;I:255–259.

17. Singh SN, Fletcher RD, Fisher SG, et al. Amiodarone in patients with congestive heart failure and asymptomatic ventricular arrhythmia. *N Engl J Med.* 1995;333:77–82.

18. SOLVD Investigators. Effect of enalapril on mortality and development of heart failure in asymptomatic patients with reduced left ventricular ejection fraction. *N Engl J Med.* 1992;327:685–691.

19. Stampfer M, Epstein SE, Beiser GD, Braunwald E. Hemodynamic effects of diuresis at rest and during intense upright exercise in patients with impaired cardiac function. *Circulation.* 1968;37:900–911.

20. Topol EJ, Traill TA, Fortuin NJ. Hypertensive hypertrophic cardiomyopathy of the elderly. *N Engl J Med.* 1985;312:2177–2287.

21. Waagstein F, Bristow MR, Swedberg K, et al. Beneficial effects of metoprolol in idiopathic cardiomyopathy. *Lancet.* 1993;342:1441–1446.

24

Cardiopulmonary Resuscitation

Cardiopulmonary arrest is usually the result of a cardiac dysrhythmia. The majority of adults (80% to 90%) with sudden, nontraumatic cardiac arrest are found to be in ventricular fibrillation when the initial electrocardiogram is obtained. When ventricular fibrillation occurs outside the hospital, it is presumed to reflect chronic myocardial ischemia with electrical instability, rather than acute myocardial infarction. In-hospital cardiac arrest most often follows acute myocardial infarction or is the result of severe multisystem disease, with asystole, bradydysrhythmias, or pulseless electrical activity.

Despite an improved understanding and management of cardiac arrest, and the widespread application *of do not resuscitate* orders in an attempt to prevent the inappropriate use of cardiopulmonary resuscitation (CPR), the success rate following in-hospital cardiac arrest has remained unchanged over the last three decades: Return of spontaneous circulation occurs in about 30% of patients, with approximately 15% being discharged neurologically intact. Patients who suffer an out-of-hospital cardiac arrest fare worse than those patients who are resuscitated in-hospital, with a hospital admission rate of between 8% and 22%, and with between 1% and 8% being discharged neurologically intact. CPR performed in-hospital is most likely to succeed in patients with primary ventricular fibrillation and ischemic heart disease; those with cardiac arrest in the absence of life-threatening conditions; and those with hypothermia, drug overdose, airway obstruction, or primary respiratory arrest. In patients suffering out-of-hospital cardiac arrest, the highest discharge rate has been achieved when CPR is initiated within 4 minutes of the arrest.

■ INITIAL MANAGEMENT OF CARDIOPULMONARY ARREST

The first and most crucial step in the management of the cardiac arrest victim is the assessment of the victim (see Figure 24-1). No victim should undergo the intrusive and potentially injurious procedures of CPR until the need has been established by an appropriate assessment. This involves determining whether the patient is unconscious, whether the patient is breathing, and whether the patient has a carotid pulse. Furthermore, the patient should be rapidly evaluated for possible injuries.

The initial management of cardiopulmonary arrest will vary depending on the availability of equipment to monitor cardiac rhythm and perform countershock. In the hospital, such equipment should be available within minutes. If ventricular fibrillation or ventricular tachycardia is documented by conventional monitoring or by "quick-look" defibrillation paddles, three sequential countershocks should be delivered as soon as possible at energy settings of 200, then 300, then 360 J. If ventricular fibrillation/ventricular tachycardia (VF/VT) is not the initially recognized rhythm or if defibrillation is not successful in establishing an effective rhythm, chest compressions should then be initiated. If the arrest occurs outside the hospital, chest compressions should be initiated and continued until defibrillation and/or cardiac monitoring equipment become available. A precordial thump may terminate VT and rarely VF and should be considered in a witnessed cardiac arrest when a defibrillator is not immediately available.

In adults, primary or unexpected sudden cardiac arrest is most often due to VF. The survival of sudden cardiac arrest secondary to VF is significantly better than that due to asystole or pulseless electrical activity. The survival following VF drops precipitously with time, with a survival rate of >70% when defibrillation is applied within 1 minute and dropping by 10% for each minute that defibrillation is delayed. Electrical defibrillation provides the single most important therapy for the treatment of these patients. Electrical defibrillation is the only effective method of terminating VF, and the chances of surviving diminish as the interval between collapse and countershock lengthens. Precordial chest compression should be regarded as the second priority, immediately after attempts at electrical defibrillation have failed. Therefore, the American Medical Association and the International Liaison Committee on Resuscitation endorse the concept that in many settings nonmedical individuals should be allowed and encouraged to use defibrillators. In a meta-analysis, Auble et al. demonstrated that defibrillation performed by basic life support providers reduced the relative risk of death for out-of-hospital cardiac arrest victims in ventricular fibrillation by 8.5%.

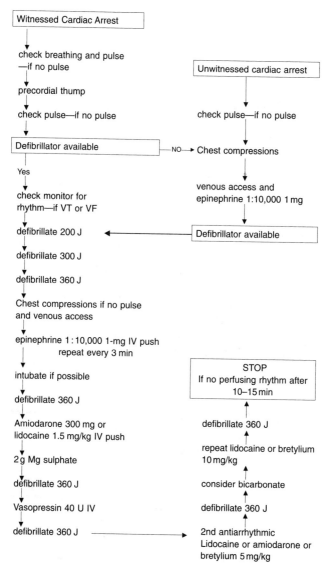

Figure 24-1. Treatment approach for ventricular fibrillation.

The aim of electrical therapy is to provide a current through the myocardium to change enough myocardial cells to the same electrical state, for sufficient time to break the reentrant circuits or produce electrical homogeneity. This allows a stable rhythm to be reestablished from the sinus node. Animal experiments have shown that the period of homogeneity needs to be 4 to 12 ms. As little as 4% of the delivered current actually traverses the heart, with most of the current taking alternative routes through the chest wall. More organized arrhythmias (e.g., atrial flutter or monomorphic tachycardia) require less energy to break the circuit (5 to 10 J internal, 20 to 100 J external) compared to disorganized rhythms (e.g., VF, 10 to 13 J internal, 200–300 J external).

The current delivered to the heart is determined by both the energy chosen (J) and the transthoracic impedance. The use of bare paddles without a couplant (gel/cream) results in very high transthoracic impedance. Impedance may be reduced by strong pressure on the paddles, anteroposterior positioning of the paddles, repetitive shocks, and delivery of the shock during expiration. The energy level chosen for the initial shock is a compromise between risking myocardial damage from excessive current and unsuccessful defibrillation from too low a current. The American Heart Association (AHA) and the European Resuscitation Council recommend 200 J for the first attempts in adults. Since thoracic impedance declines with successive shocks, the second attempt may be 200 to 300 J. If this fails, then another shock at maximum joules (360 J) is administered. The defibrillator paddles should be placed in a position that will maximize current flow through the myocardium. The most commonly employed placement is apex-anterior. The anterior electrode should be placed on the right of the upper sternum below the clavicle; the apex electrode should be placed to the left of the nipple, with the center of the electrode in the midaxillary line.

After successful defibrillation, normal electrical impulse generation is established and myocardial contraction follows. However, postresuscitation myocardial dysfunction is usual, recovering over minutes to hours, depending on the duration of the arrhythmia. Intracellular calcium overload has been postulated to be responsible for this finding.

In an experimental model, Niemann and colleagues demonstrated that resuscitation initiated after 7.5 minutes of ventricular fibrillation was substantially more effective following pretreatment with CPR and epinephrine compared with immediate defibrillation. Cobb and co-authors have recently confirmed this finding by demonstrating an improved survival in patients with out-of-hospital ventricular fibrillation who underwent 90 seconds of CPR before delivery of the first shock.

■ CHEST COMPRESSION AND VENTILATION

The overall objective of CPR is to generate adequate flow of well-oxygenated blood to the heart and brain until more definitive therapy can be applied and spontaneous, effective circulation can be restored. The basic life-support guidelines established by the AHA include a combination of external chest compression and ventilation. For resuscitative efforts and evaluation to be effective, the patient must be supine and on a firm, flat surface. Compressions are performed in the lower part of the sternum, $1\frac{1}{2}$ inches in depth in the adult, at a rate of 80 to 100 compressions per minute. Arterial pressure during chest compression is maximal when the duration of compression is 50% of the compression–release cycle. During cardiac arrest, properly performed chest compressions can produce systolic arterial blood pressure peaks of 60 to 80 mm Hg, but diastolic pressure is low.

Mean blood pressure in the carotid artery seldom exceeds 40 mm Hg. Cardiac output resulting from chest compressions is only one fourth to one third of normal. Coronary perfusion occurs during diastole, and for this reason, the diastolic pressure should be followed during CPR; the operator will have a false sense of security if only the systolic pressure is monitored. Cough CPR, deep rhythmic forceful coughing repeated 30 to 60 times per minute, has been reported to be an effective means of maintaining consciousness in patients who suffer a cardiac arrest in the cardiac catheterization laboratory or in the coronary care unit.

There is a remarkably small requirement for ventilation to maintain an optimal ventilation perfusion relationship. Arterial carbon dioxide levels are reduced to low levels of <20 mm Hg during CPR because ventilation exceeds the minute volumes required for normal gas exchange in the setting of low pulmonary flow. Ventilation is performed with a recommended tidal volume of approximately 1000 cc delivered slowly. In case of one-rescuer CPR, ventilations are performed in a cycle of 15 compressions and 2 breaths, with 1.5 to 2 seconds devoted to the 2 rescue breaths. In two-rescuer CPR, ventilations are provided at the end of each fifth compression. In the absence of sufficient muscle tone, the tongue and epiglottis may obstruct the pharynx. If there is no evidence of head or neck trauma, the rescuer should use the head-tilt chin-lift or the jaw-thrust maneuver to open the airway. If foreign material or vomitus is in the mouth, it should be removed. Rescue breathing can be provided by the mouth-to-mouth or mouth-to-nose technique. Barrier devices are available for mouth-to-mouth ventilation to prevent possible spread of pathogens to the rescuer. Supplemental oxygen should be used as soon as possible. Rescue breathing will deliver only about 16% to 17% oxygen to the patient, ideally producing an alveolar oxygen tension of 80 mm Hg. Bag-valve devices, consisting of a self-inflating bag and nonrebreathing valve, may be used with a mask or endotracheal tube.

Rescuers are frequently unwilling to perform mouth-to-mouth ventilation out of the fear of contracting an infectious disease, particularly human immunodeficiency virus. Recent evidence has suggested that ventilation may not be necessary in the initial stages of cardiac arrest. Agonal gasping during cardiac arrest has been demonstrated to achieve adequate ventilation. Chandra and colleagues found that intubated dogs maintained an arterial oxygen saturation above 90% for the first 5 minutes of VF when chest compression was performed without ventilation. In animal models of bystander CPR, no difference in hemodynamics, 48-hour survival, or neurological outcome could be detected when CPR was applied with and without ventilatory support. The Cerebral Resuscitation Group of Belgium found no statistically significant differences in outcome among patients revived by bystanders, whether or not mouth-to mouth ventilation was performed in addition to chest compressions. This postulate has recently been confirmed in a randomized, controlled clinical trial. Hallstrom and colleagues demonstrated a higher survival (14.6% vs. 10.4%; Not Significant (NS)) in victims of out-of-hospital cardiac arrest who received bystander chest compressions alone as compared to those who received chest compression and mouth-to mouth ventilation. This suggests that chest compressions alone will suffice until qualified professionals and appropriate equipment become available. This may be particularly important during one-person CPR, where the rescuer should concentrate on providing adequate chest compressions.

As soon as is practical during the resuscitative effort, the trachea should be intubated by trained personnel. Endotracheal intubation isolates the airway, keeps it patent, reduces the risk of aspiration, permits suctioning of the trachea, ensures delivery of a high concentration of oxygen, and provides a route for the administration of certain drugs. Patients with suspected or confirmed cervical spine injuries should be intubated with extreme caution, with every effort taken to avoid hyperextension of the neck. Endotracheal intubation should not be attempted by inadequately trained individuals, as this may be result in esophageal intubation or upper airway injury. Furthermore, the esophageal obturator airway, esophageal gastric tube airway, and pharyngotracheal lumen airway cannot be recommended, as these devices are associated with a higher complication rate when compared with tracheal intubation. In the absence of personnel trained in endotracheal intubation, the patient may be effectively ventilated and oxygenated with a bag and mask. The initial step is to establish an airway by placing the finger of one hand under the mandible and lifting upward and backward (extending the patient's neck) or by using the index fingers of both hands to lift the mandible from the angle of the jaw. Care should be taken not to generate excessive pressure when ventilating by bag and mask. Airway pressure >25 mm Hg is likely to overcome the resistance of the gastroesophageal sphincter and fill the patient's stomach with gas. This will increase the risk of regurgitation and gastric aspiration. When ventilation is effective, the chest rises with each squeeze of the bag. The patient should be oxygenated in this way with 100% oxygen.

Some controversy exists regarding the timing of ventilatory efforts. Simultaneous chest compressions and ventilation (asynchronous ventilation) may improve cerebral and coronary blood flow by increasing overall intrathoracic pressure. Another promising line of research has focused on the efficacy of abdominal compressions during CPR. Abdominal compressions are performed with the hands of a second or third rescuer and require no special equipment. Two different techniques have been studied; synchronized (or simultaneous) chest and abdominal compressions, and interposed abdominal compressions (alternating with chest compressions). To date, no data are available demonstrating a survival advantage with this technique.

■ DRUG THERAPY DURING CARDIAC ARREST

During cardiac arrest, medications take second place to other interventions. Basic CPR, defibrillation when indicated, and airway management remain the cornerstone of managing the cardiac arrest victim. Once these interventions are initiated, the resuscitation personnel can turn to starting an IV infusion and giving medications. The role of the standard advanced cardiac life support drugs during cardiac arrest is highly controversial, with very little data available to support their use. Indeed, in a retrospective analysis, van Walraven and colleagues demonstrated a significant association between unsuccessful resuscitation and the use of epinephrine (odds ratio [OR] 0.08), atropine (OR 0.24), bicarbonate (OR 0.31), calcium (OR 0.32), and lidocaine (OR 0.48).

If no vein has been cannulated before the arrest, the antecubital vein should be the first choice, because CPR would have to be interrupted to obtain central venous access (internal jugular or subclavian vein). The advantages of central venous access include the more rapid arrival of drugs at their site of action, the ability to give multiple medications and fluid simultaneously, rapid volume resuscitation, and less likelihood of extravasation. Extravasation of a peripheral infusion of vasoactive agents may result in severe tissue necrosis. High success rates have been reported with subclavian and internal jugular catheterization during cardiac arrest and in shocked patients. A short femoral venous line should not be used for drug administration during CPR, since little cephalad flow occurs from below the diaphragm.

Furthermore, femoral catheterization during cardiac arrest has been reported to have a higher rate of failure and misplacement when compared to subclavian vein catheterization. If an endotracheal tube has been placed and venous access is delayed, epinephrine, lidocaine, and atropine can be administered by the endotracheal tube. These medications should be administered at two times the recommended intravenous dose and should be diluted in 10 mL of normal saline.

The work of Redding and Pearson provides the basis of our modern understanding of the effects of adrenergic stimulation during cardiac arrest. These investigators showed that adrenergic drugs that were clinically effective in improving rates of resuscitation shared the common property of alpha-agonist activity. Drugs that had purely beta-agonist activity (i.e., isoproterenol) had either no effect on resuscitation outcomes or actually resulted in fewer survivors. When used early in resuscitation, agents such as epinephrine and methoxamine resulted in significantly higher rates of resuscitation. The addition of adrenergic agents improves the arterial pressures generated during CPR and selectively increases blood flow to the heart and brain. The degree to which an individual agent can increase flow to these areas is a critical determinant of success in resuscitation.

The current AHA-recommended alpha-agonist is epinephrine, which has been in clinical use since 1906. It was formally incorporated into the AHA guidelines for resuscitation in 1973. Early work with epinephrine showed that doses of 0.1 mg/kg clearly improved resuscitation rates and survival in 10-kg dogs. This 1-mg dose was applied unchanged to clinical use in humans, without any evidence of comparable clinical efficacy. After 30 years of clinical use, studies in both animals and humans suggested that the standard 1-mg dose of epinephrine was inadequate. In 1992, the results of three large-scale clinical studies comparing standard-dose to high-dose epinephrine were reported. No statistically significant differences in rates of return of spontaneous cardiorespiratory function, short-term survival, or survival to hospital discharge were demonstrated. Recently, vasopressin has been used for victims of cardiac arrest with encouraging results. Vasopressin should be considered in patients in VF who have not responded to epinephrine after 5 minutes of continuous CPR.

Studies in victims of out-of-hospital VF have shown that bretylium and lidocaine are equally effective in their ability to restore an organized rhythm in patients with VF not responsive to defibrillation and epinephrine. The standard of care at the present time is to administer them to the patient with VT/VF refractory to defibrillation, intubation, and epinephrine. Current AHA recommendations categorize bretylium and lidocaine as medications that are of probable benefit; conclusive scientific evidence supporting their use is lacking. In addition, considerable clinical and experimental evidence shows that magnesium may be helpful in the suppression of refractory ventricular dysrhythmias.

Amiodarone is an antiarrhythmic agent that has been shown to be effective in the treatment of refractory ventricular dysrhythmias. The ARREST study randomized 504 patients with nontraumatic out-of-hospital cardiac arrest who had not responded to three initial shocks to receive a bolus of amiodarone or placebo. In this study, survival to hospital was significantly higher in the amiodarone group (44% vs. 35%). Amiodarone may become the antidysrhythmic agent of choice in patients who have failed initial attempts at defibrillation.

The use of buffer therapy during CPR has been a contentious issue. However, the bulk of current evidence suggests that the patient who is receiving optimal CPR derives no clinical benefit from early administration of buffers. In the absence of a preexisting acidosis, arterial pH is usually within normal limits during the first 5 to 10 minutes of CPR. In fact, in a ventilated animal model, the arterial sample often shows a respiratory alkalosis. However, a mixed venous sample drawn at the same time is likely to show an acidosis, which is typically due to venous hypercarbia. This paradoxical difference between arterial and venous samples is due to the low flow state that exists during CPR. Correction of the acidosis through measures other than ventilation and restoration of flow have not been shown to favorably impact on arrest outcome. To date, the body of experimental evidence has failed to show a survival benefit to administration of sodium bicarbonate during CPR. Although calcium ions play a critical role in the myocardial contractile performance and impulse formation, retrospective and prospective studies in the cardiac arrest setting have not demonstrated benefit from the use of calcium. Because of the potential role of intracellular calcium accumulation in irreversible ischemic cell injury, calcium is now recommended only in selected situations (e.g., hyperkalemia, calcium channel blocker toxicity, and hypocalcemia).

■ SELECTED REFERENCES

1. American Heart Association's standard and guidelines for cardiopulmonary resuscitation (CPR) and emergency care. *JAMA*. 1992;268:2184–2241.
2. Auble TE, Menegazzi JJ, Paris PM. Effect of out-of-hospital defibrillation by basic life support providers on cardiac arrest mortality: a meta-analysis. *Ann Emerg Med*. 1995;25:642–648.
3. Callahan M, Madsen CD, Barton CW. A randomized clinical trial of high-dose epinephrine and norepinephrine vs. standard dose epinephrine in prehospital cardiac arrest. *JAMA*. 1992;268:2667–2672.
4. Chandra NN, Gruben KG, et al. Ventilation during CPR [abstract]. *Circulation*. 1991;84(suppl 2):11–19.

5. Cobb LA, Fahrenbruch CE, Walsh TR, et al. Influence of cardiopulmonary resuscitation prior to defibrillation in patients with out-of-hospital ventricular fibrillation. *JAMA*. 1999;281:1182–1188.

6. Criley JM, Blaufuss AH, Kissel GL. Cough-induced cardiac compression: self administered form of cardiopulmonary resuscitation. *JAMA*. 1976;236:1246–1250.

7. Gueugniaud PY, Mols P, Goldstein P, et al. A comparison of repeated high doses and repeated standard doses of epinephrine for cardiac arrest outside the hospital. European Epinephrine Study group. *N Engl J Med*. 1998;339:-1595–1601.

8. Hallstrom A, Cobb L, Johnson E, Copass M. Cardiopulmonary resuscitation by chest compression alone or with mouth-to-mouth ventilation. *N Engl J Med*. 2000;342:1546–1553.

9. Kudenchuk PJ, Cobb LA, Copass MK, et al. Amiodarone for resuscitation after out-of-hospital cardiac arrest due to ventricular fibrillation. *N Engl J Med*. 1999;341:871–878.

10. Lindner KH, Dirks B, Strohmenger HU, et al. Randomised comparison of epinephrine and vasopressin in patients with out-of-hospital ventricular fibrillation. *Lancet*. 1997;349:535–537.

11. Niemann JT, Cairns CB, Sharma J, Lewis RJ. Treatment of prolonged ventricular fibrillation: immediate countershock versus high-dose epinephrine and CPR preceding countershock. *Circulation*. 1992;85:281–287.

12. Redding JS, Pearson JW. Evaluation of drugs for cardiac resuscitation. *Anaesthesia*. 1963;24:203–207.

13. Van Hoeyweghen RJ, Bossaert LL, Mullie A, et al. Quality and efficiency of bystander CPR. Belgian Resuscitation Study Group. *Resuscitation*. 1993;26:47–52.

14. Van Walraven C, Stiell IG, Wells GA, Hebert PC, Vandemheen K. Do advanced cardiac life support drugs increase resuscitation rates from in-hospital cardiac arrest? The OTAC Study Group. *Ann Emerg Med*. 1998;-32:544–553.

Part 3

The Gastrointestinal Tract

25

Stress Ulcer Prophylaxis

Stress ulcers are superficial erosions in the gastric mucosa that are common in patients with acute, life-threatening diseases. These lesions are usually shallow and well demarcated, primarily involving the superficial layers of the gastric epithelium. Infrequently, erosions may penetrate the muscularis mucosa, resulting in a lesion that resembles a true gastric ulcer. Endoscopic studies have shown that nearly all critically ill patients develop upper gastrointestinal erosions after critical illness or major surgery. Although gastric erosions are common in critically ill patients, they are usually clinically silent. In addition, the incidence of clinically important bleeding from stress ulceration has declined over the last two decades, probably due to earlier and more effective resuscitation.

Not all ICU patients are at an equal risk for stress ulceration. It is therefore important to identify those patients at minimal risk so that they are not subjected to the costs and potential complications of prophylaxis without a reasonable chance of benefit. A number of studies have evaluated those risk factors that increase the chances of bleeding from stress ulceration. These are listed in Table 25-1. Respiratory failure and coagulopathy are the most important risk factors for clinically important bleeding from stress ulceration. The risk of bleeding is also related to the number of risk factors present. Stress ulcer prophylaxis is *only* recommended in those patients with risk factors for bleeding from stress ulceration, particularly, those patients receiving mechanical ventilation and patients with a coagulopathy.

Although the effectiveness of stress ulcer prophylaxis has been questioned, a review of the published data suggests that stress ulcer prophylaxis with antacids, H_2-blockers, and sucralfate does indeed reduce the risk of both overt bleeding as well as clinically important bleeding. Preliminary data suggest that early enteral alimentation may afford some degree of protection against overt bleeding from stress

Table 25-1. Risk factors for stress ulceration.

Mechanical ventilation > 48 h
Coagulopathy
Acute hepatic failure
Significant hypotension
Sepsis
Chronic renal failure
Alcoholism
Glucocorticoid administration
Prolonged nasogastric tube placement
Severe head injury
Burns > 30% body surface area

ulceration. However, in patients with multiple risk factors for stress ulceration, it may be prudent to add an antiulcer agent. It should be emphasized that postpyloric alimentation may increase the risk for bleeding from stress ulceration, as this mode of feeding stimulates gastric acid secretion without buffering the gastric contents.

■ SPECIFIC PROPHYLACTIC AGENTS

Prophylaxis with antacids, H_2-blockers, and sucralfate reduces the risk of both overt and clinically important bleeding when compared to placebo. There is no clear-cut evidence that sucralfate, antacids, or H_2-blockers differ with respect to the prevention of clinically important bleeding.

The choice of a prophylactic agent is therefore largely determined by economic factors and the risk of drug-associated complications (Figure 25-1). Sucralfate is the most cost-effective agent for stress ulcer prophylaxis. In mechanically ventilated patients, sucralfate suspension is best administered via a gastric tube. Antacids have fallen from favor because of the need for frequent dosing and gastric aspiration. Furthermore, the large volume of antacids required may be associated with complications such as aspiration pneumonitis, diarrhea, and electrolyte disturbances. In patients who are unable to take medication orally, prophylaxis with parenteral H_2-blockers is indicated. The H_2-blocker of choice will depend on the acquisition cost of the drug as well as the use of concomitant medications (see below). There are no conclusive data that titrating H_2-blockers to intragastric pH is a useful exercise. Furthermore, while studies have demonstrated that a continuous infusion of an H_2-blocker results in a significantly lower intragastric pH than when the drug is given by

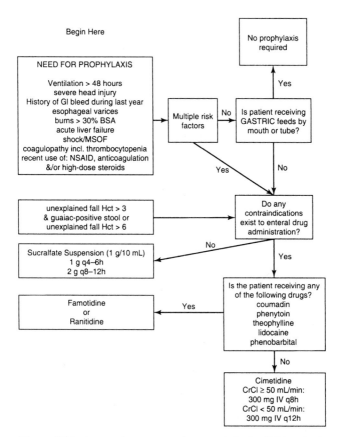

Figure 25-1. Approach to stress ulcer prophylaxis. (BSA = body surface area; MSOF = multisystem organ failure; NSAID, non-steroidal anti-inflammatory drug.)

intermittent boluses, this has not been demonstrated to be clinically important. The recommended dosages of these drugs and the dosage adjustment in patients with renal dysfunction are listed in Table 25-2. Recently, omeprazole and misoprostol have been shown to prevent stress ulceration. However, the role of these agents has yet to be determined.

Table 25-2. Dosages of agents recommended for prophylaxis of stress ulceration.

Drug		Loading Dose Renal Function	Maintenance Dose Intermittent Dosing	Continuous Infusion
Cimetidine	300 mg IV	CrCl > 50 mL/min CrCl < 50 mL/min	300 mg q8 h 300 mg q12 h	900 mg/day 600 mg/day
Ranitidine	150 mg IV	CrCl > 50 mL/min CrCl < 50 mL/min	50 mg q8 h 50 mg q12 h	150 mg/day 100 mg/day
Famotidine˙	20 mg IV	CrCl > 50 mL/min CrCl < 50 mL/min	20 mg q12 h 10 mg q12 h	
Sucralfate suspension (2 g/10 ml)			2 g q8–12 h or 1 g q4–6 h	

Drug Side Effects and Interactions

Sucralfate has few if any side effects; administration of long-term sucralfate has not been documented to result in an increase in plasma aluminum concentration, even in critically ill patients with impaired renal function. Sucralfate reduces the bioavailability and absorption of certain drugs when given simultaneously with them. Important drugs involved in this interaction include quinolone antibiotics, theophylline, tetracycline, phenytoin, digoxin, and amitriptyline. The effect of combined therapy of sucralfate with H_2-blockers has not been evaluated. However, since sucralfate requires an acid medium to be activated, this combination should be avoided.

H_2-blockers have a wide therapeutic index; however, adverse reactions occur on average in 4.4% of outpatients and 7% of hospitalized patients. The failure to reduce the dose of H_2-blockers in patients with renal dysfunction doubles the likelihood of an adverse drug reaction. Those reactions of most concern in critically ill patients include altered mental status, neutropenia, and thrombocytopenia. H_2-blockers may rarely cause a sinus bradycardia with rapid infusion. The central nervous system reactions include confusion, delirium, disorientation, hallucinations, and obtundation. These reactions have been reported to occur in between 2% to 3% of hospitalized patients. While an altered mental status is common in ICU patients, treatment with H_2-blockers is associated with a significant increase in central nervous system dysfunction, having been reported in up to 80% of patients. Considering the frequency of this reaction, H_2-blockers should be avoided in ICU patients with an altered mental status and patients at high risk of developing this complication. While H_2-blockers have been associated with neutropenia and thrombocytopenia, the incidence of this reaction is probably less than 0.1%; furthermore, contrary to popular belief, there is no clear evidence that the rate of any of these reactions is higher with one H_2-blocker as compared with another. Cimetidine has a high affinity for the cytochrome P-450 system and interferes with the metabolism of a large number of drugs. However, the most clinically important drug interactions occur with theophylline, phenytoin, lidocaine, procainamide, quinidine, warfarin, and phenobarbitone. Cimetidine should therefore be substituted for another H_2-blocker in patients receiving any of these drugs.

■ SELECTED REFERENCES

1. Cook DJ, Fuller HD, Guyatt GH, et al. Risk factors for gastrointestinal bleeding in critically ill patients. Canadian Critical Care Trials group. *N Engl J Med*. 1994;330:377–381.
2. Cook DJ, Reeve BK, Guyatt GH, et al. Stress ulcer prophylaxis in critically ill patients. Resolving discordant meta-analyses. *JAMA*. 1996;275:308–314.
3. Cook DJ, Witt LG, Cook RJ, Guyatt GH. Stress ulcer prophylaxis in the critically ill: a meta-analysis. *Am J Med*. 1991;1991:519–527.
4. Ephgrave KS, Kleiman-Wexler RL, Adair CG. Enteral nutrients prevent stress ulceration and increase intragastric volume. *Crit Care Med*. 1990;18: 621–624.
5. Marik PE. Stress ulcer prophylaxis: a practical approach. *J Intensive Care Med*. 1999;14:1–8.

26

Management of Gastrointestinal Bleeding

■ INITIAL ASSESSMENT

- The urgency with which gastrointestinal (GI) bleeding is managed is dictated by the rate of bleeding.

    The patient with trace heme-positive stools and without severe anemia can be managed as an outpatient.

    Visible blood requires hospitalization and inpatient evaluation.

    Persistent bleeding or rebleeding with hemodynamic instability necessitates ICU admission.

    Massive bleeding is defined as loss of ≥30% of estimated blood volume or bleeding requiring blood transfusion of ≥6 U/24 hours.

- Hemodynamic assessment: blood pressure, pulse, postural changes and assessment of peripheral perfusion.

- The presence of comorbid disease must be determined.

- *Estimating blood loss*. This can be estimated by measuring the return from a nasogastric (NG) tube. An approximate estimate of blood loss can be made by the hemodynamic response to a 2-L crystalloid fluid challenge:

    If blood pressure (BP) returns to normal and stabilizes, blood loss of 15% to 30% has occurred.

    If BP rises but falls again, blood volume loss of 30% to 40% has occurred.

    If BP continues to fall, blood volume loss of >40% has probably occurred.

- *History and examination*: Attempt to localize most likely source of bleeding.

    The presence of melena indicates upper GI bleeding.

Hematemesis indicates upper GI bleeding.

When small amounts of bright red blood are passed per rectum, the lower GI tract can be assumed to be the source.

In patients with large-volume maroon stools, NG tube aspiration should be performed to exclude upper GI hemorrhage. It should be noted that in about 15% of patients with upper GI bleeding, NG aspirate will fail to obtain blood or "coffee-ground" material. In most cases, concerns that placement of an NG tube may induce bleeding in patients with coagulopathies are outweighed by the benefits of the information obtained.

- *An NG tube should be inserted in **all** patients with upper GI bleeding* to decompress the stomach. No data suggest that NG tube placement may initiate or potentiate bleeding in patients with esophageal varices. NG tube placement is essential to monitor ongoing bleeding and to decompress the stomach.

■ INITIAL RESUSCITATION

- Establish two large-bore intravenous lines or a large-bore central line.
- Insert the NG tube and aspiration (by hand).
- Volume expansion with colloid and crystalloid.
- Crossmatch blood: Transfuse in the presence of large blood loss or if the patient is hemodynamically unstable. Blood products are the most efficient volume expanders and should be infused as soon as possible in patients with significant bleeding. Packed red blood cells (RBCs) should be transfused to maintain the hematocrit at about 30%. However, it is *very* important to note that it takes up to 72 hours for the hematocrit to reach its nadir after a single episode of bleeding. Therefore, a normal or moderately low hematocrit does not exclude significant bleeding. *Blood transfusion should not be withheld from actively bleeding patients based on their hematocrit.* Conversely, a falling hematocrit does not imply continued bleeding but, rather, may represent equilibration of fluid between the intravascular and extracellular extravascular compartment.
- In patients with active bleeding, fresh-frozen plasma (FFP) should be given if the prothrombin time is at least 1.5 times the control value. Platelet transfusion is indicated if the platelet count is <50,000/mm^3. In addition, FFP should be given after 6 U of RBCs and platelets after 10 U.
- Monitor BP, pulse, and urine output.

- Airway protection: The risk of aspiration is especially high in patients with massive bleeding or in those who have an altered mental status. Endotracheal intubation is recommended in these patients. In addition, endotracheal intubation facilitates endoscopy.
- In patients with severe upper GI bleeding and clinical evidence or a history of advanced liver disease or a history of previous variceal bleeding, an octreotide infusion should be commenced before endoscopy (see treatment of variceal hemorrhage, below).

■ TRIAGE OF PATIENTS: WHOM TO ADMIT TO THE ICU?

At the time of triage, the following criteria can stratify patients into a high-risk group (high risk of rebleeding, requiring surgery, and dying).

- A systolic blood pressure of <100 mm Hg on admission
- Severe comorbid disease
- Evidence of *active, ongoing GI hemorrhage* at the time of triage
- Prothrombin time >1.5 times normal

The rate of rebleeding is approximately 3% in the low-risk group as compared to 25% in the high-risk group. Patients in the low-risk group therefore do not require admission to an ICU and can be adequately managed on a general medical floor.

■ FURTHER MANAGEMENT OF UPPER GI BLEEDING

Early upper GI endoscopy is the cornerstone of management of upper GI bleeding. Endoscopy within 12 to 24 hours of presentation is generally recommended. Early endoscopy serves three vital roles—diagnosis, treatment, and risk stratification—discussed next.

Diagnosis

Early endoscopy is the most accurate method available for identifying the site and source of bleeding.

Treatment

Nonvariceal Bleeding

Endoscopic therapy has been shown to improve outcomes in patients with nonvariceal bleeding. The endoscopic methods of controlling bleeding include thermal coagulation of a bleeding vessel, injection of a bleeding site with epinephrine or a sclerosing agent, and laser therapy to produce tissue coagulation. Endoscopic therapy has been shown to benefit patients with actively bleeding lesions or lesions that have a protuberance in the ulcer crater (i.e., a visible vessel) seen on endoscopy. The rate of rebleeding in patients with active bleeding or a nonbleeding visible vessel is reduced by about 50% with endoscopic therapy. However, in about 20% of such patients, bleeding recurs.

Variceal Bleeding

Since 1990, endoscopic sclerotherapy has been the method of choice in controlling active variceal hemorrhage. Recently, an alternative endoscopic treatment, band ligation, has been introduced. Clinical trials have demonstrated that band ligation reduces rebleeding, mortality, and complications and achieves obliteration more rapidly than sclerotherapy.

Risk Stratification

Establishing an endoscopic diagnosis of the lesion and associated stigmata greatly enhances the ability to predict outcomes (i.e., the risk of rebleeding). Both clinical findings and endoscopic findings are therefore required for accurate risk assessment.

As discussed previously, a falling hematocrit does not imply rebleeding, as it may take up to 72 hours for the hematocrit to stabilize after a bleed. Furthermore, due to abnormalities of RBCs with storage, up to 20% of transfused RBCs are removed from the circulation within the first 24 hours. It therefore follows that tracking the hematocrit over time is not a particularly reliable sign of rebleeding. Repeating the hematocrit every 4 to 6 hours therefore does not make much sense.

Because of the laxative properties of fresh blood in the GI tract, repeated passage of liquid blood per rectum implies ongoing or recurrent bleeding. As bleeding stops, the stool will change from liquid to formed stool and from red to maroon blood to darker stool and eventually to brown guaiac-positive stool. The stool may remain guaiac positive for as long as 2 weeks after GI bleeding has ceased.

■ FURTHER MANAGEMENT OF BLEEDING PEPTIC ULCERS

- No evidence that gastric lavage will stop bleeding or prevent rebleeding.
- No evidence that vasoconstrictors such as vasopressin or somatostatin are of any benefit.
- No evidence that H_2 blockers have any impact on actively bleeding ulcers or on the risk of rebleeding.
- Omeprazole administered orally (40 mg q12h for 5 days) reduces the risk of rebleeding and surgery in hospitalized patients with peptic ulcers.
- Recent studies indicate that patients who rebleed after endoscopic therapy are best treated by a second "sitting" of endoscopic therapy as compared to emergency surgery.

■ FURTHER MANAGEMENT OF ESOPHAGEAL VARICES

- Volume resuscitation: use colloids, as excess crystalloids will exacerbate ascites; avoid overhydration.
- Correct clotting factors.
- NG intubation: Evacuate blood and monitor bleeding.
- In patients with variceal hemorrhage, there remains a 40% chance of recurrent variceal bleeding within 72 hours and a 60% chance within 10 days if no additional treatment is persued.
- Octreotide, 50-μg bolus, followed by an infusion at a rate of 50 μg/h has been demonstrated to reduce the risk of early rebleeding. Endoscopic banding in combination with an octreotide infusion is more effective than endoscopic therapy alone for controlling bleeding and reducing the incidence of rebleeding.
- Balloon tamponade with a Minnesota or Sengstaken-Blackmore tube can be lifesaving in the presence of severe ongoing bleeding when carried out by experienced staff. However, placement by inexperienced staff is associated with an increased risk of death, due largely to esophageal perforation and pulmonary aspiration.
- Transjugular intrahepatic portosystemic shunt (TIPS) is a radiological intervention that creates a portosystemic tract through the liver parenchyma, through which an 8- to 12-mm expandable metal stent is inserted. TIPS has become the treatment of choice

as rescue therapy for the 10% to 20% of patients with variceal hemorrhage unresponsive to endoscopic management. TIPS has largely replaced emergency surgical shunting. The main limitations of TIPS is the development of encephalopathy in about 20% of patients and progressive development of shunt insufficiency (thrombosis).

- Gastric varices are the source of bleeding in 10% to 36% of patients with variceal hemorrhage. Unless the gastric varices are located on the proximal lesser curve, they are not amenable to endoscopic ligation; early TIPS therefore is generally recommended.
- The combination of a nonselective beta-blocker in combination with nitroglycerin has been demonstrated to reduce the risk of rebleeding.
- Urgent TIPS is recommended in patients who continue to bleed despite banding/sclerotherapy and pharmacological therapy.
- The role of TIPS in preventing recurrent bleeding is unclear, with studies showing discordant results, with no clear survival benefit.
- Bacterial infection: Patients with cirrhosis who are admitted with acute GI bleeding have a high risk of developing bacterial infection. A recent meta-analysis demonstrated that antibiotic prophylaxis resulted in fewer episodes of bacterial infection, bacteremia and spontaneous bacterial peritonitis and resulted in improved survival compared with untreated patients. On the basis of these data, prophylactic antimicrobial agents with gram-negative activity are recommended in patients with variceal bleeds. Ciprofloxacin, levofloxacin, ceftazidime, amoxicillin-clavulanic acid, and aztreonam are appropriate choices.

■ MANAGEMENT OF PATIENTS WITH LOWER GI BLEEDING

Angiodysplasia and diverticular disease of the right colon account for the vast majority of episodes of acute lower GI bleeding. The spontaneous remission rate, even with massive bleeding, is approximately 80%. In patients with ongoing lower GI bleeding, a radionuclide bleeding scan is indicated. There are two types of bleeding scans. The first is a technetium-labeled sulphur colloid scan, which although very sensitive, can only detect bleeding that occurs during the 1 to 2 hours following infection of the isotope. Alternatively, a technetium-labeled ("tagged") RBC bleeding scan can detect bleeding sites for up to 24 hours after the cessation of bleeding. If the result of either type of bleeding scan is positive, angiography should then be performed.

Selective mesenteric angiography detects arterial bleeding that occurs at a rate of 0.5 mL/min or faster. It can be both diagnostic and therapeutic. When active bleeding is seen, selective arterial infusion of vasopressin arrests the hemorrhage in 90% of patients; adding sterile, absorbable gelatin powder further increases the efficacy of vasopressin.

If bleeding continues and no source has been found, surgical intervention is warranted. Surgical intervention is also recommended in patients with recurrent diverticular bleeding.

■ SELECTED REFERENCES

1. Barange K, Peron JM, Imani K, et al. Transjugular intrahepatic porosystemic shunt in the treatment of refractory bleeding from ruptured gastric varices. *Hepatology.* 1999;30:1139–1143.
2. Bernard B, Grange JD, Khac EN, et al. Antibiotic prophylaxis for the prevention of bacterial infections in cirrhotic patients with gastrointestinal bleeding: a meta-analysis. *Hepatology.* 1999;29:1655–1661.
3. Chung SS, Lau JY, Sung JJ, et al. Randomised comparison between adrenaline injection alone and adrenaline injection plus heat probe treatment for actively bleeding ulcers. *BMJ.* 1997;314:1307–1311.
4. Corley DA, Stefan AM, Wolf M, Cook EF, Lee TH. Early indicators of prognosis in upper gastrointestinal hemorrhage. *Am J Gastroenterol.* 1998; 93:336–340.
5. Khuroo MS, Yattoo GN, Javid G, et al. A comparison of omeprazole and placebo for bleeding peptic ulcer. *N Engl J Med.* 1997;336:1054–1058.
6. Kollef MH, Canfield DA, Zuckerman GR. Triage considerations for patients with acute gastrointestinal hemorrhage admitted to a medical intensive care unit. *Crit Care Med.* 1995;23:1048–1054.
7. Lin HJ, Lo WC, Lee FY, Perng CL, Tseng GY. A prospective randomized comparative trial showing that omeprazole prevents rebleeding in patients with bleeding peptic ulcer after successful endoscopic therapy. *Arch Intern Med.* 1998;158:54–58.
8. Peterson WL, Cook DJ. Antisecretory therapy for bleeding peptic ulcer. *JAMA.* 1998;280:877–878.
9. Rockall TA, Logan RF, Devlin HB, Northfield TC. Selection of patients for early discharge or outpatient care after acute upper gastrointestinal haemorrhage. National Audit of Acute Upper Gastrointestinal Haemorrhage. *Lancet.* 1996;347:1138–1140.
10. Sanyal AJ, Freedman AM, Luketic VA, et al. Transjugular intrahepatic portosystemic shunts for patients with active variceal hemorrhage unresponsive to sclerotherapy. *Gastroenterology.* 1996;111:138–146.
11. Sung JJ, Chung SC, Yung MY, et al. Prospective randomised study of effect of octreotide on rebleeding from oesophageal varices after endoscopic gation. *Lancet.* 1995;346:1666–1669.

12. Tait IS, Krige JE, Terblanche J. Endoscopic band ligation of oesophageal varices. *Br J Surg.* 1999;86:437–446.
13. Villanueva C, Balanzo J, Novella MT, et al. Nadolol plus isosorbide mononitrate compared with sclerotherapy for the prevention of variceal rebleeding. *N Engl J Med.* 1996;334:1624–1629.

27

Pancreatitis

Calculi in the common bile duct (choledocholithiasis) and alcohol account for 80% of cases of acute pancreatitis. Other conditions associated with pancreatitis include drugs, trauma, major abdominal surgery, cardiopulmonary bypass, hypercalcemia, hyperlipidemia, and viral infections. In about 10% of cases of acute pancreatitis, no underlying cause can be identified. A number of studies suggest that about two thirds of these cases are related to small gallstones or biliary sludge.

■ DIAGNOSIS

Serum amylase and serum lipase are the initial diagnostic tests of choice. The simultaneous determination of amylase and lipase offers a sensitivity and specificity of 90% to 95% for detecting acute pancreatitis in patients presenting with acute abdominal pain. Contrast-enhanced abdominal computed tomography is the gold standard for the noninvasive diagnosis of pancreatic necrosis, with an accuracy of more than 90% when there is more than 30% glandular necrosis. Because the normal pancreatic microcirculation is disrupted during acute necrotizing pancreatitis, affected portions of the pancreas do not show normal contrast enhancement. The presence of radiographically detected pancreatic necrosis markedly increases the morbidity and mortality associated with acute pancreatitis. Distinguishing between the two most common causes of acute pancreatitis, gallstones and alcohol, has important implications for treatment. Isolated hyperbilirubinemia is a nonspecific sign. Ultrasonography, while helpful in distinguishing gallstone from alcoholic pancreatitis, has technical limitations.

■ ASSESSMENT OF SEVERITY

The most useful classification of acute pancreatitis distinguishes between mild and severe disease. Severe disease is characterized by organ failure or local complications such as necrosis, pseudocyst, or fistula. Scoring systems use prognostic signs to stratify patients and help in the early recognition of patients with a high probability of developing severe pancreatitis. The Ranson Criteria and the APACHE II scoring systems are the most frequently cited methods for assessing the severity of pancreatitis. The mortality increases with the number of Ranson's signs.

Ranson Criteria for Grading the Severity of Pancreatitis

On Admission

- Age >55
- Blood glucose >200 mg/dL
- White blood cell count >16*10^9/L
- Serum glutamate oxaloacetate transaminase >120 IU/L
- Lactic dehydrogenase >350 IU/L

During the First 48 Hours

- Fall in hematocrit >10%
- Serum calcium <8.0 mEq/L
- Base deficit >4 mEq/L
- Blood urea increase >5 mg/dL
- Fluid sequestration >6 L
- Arterial Po$_2$ <60 mm Hg

Treatment

- Vigorous fluid resuscitation with monitoring of intravascular volume (see Chapters 17 and 18).
- Correct electrolytes imbalances.
- Treat pain with fentanyl (meperidine has a neurotoxic metabolite and should be avoided, especially in patients with renal dysfunction).
- Nasogastric suction; only in patients with an ileus or vomiting.
- Monitor arterial blood gasses and/or pulse oximetry.
- Therapeutic peritoneal lavage is of no value.
- The results of randomized, controlled clinical trials (RCTs) restricted to patients with prognostically severe acute pancreatitis have demonstrated improvement in outcome associated

with antibiotic treatment. Broad-spectrum antibiotics with anaerobic cover reduce the risk of pancreatic abscess. Imipenem or piperacillin/tazobactam are recommended.

- Endoscopic detection and extraction of common bile duct stones by endoscopic retrograde cholangiopancreatography (ERCP) is indicated in the acute setting only when severe pancreatitis is complicated by progressive jaundice or cholangitis. ERCP has no role in the treatment of patients with acute gallstone pancreatitis in the absence of cholangitis.
- Surgical necrosectomy and lavage if the pancreas is necrotic or if abscess develops: Percutaneous methods of debridement of the necrotic pancreas have recently been described. These techniques require considerable technical expertise. The role of these techniques in the management of necrotizing pancreatitis has yet to be determined.

■ NUTRITIONAL SUPPORT IN PANCREATITIS

Despite the lack of prospective data, conventional wisdom dictates that gut rest with or without the provision of parenteral nutrition remains the treatment of choice in acute pancreatis. However, the results of a number of RCTs challenge this standard dogma. These studies have clearly demonstrated that oral feeds in mild-to-moderate pancreatitis and enteral feeding via a nasoenteric tube placed distal to the ligament of Treitz in patients with severe pancreatitis reduces indices of pancreatic and systemic inflammation and reduces the incidence of intra-abdominal sepsis, multiple organ failure, need for operative intervention, and mortality when compared with the parenterally fed patients. Total parenteral nutrition consequently appears to have little role in the management of patients with acute pancreatitis. Where expertise for placement of nasoenteric tubes does not exist (such hospitals should not be treating severe pancreatitis), patients should be kept NPO (nothing by mouth) until the pain resolves; however, such patients should be transferred to another facility. Oral refeeding is only recommended once pain has subsided **and** the serum amylase has approached normal levels.

Complications

Abdominal

- Pancreatic necrosis
- Pancreatic abscess
- Pseudocyst

- Intraperitoneal hemorrhage
- Splenic vein thrombosis
- Obstructive jaundice

Systemic

- Pulmonary: acute respiratory distress syndrome, pleural effusion, atelectasis, pneumonia
- Disseminated intravascular coagulation/coagulopathy
- Upper gastrointestinal bleeding
- Acute renal failure
- Metabolic: hypocalcemia, hyperglycemia, hypertriglyceridemia

■ SELECTED REFERENCES

1. Banks PA. Practice guidelines in acute pancreatitis. *Am J Gastroenterol.* 1997; 92:377–386.
2. Baron TH, Morgan DE. Acute necrotizing pancreatitis. *N Engl J Med.* 1999; 340:1412–1417.
3. Folsch UR, Nitsche R, Ludtke R, et al. Early ERCP and papillotomy compared with conservative treatment for acute biliary pancreatitis. The German Study Group on Acute Biliary Pancreatitis. *N Engl J Med.* 1997;336:237–242.
4. Kalfarentzos F, Kehagias J, Mead N, Kokkinis K, Gogos CA. Enteral nutrition is superior to parenteral nutrition in severe acute pancreatitis: results of a randomized prospective trial. *Br J Surg.* 1997;84:1665–1669.
5. Levy P, Heresbach D, Pariente EA, et al. Frequency and risk factors of recurrent pain during refeeding in patients with acute pancreatitis: a multivariate multicentre prospective study of 116 patients. *Gut.* 1997;40:262–266.
6. Powell JJ, Miles R, Siriwardena AK. Antibiotic prophylaxis in the initial management of severe acute pancreatitis. *Br J Surg.* 1998;85:582–587.
7. Windsor AC, Kanwar S, Li AG, et al. Compared with parenteral nutrition, enteral feeding attenuates the acute phase response and improves disease severity in acute pancreatitis. *Gut.* 1998;42:431–435.

28

Liver Failure and Jaundice in the Intensive Care Unit

Liver disease has two major components: hepatocyte failure and portal hypertension. The clinical picture of chronic liver disease is frequently dominated by the compilations of portal hypertension. On the other hand, the clinical picture of acute/fulminant hepatic failure is dominated by hepatocyte failure (Table 28-1). Fulminant hepatic failure (FHF) is potentially reversible and must be distinguished from chronic liver failure, an irreversible condition that develops over months to years. Patients with FHF are best managed in tertiary care facilities that have extensive experience in treating such patients, with facilities for orthotopic liver transplantation.

■ CAUSES OF FULMINANT HEPATIC FAILURE

Viral Hepatitis

- Hepatitis B, C, and E, and rarely, A and D infection
- Cytomegalovirus infection
- Viral hemorrhagic fevers

Drugs and Toxins

- Acetaminophen
- Alcohol
- Isoniazid
- Valproic acid

Table 28-1. Liver failure: acute vs. chronic.

Chronic Liver Failure	Acute Liver Failure
Long course	Short course (<8 weeks)
Portal hypertension	Portal hypertension rare
Encephalopathy	Encephalopathy
Cerebral edema does not occur	Cerebral edema frequent
Irreversible	Reversible

- Phenytoin
- Amanita phalloides
- Carbon tetrachloride
- Methylenedioxymethamphetamine ("ecstasy")

Miscellaneous

- Fatty liver of pregnancy
- Reye's syndrome
- Wilson's disease
- Autoimmune chronic active hepatitis
- Budd-Chiari syndrome (especially in patients with underlying hepatic disease)

■ CEREBRAL COMPLICATIONS

It is important to distinguish between hepatic encephalopathy and cerebral edema. Encephalopathy is a reversible chemical state that occurs when hepatic function falls below a critical level. Hepatic encephalopathy is usually graded into 4 stages (Table 28-2). Cerebral edema is a physical condition in which brain water is increased. It begins early in the course of FHF but does not pose a danger until intracerebral pressure (ICP) increases. An increased ICP has been reported in 75% to 80% of cases that progress to grade IV encephalopathy. If left unchecked, cerebral edema leads to cerebral ischemia or herniation of the brain stem. Either of these is likely to be fatal, so much of the management of FHF attempts to delay these complications in the hope of recovery or emergency orthotopic liver transplantation. Both clinical signs and computed tomography are unreliable for detecting raised ICP in patients with FHF. Consequently, ICP monitoring is used in most liver transplant centers in the United States. However, therapeutic interventions based on ICP monitoring have not been shown to change the outcome of FHF. ICP monitoring may, however, be useful in patients who are being considered for liver transplant.

Table 28-2. Clinical stages of acute hepatic encephalopathy

Stage	Mental State	Neuromuscular	Changes on Electroencephalogram
Stage I	Euphoria, mild confusion, slowness of mentation, slurred speech	Slight asterixis, normal tone and reflexes	Usually lacking
Stage II	Drowsy but speaking, inappropriate behavior, incontinence	Asterixis, brisk reflexes, increased muscle tone	Abnormal generalized slowing
Stage III	Sleeps most of the time but rousable, incoherent or no speech, marked confusion	Asterixis, upgoing plantar/clonus, flexion response to pain	Always abnormal
Stage IV	Coma, may or may not respond to painful stimuli	Asterixis usually absent, sustained clonus, extension response to pain	Always abnormal

■ MANAGEMENT OF HEPATIC FAILURE

- Elevate head of bed 20 to 35 degrees.
- Monitor blood glucose; 5% to 10% dextrose in water to prevent hypoglycemia.
- Monitor volume status, urine output.
- Exclude/treat sepsis.
- Exclude/treat upper gastrointestinal bleeding.
- The use of protein restriction in hepatic encephalopathy/liver failure is controversial. No controlled studies have been performed. Intolerance of dietary protein should be balanced against the increasing evidence that adequate nutrition, including fair amounts of protein, can improve clinical outcome in patients with hepatic encephalopathy. Therefore, in patients with liver cirrhosis and hepatic encephalopathy, one should initially restrict daily protein intake to 0.5 g/kg/day and slowly increase the intake to 1.0 g/kg/day. In patients with alcoholic hepatitis who can be treated with standard antiencephalopathy medications (e.g., lactulose), low protein intake may be associated with worsening hepatic encephalopathy while a higher protein intake correlates with improvement in hepatic encephalopathy.
- Enteral formulations supplemented with ornithine aspartate reduce ammonia levels and have useful therapeutic effects in patients with mild encephalopathy. L-ornithine–L-aspartate can be administered three times daily in a total dose of 18 g/day.
- Zinc deficiency is common in patients with cirrhosis. Zinc is required for the metabolism of ammonia to urea. Zinc supplementation (600 mg zinc sulphate daily) should be considered.
- *Avoid sedative/hypnotic drugs* (benzodiazepines are notorious for precipitating hepatic encephalopathy).
- Iatrogenic hyperventilation decreases cerebral blood flow and perfusion, and should be avoided.
- Lactulose titrated to produce two to four loose stools/day.
- Vitamin K 5 mg subcutaneously for first 3 days.
- Fresh-frozen plasma/fibrinogen—for active bleeding only.
- Treatment with prednisolone (40 mg daily) has been demonstrated to improve the short-term survival of patients with severe alcoholic hepatitis.

■ ADDITIONAL THERAPEUTIC OPTIONS IN FHF

- Mannitol 0.5 mg/kg in patients in stage IV encephalopathy (who do not have renal failure/azotemia). Monitor volume status, electrolytes, and osmolarity very carefully. Keep osm <320 mOsml/L.

- Pulmonary artery catheterization is recommended in patients who remain hypotensive despite fluid administration. FHF results in a hemodynamic profile that is typical of septic shock. Norepinephrine infusion is recommended for blood pressure support; dobutamine may be required *in addition* for inotropic support.
- Oliguric renal failure (hepatorenal syndrome) is a common complication of FHF. There is no specific therapy for this disorder; low-dose dopamine is probably ineffective. To delay the development of renal failure, aggressive fluid and pressor resuscitation are recommended as well as the avoidance of nephrotic drugs (e.g., aminoglycosides).
- Moderate hypothermia is useful in the treatment of uncontrolled increase in intracranial pressure in patients with acute liver failure and may serve as a bridge to liver transplantation.
- Extracorporeal liver assist devices hold promise for temporary hepatic support.

■ CAUSES OF JAUNDICE IN THE ICU PATIENT

Prehepatic (<15% Conjugated Bilirubin)

- Blood transfusions
- Blood resorption from hematomas
- G6PD deficiency
- Sickle cell disease
- Hemolysis secondary to sepsis
- Hemolysis secondary to hypophosphatemia

"Noncholestatic" Hepatocellular Dysfunction

- "Shock liver" from prolonged hypotension especially if underlying cardiac failure
- Postcardiopulmonary bypass
- Drugs
    Direct hepatotoxicity
    Hypersensitive reactions
- Hepatitis
    Viral
    Alcoholic

Cholestatic/Hepatocellular Dysfunction

- Benign postoperative cholestasis
- Total parenteral nutrition (see Chapter 49)
- Sepsis/multisystem organ failure

Obstructive (>40% Conjugated Bilirubin)

- Acalculous cholecystitis
- Choledocholithiasis
- Pancreatitis

■ SELECTED REFERENCES

1. Canalese J, Gimson AE, Davis C, et al. Controlled trial of dexamethasone and mannitol for the cerebral oedema of fulminant hepatic failure. *Gut.* 1982;23:625–629.
2. Jalan R, Damink SW, Deutz NE, Lee A, Hayes PC. Moderate hypothermia for uncontrolled intracranial hypertension in acute liver failure. *Lancet.* 1999;354:1164–1168.
3. Mas A, Rodes J. Fulminant hepatic failure. *Lancet.* 1997;349:1081–1085.
4. Morgan TR, Moritz TE, Mendenhall CL, Haas R. Protein consumption and hepatic encephalopathy in alcoholic hepatitis. VA Cooperative Study group. *J Am Coll Nutr.* 1995;14:152–158.
5. Ramond MJ, Poynard T, Rueff B, et al. A randomized trial of prednisolone in patients with severe alcoholic hepatitis. *N Engl J Med.* 1992;326:507–512.
6. Reding P, Duchateau J, Bataille C. Oral zinc supplementation improves hepatic encephalopathy. Results of a randomised controlled trial. *Lancet.* 1984;2:493–495.
7. Riordan SM, Williams R. Treatment of hepatic encephalopathy. *N Engl J Med.* 1997;337:473–479.
8. Shakil AO, Mazariegos GV, Kramer DJ. Fulminant hepatic failure. *Surg Clin North Am.* 1999;79:77–108.
9. Staedt U, Leweling H, Gladisch R, et al. Effects of ornithine aspartate on plasma ammonia and plasma amino acids in patients with cirrhosis. A double-blind, randomized study using a four-fold crossover design. *J Hepatol.* 1993;19:424–430.
10. Stauch S, Kircheis G, Adler G, et al. Oral L-ornithine-L-aspartate therapy of chronic hepatic encephalopathy: results of a placebo-controlled double-blind study. *J Hepatol.* 1998;28:856–864.

Part 4

Renal and Metabolic Issues

29

Acid–Base Disturbances

■ AN APPROACH TO ARTERIAL BLOOD GAS ANALYSIS

Step 1: Is There an Acid–Base Disorder?

Look at the $Paco_2$ and the HCO_3 to determine whether they are in the normal range (Table 29-1). If abnormal go to Step 2, if normal go to Step 5.

Step 2: Is the Patient Acidemic or Alkalemic?

Look at the pH. If the pH is normal (i.e., pH between 7.35 and 7.45), is the pH on the acidemic or alkalemic side of 7.40?

Step 3: What Is the Primary Acid–Base Disorder?

From an analysis of the pH, $Paco_2$, and HCO_3, determine the primary defect (Table 29-2):

1. If the pH is decreased, the patient has an acidemia, which may be either
   a. Metabolic acidosis—characterized by a low HCO_3
   b. Respiratory acidosis—characterized by an increased Pco_2

2. If the pH is increased, the patient has an alkalemia, which may be either
   a. Metabolic alkalosis—characterized by an increase in plasma HCO_3
   b. Respiratory alkalosis—characterized by a decreased Pco_2

Table 29-1. Normal acid–base ranges.

	Mean	1 SD	2 SD
$Paco_2$ (mm Hg)	40	38–42	35–45
pH	7.40	7.38–7.42	7.35–7.45
HCO_3	24	23–25	22–26

Table 29-2. Acid–base terminology.

Clinical Terminology	Criteria
Respiratory failure/respiratory acidosis	$Paco_2 > 45$ mm Hg
Alveolar hyperventilation (resp. alkalosis)	$Paco_2 < 35$ mm Hg
Acute respiratory failure	$Paco_2 > 45$ mm Hg; pH < 7.35
Chronic respiratory failure	$Paco_2 > 45$ mm Hg; pH 7.36–7.44
Acute respiratory alkalosis	$Paco_2 < 35$ mm Hg; pH > 7.45
Chronic respiratory alkalosis	$Paco_2 < 35$ mm Hg; pH 7.36–7.44
Acidemia	pH < 7.35
Alkalemia	pH > 7.45
Acidosis	$HCO_3 < 22$ mEq/L
Alkalosis	$HCO_3 > 26$ mEq/L

Step 4: Expected Compensatory Response

Determine whether the compensatory response is of the magnitude expected (Tables 29-3 and 29-4); i.e., is there a secondary (uncompensated) acid–base disturbance?

Step 5: How to Recognize Mixed Acid–Base Disorders

Acid–base disorders may present as two or three coexisting disorders. It is possible for a patient to have an acid–base disorder with a normal pH, Pco_2, and HCO_3, and with the only clue to an acid–base disorder being an increased anion gap (AG).

$AG = [Na] – ([Cl] + [HCO_3])$: Normal 12 ± 2 mEq/L

1. Calculate the plasma anion gap; if it is increased by >5 mEq/L, the patient most likely has a *metabolic acidosis*.
2. Compare the fall in plasma HCO_3 ($25\text{-}HCO_3$) with the increase in the plasma AG; these should be of similar magnitude. If there is a gross discrepancy (5 mEq/L), a mixed disturbance is present:
   a. An increase in AG that exceeds the fall in HCO_3 suggests that a component of the metabolic acidosis is due to HCO_3 loss.

Table 29-3. Traditional acid–base definitions.

		pH	$PaCO_2$	HCO_3	Base Excess
Respiratory acidosis (defined as increased $PaCO_2$)	Uncompensated	↓	↑	N	N
	Partly compensated	↓	↑	↑	↑
	Compensated	N	↑	↑	↑
Respiratory alkalosis (defined as decreased $PaCO_2$)	Uncompensated	↑	↓	N	N
	Partly compensated	↑	↓	↓	↓
	Compensated	N	↓	↓	↓
Metabolic acidosis (defined as decreased HCO_3)	Uncompensated	↓	N	↓	↓
	Partly compensated	↓	↓	↓	↓
	Compensated	N	↓	↓	↓
Metabolic alkalosis (defined as decreased HCO_3)	Uncompensated	↑	N	↑	↑
	Partly compensated	↑	↑	↑	↑
	Compensated	N	↑	↑	↑

Table 29-4. Compensation for acid–base disorders.

Primary Disorder	Primary Change	Compensatory Change	Expected Compensation
Metabolic acidosis	↓ HCO_3	↓ $Paco_2$	$\Delta Paco_2 = 1.0 \Delta HCO_3$
Metabolic alkalosis	↑ HCO_3	↑ $Paco_2$	$\Delta Paco_2 = 0.7 \Delta HCO_3$
Respiratory acidosis	↑ $Paco_2$	↑ HCO_3	Acute: $\Delta HCO_3 = 0.1 \Delta Paco_2$ $\Delta pH \approx \Delta Paco_2 \times 0.01$ Chronic: $\Delta HCO_3 = 0.35 \Delta Paco_2$ $\Delta pH \approx \Delta Paco_2 \times 0.003$
Respiratory alkalosis	↓ $Paco_2$	↓ HCO_3	Acute: $\Delta HCO_3 = 0.2 \Delta Paco_2$ $\Delta pH \approx \Delta Paco_2 \times 0.01$ Chronic: $\Delta HCO_3 = 0.5 \Delta Paco_2$ $\Delta pH \approx \Delta Paco_2 \times 0.002$

  b. An increase in AG that is less than the fall of the HCO_3
     suggests coexistent metabolic alkalosis.

Step 6: Calculate the Osmolar Gap (in Patients With an Unexplained AG Metabolic Acidosis)

Estimated serum osmolality = $2 \times Na$ + glucose/18 + BUN/2.8
  Normal $\approx 290\,mOsm/kg \cdot H_2O$

Osmolal gap = osm (measured) − osm (calculated)
  Normal < 10

Causes of an Increased Osmolal Gap (Table 29-5)

- Alcohol (ethanol)
- Methanol
- Isopropyl alcohol (does not cause an AG or an acidosis)
- Ethylene glycol
- Mannitol
- Sorbitol
- Paraldehyde
- Acetone

Table 29-5. Osmolal gap and lethal intoxications.

Substance	Mol Wt	Lethal Level (mg/dL)	Osm Gap at That Level
Ethanol	46	350	80
Isopropyl alcohol	60	340	60
Methanol	32	80	27
Acetone	58	55	10
Ethylene glycol	62	21	4

■ METABOLIC ACIDOSIS

The manifestations of metabolic acidosis depend largely on the underlying cause and the rapidity with which the condition developed. An acute severe metabolic acidosis results in myocardial depression with a reduction in cardiac output, decreased blood pressure, and decreased hepatic and renal blood flow. Reentrant arrhythmia and a reduction in the ventricular fibrillation threshold can occur. Brain metabolism becomes impaired with progressive obtundation and coma. See Figure 29-1 for an approach to the diagnosis of metabolic acidosis. Metabolic acidosis in the critically ill patient is an ominous sign and warrants an aggressive approach to the diagnosis and management of the cause(s) of the disorder. In almost all circumstances, the treatment of metabolic acidosis involves the treatment of the underlying disorder. The role of bicarbonate in the management of patients with acute metabolic acidosis is very controversial with a paucity of data on which to make rational decisions. However, in most circumstances, bicarbonate seems to cause more harm than benefit. *Except in specific circumstances (outlined below), there is no scientific evidence to support treating a metabolic or respiratory acidosis with sodium bicarbonate.* Furthermore, it is the intracellular pH that is of importance in determining cellular function. The intracellular buffering system is much more effective in restoring pH to normal than the extracellular buffers. Consequently, patients have tolerated a pH as low as 7.0 during sustained hypercapnia without obvious adverse effects.

The infusion of bicarbonate can lead to a variety of problems in patients with acidosis, including fluid overload, a postrecovery metabolic alkalosis, and hypernatremia. Furthermore, studies in both animals and humans suggest that alkali therapy may only transiently raise the plasma bicarbonate concentration. This finding appears to be related in part to the CO_2 generated as the administered bicarbonate buffers excess hydrogen ions. This CO_2 is normally eliminated via the lungs. However, critically ill patients often have a reduction in pulmonary blood flow. As a result, mixed venous P_{CO_2} may continue to

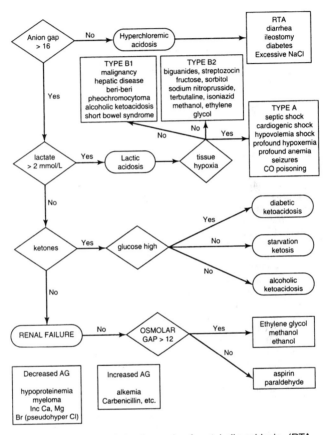

Figure 29-1. Approach to diagnosis of metabolic acidosis. (RTA = renal tubular acidosis.)

rise until the product of the greater than normal mixed venous Pco_2 and the less than normal pulmonary blood flow is sufficient to eliminate the CO_2 that is produced. In addition, unless the minute ventilation is increased (in ventilated patients), CO_2 elimination will not be increased.

Indications for Bicarbonate Therapy

No data support the use of bicarbonate in patients with lactic acidosis. The prognosis is related to the underlying disorder causing the acidosis. In hyperchloremic acidosis (e.g., that produced by severe diarrhea), endogenous regeneration of bicarbonate cannot occur (as bicarbonate has been lost, rather than buffered). Therefore, even if the cause of the acidosis can be reversed, exogenous alkali is often required for prompt attenuation of severe acidemia. Bicarbonate therapy is therefore indicated in patients with severe hyperchloremic acidosis in when the pH is <7.2; this group of patients is largely composed of patients with severe diarrhea, high-output fistulas, and renal tubular acidosis. To prevent sodium overload, I suggest that 2×50-ml ampoules of $NaHCO_3$ (each containing 50 mmol of $NaHco_3$) be added to 1 L of 5% dextrose in water, and infused at a rate of 100 to 200 mL/h.

Methanol and ethylene glycol intoxication can produce a severe, acute, high-AG metabolic acidosis caused by the accumulation of toxic metabolites. Large amount of alkali are often required to control the severe acidemia. Bicarbonate may have a role in patients with a metabolic acidosis who are unable to compensate for this disorder, i.e., patients with chronic obstructive pulmonary disease who have a limited ability to increase CO_2 elimination. In these patients, *small* amounts of bicarbonate may avert respiratory failure and the need for intubation and mechanical ventilation.

Bicarbonate and Ketoacidosis

Bicarbonate is frequently administered to "correct the acidosis" in patients with diabetic ketoacidosis. However, paradoxically, bicarbonate has been demonstrated to increase ketone production. Studies have demonstrated an increase in acetoacetate levels during alkali administration, followed by an increase in 3-hydroxybutyrate levels after its completion. In pediatric patients, treatment with bicarbonate has been demonstrated to prolonged hospitalization. In addition, bicarbonate may decrease cerebrospinal fluid pH, as increased CO_2 produced by buffering acid crosses the blood–brain barrier, combines H_2O, and regenerates H^+. It is generally believed that adjunctive bicarbonate is unnecessary and potentially disadvantageous in severe diabetic ketoacidosis.

D-Lactic Acidosis

Certain bacteria in the gastrointestinal tract may convert carbohydrate into organic acids. The two factors that make this possible are slow gastrointestinal transit (blind loops, obstruction) and change of the normal flora (usually with antibiotic therapy). The most prevalent organic acid is D-lactic acid. Since humans metabolize this isomer more slowly than L-lactate and production rates can be very rapid, life-threatening acidosis can be produced. This usual laboratory test for lactate is specific for the L-lactate isomer. Therefore, to confirm the diagnosis, the plasma D-lactate must be measured.

■ METABOLIC ALKALOSIS

Metabolic acidosis (MA) is a common acid–base disturbance in ICU patients, characterized by an elevated serum pH (>7.45) secondary to plasma bicarbonate (HCO_3.) retention. The MA is usually the result of several therapeutic interventions in the critically ill patient. Nasogastric drainage, diuretic-induced intravascular volume depletion, hypokalemia, and the use of corticosteroids are common causes of MA in these patients. In addition, the citrate in transfused blood is metabolized to bicarbonate, which may compound the MA. Overventilation in patients with type 2 respiratory failure may result in a posthypercapnic MA (Figure 29-2). In many patients, the

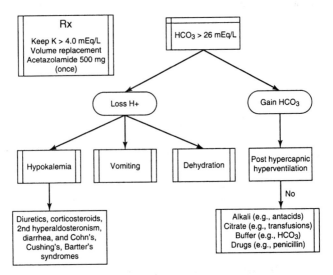

Figure 29-2. Approach to diagnosis of metabolic alkalosis.

events that generated the MA may not be present at the time of diagnosis.

MA may have adverse effects on cardiovascular, pulmonary, and metabolic function. It can decrease cardiac output, depress central ventilation, shift the oxyhemoglobin saturation curve to the left, worsen hypokalemia and hypophosphatemia, and negatively affect the ability to wean patients from mechanical ventilation. Increasing serum pH has been shown to correlate with ICU mortality. Correction of MA has been shown to increase minute ventilation, increase arterial oxygen tension, and mixed venous oxygen tension, and decrease oxygen consumption. It is therefore important to correct MA in all critically ill patients.

The first therapeutic maneuver in patients with MA is to replace any fluid (with normal saline) and electrolyte deficits. Aggressive potassium supplementation is warranted to achieve a $K^+ > 4.5\,mEq/L$. If these interventions fail, ammonium chloride, hydrochloric acid, or arginine hydrochloride may be given. The disadvantage of these solutions is that they are difficult to use and require the administration of a large volume of hypotonic fluid. Extravasation of hydrochloric acid may result in severe tissue necrosis, mandating administration through a well-functioning central line. Acetazolamide is a carbonic anhydrase inhibitor that promotes the renal excretion of bicarbonate and has been demonstrated to be very effective in treating MA in ICU patients. A single dose of 500 mg is recommended. The onset of action is within 1.5 hours with a duration of approximately 24 hours. Repeat doses may be required as necessary.

■ SELECTED REFERENCES

1. Kannan CR. Bicarbonate therapy in the management of severe diabetic ketoacidosis. *Crit Care Med.* 1999;27:2833–2834.
2. Marik PE, Kussman BD, Lipman J, Kraus P. Acetazolamide in the treatment of metabolic alkalosis in critically ill patients. *Heart Lung.* 1991;20:455–459.
3. Mazur JE, Devlin JW, Peters MJ, et al. Single versus multiple doses of acetazolamide for metabolic alkalosis in critically ill medical patients: a randomized, double-blind trial. *Crit Care Med.* 1999;27:1257–1261.
4. Viallon A, Zeni F, Lafond P, et al. Does bicarbonate therapy improve the management of severe diabetic ketoacidosis? *Crit Care Med.* 1999;27:2690–2693.

30

Electrolyte Disturbances

■ SODIUM AND WATER

Rules of the Game

Sodium balance determines volume status.
Water balance determines tonicity, i.e., Na^+ concentration.

Volume overload = increased total body sodium (regardless of serum sodium concentration)
Euvolemia = normal total body sodium (regardless of serum sodium concentration)
Volume depletion = decreased total body sodium (regardless of serum sodium concentration)

Hyponatremia = relative water excess
Hypernatremia = relative water deficit

In volume-depleted patients, ***volume*** should be corrected before correction of tonicity; i.e., patients should initially be volume resuscitated with 0.9% NaCl or Ringer's lactate regardless of serum sodium concentration.

Hyponatremic dehydration: volume replacement with 0.9% NaCl
Hypertonic dehydration: volume replacement with Ringer's lactate or 0.9% NaCl, then change to 0.45% NaCl

■ HYPONATREMIA

Assessment of volume status (fluid overload, euvolemia, or dehydration) is central to the evaluation and management of patients with hyponatremia (Figure 30-1). Most patients with hyponatremia are asymptomatic and have a plasma sodium concentration above

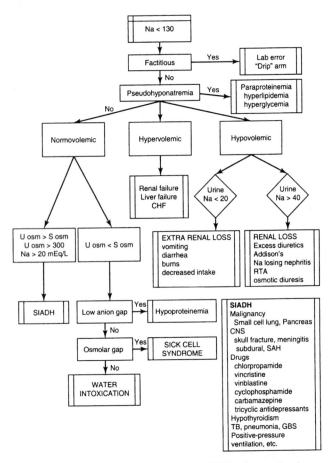

Figure 30-1. Approach to hyponatremia. (CHF = Congestive heart failure; GBS = Guillain-Barré syndrome; RTA = renal tubular acidosis; SAH = Subarachnoid hemorrhage; SIADH = syndrome of inappropriate secretion of antidiuretic hormone; TB = tuberculosis.)

120 mEq/L. In these patients, there is no urgency in correcting the serum sodium concentration, and treatment should occur over a number of days. Treatment typically consists of isotonic saline if the patient has true volume depletion or water restriction in the syndrome of inappropriate anti-diuretic hormone (ADH) secretion. More

aggressive therapy is indicated in those patients who have symptomatic or severe hyponatremia (plasma sodium concentration <110 mEq/L). In this setting, hypertonic saline can be given initially to raise the plasma sodium concentration (to ~120 mEq/L), although the rate at which this occurs must be carefully monitored to minimize the risk of central demyelinating lesions (see below). Hyponatremia in the setting of effective intravascular volume depletion and edema (congestive cardiac failure and cirrhosis) results from release of ADH in response to "hypovolemia" and carries a poor prognosis (see Chapter 17). Such patients require colloid and pressor resuscitation in an attempt to correct the effective intravascular volume deficit.

The optimal rate of correction varies with the clinical state of the patient. Acute symptomatic hyponatremia primarily results from cerebral edema due to water movement into the brain. In contrast, chronic hyponatremia gives time for cerebral adaption to occur, resulting in the return of brain volume toward normal and usually causes no neurological symptoms. Rapid initial correction of hyponatremia is warranted in symptomatic patients, but overly rapid correction can be deleterious (central pontine demyelinosis), particularly in patients with chronic hyponatremia. In general, the sodium concentration should initially be corrected to a level of 120 mEq/L. The rate at which this correction should occur will depend on the presence of symptoms and the rate at which the disorder occurred. Alcoholic patients are particularly prone to pontine demyelinosis, and therefore the serum sodium should be diligently monitored.

- In asymptomatic patients, the plasma sodium concentration should be raised at a maximal rate <0.5 mEq/L/h, and more important, <10 mEq/L in the first day and <18 mEq/L over the first 2 days; a more rapid elevation can increase the risk of osmotic demyelination.
- More rapid correction is indicated in patients with symptomatic hyponatremia who present with seizures or other severe neurologic manifestations; these findings are primarily due to cerebral edema induced by acute hyponatremia. In this setting, the plasma sodium concentration can be raised at an initial rate of 1.5 to 2 mEq/L/h for the first 3 to 4 hours, since the risk of persistent severe hyponatremia is greater than the possible danger of overly rapid correction. Despite the more rapid initial rate of correction with symptomatic hyponatremia, the total increase in the plasma sodium concentration over the first 24 hours probably should not exceed 10 to 12 mEq/L, the same limit noted with asymptomatic patients.
- Hyponatremia occurring after transurethral resection of the bladder or prostate is one setting in which even more rapid correction may be warranted. The dilutional fall in plasma sodium concentration induced by absorption of nonelectrolyte irrigation

fluids occurs over a very short period of time, before significant cerebral adaption has begun.

The amount of Na^+ required to raise the plasma Na^+ concentration to a safe level (120 mEq/L) can be calculated from the following formula:

Na^+ deficit = 0.6 × lean body weight (kg) × (120 − plasma [Na^+])
(Substitute 0.6 for 0.5 in women)

Since 3% saline contains ~500 mEq/L, the total amount of this solution (in liters) required to increase the serum sodium to 120 mEq/L can be calculated as follows:

Total volume of 3% saline (liters) = Na^+ deficit/500

■ HYPERNATREMIA

Hypernatremia is not uncommon in ICU patients primarily due to excessive resuscitation with 0.9 NaCl ([Na^+] 154 mEq/L). Hypernatremia may also occur in dehydrated patients in whom thirst is impaired (e.g., bedridden or altered mental status). The treatment of the former is free water (e.g., 200 mL water orally q4–6 h). In hypertonic dehydration, volume status should be corrected first (0.9% saline) followed by correction of tonicity (0.45% saline and/or free water). Rapid correction of hypernatremia can induce cerebral edema, seizures, permanent neurological damage, and death. To minimize these risks, the plasma Na^+ concentration should be corrected slowly. The maximum rate at which the plasma Na^+ should be corrected is 0.5 mEq/L/h, or 12 mEq/p/L per day, a rate equivalent to that of hyponatremia. The water deficit can be calculated using the following formula:

Water deficit = 0.5 × (([Na^+]/140) − 1)
(substitute 0.5 with 0.4 in women)

■ HYPOKALEMIA

Only a small fraction of the total body K^+ is extracellular. Therefore serum K^+ levels do not accurately reflect the total body K^+. The degree of K^+ deficit is dependent on the duration of the precipitating cause (time for equilibration) and the serum K^+ level. In patients with chronic hypokalemia, a 1-mEq fall in serum K^+ is approximately equal to a 200-mEq total body deficit. In critically ill ICU patients, it is generally recommended to keep the serum [K+] ≥ 4.0 mEq/L For approach to diagnosis see Figure 30-2.

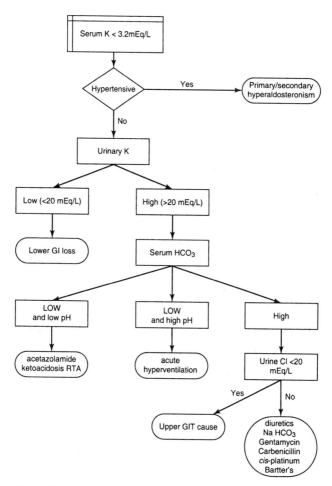

Figure 30-2. Approach to hypokalemia. (GIT = gastrointestinal tract; RTA = renal tubular acidosis.)

IV Replacement Therapy of KCl

- No more than 20 mEq/h should be given
- central line infusion
    20 mEq in 50 mL over 1 hour
    40 mEq in 100 mL over 2 hours
- peripheral line infusion
    10 mEq in 100 mL over 1 hour
    20 mEq in 200 mL over 2 hours

■ HYPERKALEMIA

Acute hyperkalemia is usually the result of renal failure. Hyperkalemia may also occur with overzealous potassium replacement and in patients receiving angiotensin-converting enzyme inhibitors and potassium-spacing dietetics. Factors such as the duration of hyperkalemia, the plasma Ca^{++} concentration, and the acid–base balance modify the toxicity of hyperkalemia. However, a $K^+ > 7.5$ mEq/L or hyperkalemia associated with electrocardiogram (ECG) changes should be regarded as life-threatening, requiring immediate treatment (Table 30-1).

- Clinical features usually occur when the $K^+ > 6.5$ mEq/L: weakness, paresthesia, ileus, paralysis, cardiac arrest
- ECG changes:
    Peaked T waves
    Flattened P
    Prolonged PR interval
    Widening of the QRS complex
    Sine wave leading to ventricular fibrillation or asystole

Table 30-1. Agents used in the treatment of hyperkalemia.

Agent	Mechanism	Dosage	Onset of Action
10% Ca gluconate	Direct antagonism	10–20 mL IV over 2–5 min	Immediate
Sodium bicarbonate	Redistribution	50 mL IV over 2–5 min	Minutes
Glucose/insulin	Redistribution	2–3 g glucose/U regular insulin 50 mL 50% D/W + 10 U insulin	Minutes
Sodium polystyrene Sulfonate (Kayexalate)	Increased elimination	15–60 g po or rectally	2–12 h

- The rate of progression of the ECG changes is not predictable, and patients may progress from minor ECG changes to dangerous conduction disturbances or arrhythmias within minutes. The ECG changes are exacerbated by coexisting hyponatremia, hypocalcemia, hypermagnesemia, and acidosis.
- Patients should be treated when the K^+ is >5.5 mEq/L; urgent treatment is required when the K^+ > 7.5 mEq/L.
- The goals of treatment are to
    Protect the heart from the effects of K^+ by antagonizing the effect on cardiac conduction (calcium)
    To shift the K^+ from the extracellular to intracellular compartment
    Reduce the total body potassium
- Life-threatening arrhythmia may occur at any time during therapy; hence, continuous ECG monitoring is required.
- Patients with a serum K^+ > 7.5 mEq/L and/or significant ECG changes should be treated immediately with calcium gluconate, followed by a glucose/insulin infusion and then an iron-exchange resin.

■ HYPOPHOSPHATEMIA

Phosphorus is an essential component of phospholipid, nucleic acids and plays an essential role in energy metabolism. Only about 1% of the total body phosphorus is extracellular, with the major phosphate store being in bone and the intracellular compartment. The normal range of serum phosphorus concentration in the serum is between 2.2 and 4.4 mg/dL, of which about 55% is in an ionized form that is physiologically active. The serum phosphate concentration is a poor indicator of the total body phosphorus, and rapid shifts of phosphate between the extracelluar and intracellular compartments only confound this situation. Interpretation of the serum phosphate is further complicated by a normal diurnal variation, which may be as large as 0.5 mg/dL. However, hypophosphatemia may cause severe life-threatening complications, particularly in patients with depleted phosphate stores.

Causes of Severe Hypophosphatemia

- Alcohol abuse and withdrawal
- Refeeding after starvation
- Respiratory alkalosis
- Malabsorption
- Oral phosphate binders
- Hyperalimentation

- Severe burns
- Therapy of diabetic ketoacidosis

There is a poor correlation between serum phosphate levels and symptoms. Although hypophosphatemia becomes life-threatening when the serum levels are less than 1 mg/dL, symptoms may develop when the serum phosphate is less than 2 mg/dL.

Manifestations Include

- Myocardial depression
- Weakness, rhabdomyolysis, and respiratory failure
- Confusion, stupor, coma, seizures
- Hemolysis, platelet dysfunction, leukocyte dysfunction

Management

- Therapy is usually empiric, and levels must be closely followed to prevent hyperphosphatemia.
- It has been recommended that patients with severe hypophosphatemia (serum phosphate level less than 1 mg/dL) be given an infusion of phosphate at a rate of 6 mg/kg/h (or 0.1 mmol phosphate/kg in 500 mL 0.45 normal saline (NS) over 6 hours), with serum levels being checked every 6 hours and discontinued when the serum phosphate level exceeds 2 mg/dL. Thereafter, the patients should receive oral phosphate to replace the intracellular stores. Phosphate solutions should be used with extreme caution in patients with renal failure.
- Patients with mild-to-moderate hypophosphatemia (serum phosphate between 1.0 and 2.2 mg/dL) should receive oral supplementation (1 g Neutra-Phos/day) unless diarrhea precludes using this route of supplementation.

■ HYPOMAGNESEMIA

Magnesium is the fourth most abundant cation in the body and the second most prevalent intracellular cation. Mg^{++} is essential for the function of important enzymes, including those related to the transfer of phosphate groups, all reactions that require adenosine triphosphate (ATP), for the replication and transcription of DNA, as well as cellular energy metabolism, membrane stabilization, nerve conduction, and calcium channel function. Magnesium plays an essential role in the function of the cell membrane sodium–potassium ATPase pump. Hypomagnesemia is reported to be common in ICU patients

(~60%) and an important prognostic marker. The causes of hypomagnesemia include

- Alcoholism and alcohol withdrawal
- Emesis
- Diarrhea
- Nasogastric suction
- Parenteral nutrition
- Refeeding syndrome
- Diabetes
- Drugs
    Loop diuretics
    Aminoglycosides
    Amphotericin B
    Cis-platinum
    Cyclosporin

The reported manifestations of hypomagnesemia include

- Hypokalemia and hypocalcemia
- Lethargy, confusion, coma, seizures, ataxia, nystagmus
- Prolonged PR and QT interval on ECG
- Atrial and ventricular arrhythmias

The diagnosis of magnesium deficiency is controversial. As only 1% of total body magnesium is extracellular, the value of measuring the serum levels has been questioned. Using the magnesium-loading test, Hebert and colleagues demonstrated that 63% of their ICU patients were "functionally magnesium deficient." However, in this study both the total serum magnesium and the ionized serum magnesium were poor predictors of functional magnesium deficiency.

Management of Hypomagnesemia

In light of the above information, the value of routinely measuring the serum magnesium is in question. However, it is probably prudent to measure the serum magnesium level in patients at risk of magnesium deficiency and to treat those who have severe hypomagnesemia (<1.2 mg/dL). Treatment of hypomagnesemia (aiming for a serum magnesium level of ~2.5 mg/dL) may be particularly important in patients with arrhythmias and those with seizures. Magnesium should be replaced cautiously in patients with renal impairment. The recommended dose is 2 g $MgSO_4$ over 10 minutes intravenously, followed either by an infusion at 0.5 g/h for 6 hours or a 1-g bolus hourly for 4 hours; this is followed by a repeat serum magnesium level. In renal failure, the dose should be halved.

■ HYPOCALCEMIA

Total serum levels of calcium have been found to be decreased in 70% to 90% of ICU patients. However, when ionized calcium (Ca^{++}) is measured, hypocalcemia is found in 15% to 50%. Ionized hypocalcemia and increased levels of parathyroid hormone (PTH) are particularly common in patients with sepsis and inflammation. Hypocalcemia in critically ill patients has been demonstrated to be of prognostic significance; hypocalcemia is associated with severity of disease and increased mortality. Many factors interact to lower the serum calcium, including an impaired ability to mobilize skeletal calcium, accumulation of calcium in the extracellular and intracellular space, impaired action of PTH, and vitamin D deficiency. Magnesium deficiency may cause severe hypocalcemia.

Cardiovascular manifestations are the most commonly encountered features of severe hypocalcemia. Patients may develop hypotension, decreased cardiac output, bradycardia, and arrhythmias. In addition, patients may fail to respond to drugs that act through calcium-regulated mechanisms (digoxin, catecholamines). It is important to note that mild degrees of hypocalcemia (ionized calcium >0.8mmol/L) are rarely associated with cardiovascular compromise. The fact that hypocalcemia is related to increased mortality does not imply that calcium supplementation will be beneficial. Indeed, current data suggest that mild ionized hypocalcemia is protective during states of systemic inflammation, ischemia, and sepsis. Since hypocalcemic symptoms are unusual unless the ionized calcium level is <0.8mmol/L, most experts do not routinely recommend treating ionized calcium levels in critically ill patients unless levels are <0.8mmol/L.

A large body of evidence suggests that cellular calcium overload contributes to cellular dysfunction and death in patients with tissue ischemia. Critically ill patients may have increased intracellular free-calcium concentrations, even when the circulating ionized calcium is low. Administration of calcium to these patients may be detrimental by activating autolytic intracellular enzymes. Thus, calcium should be given only after confirmation of ionized hypocalcemia so as to prevent further tissue damage.

Hypocalcemia is a common complication of rhabdomyolysis. Release of phosphate from injured muscle results in the local precipitation of calcium salts. Hyperphosphatemia also impairs the 1-hydroxylation of vitamin D, thereby decreasing the sensitivity of bone to PTH. Administration of calcium may result in severe soft tissue calcification. Calcium supplementation should be reserved for patients with clear clinical signs of hypocalcemia.

■ HYPERCALCEMIA

Patients with severe hypercalcemia may require admission to the ICU for management of this life-threatening disorder. Malignancy is the most common cause of hypercalcemia in hospitalized patients. The common causes of hypercalcemia are listed below:

- Malignant
  Lung
  Breast
  Multiple myeloma
  Lymphoma, other
- Primary hyperparathyroidism
- Immobilization
- Drugs
  Thiazides
  Lithium
  Theophylline, other
- Granulomatous diseases
  Sarcoid
  Tuberculosis
- Hypervitaminosis A and D
- Hyperthyroidism
- Milk alkali syndrome

Table 30-2. Treatment of hypercalcemia.

Agent	Dose	Indication/Toxicity
Normal saline	200–400 mL/h	First-line therapy; especially for dehydration
Furosemide	10–40 mg IV q4–6 h	Once patient rehydrated
Etidronate	7.5 mg/kg/day IV; up to 7 days	Avoid in renal failure
Pamidronate	single dose 60–90 mg over 24 h (can be given over 4 h)	Avoid in renal failure
Mithramycin	25 µg/kg IV	Bone marrow suppression
Calcitonin	2–8 IU/kg IM q6 h	Acts rapidly; effect not complete, and wears off rapidly
Steroids; prednisone	40–100 mg/day	Hematologic malignancies, breast cancer

The aim of treatment of hypercalcemia is to minimize its effects on central nervous system, renal, and cardiovascular function. The treatment of hypercalcemia involves attempts to (1) increase renal calcium clearance and (2) decrease bone reabsorption and decrease intestinal calcium absorption (Table 30-2) Hydration plays a critical role in the initial management of hypercalcemia, as the onset of the therapeutic response is rapid. The aim of treatment is to achieve a urine output of 3 to 5 L in 24 hours. Loop diuretics promote urinary calcium loss and prevent volume overload.

■ SELECTED REFERENCES

1. Desai TK, Carlson RW, Geheb MA. Prevalence and clinical implications of hypocalcemia in acutely ill patients in a medical intensive care setting. *Am J Med*. 1988;84:209–214.
2. Hebert P, Mehta N, Wang J, et al. Functional magnesium deficiency in critically ill patients identified using a magnesium-loading test. *Crit Care Med*. 1997;25:749–755.
3. Lind L, Carlstedt F, Rastad J, et al. Hypocalcemia and parathyroid hormone secretion in critically ill patients. *Crit Care Med*. 2000;28:93–99.
4. Rubeiz GJ, Thill-Baharozian M, Hardie D, Carlson RW. Association of hypomagnesemia and mortality in acutely ill medical patients. *Crit Care Med*. 1993;21:203–209.
5. Weisinger JR, Bellorin-Font E. Magnesium and phosphorus. *Lancet*. 1998; 352:391–396.
6. Zaloga GP. Ionized hypocalcemia during sepsis. *Crit Care Med*. 2000;28: 266–268.

31

Diabetic Ketoacidosis, Hyperosmolar Nonketotic States, and Stress-Induced Hyperglycemia

■ DIABETIC KETOACIDOSIS

Diabetic ketoacidosis (DKA) remains a major problem of uncontrolled diabetes with significant morbidity and mortality. In the pathogenesis of ketoacidosis, relative insulin deficiency and counterregulatory hormone excess lead to overproduction and underutilization of glucose, resulting in hyperglycemia. Increased lipolysis leads to excessive formation of ketone bodies, which accumulate to produce a metabolic acidosis. Insulin therapy promotes a reversal of these metabolic derangements by suppressing hepatic production of both glucose and ketones, in addition to increasing glucose utilization and ketone body clearance. Common precipitating factors include discontinuation of insulin therapy (noncompliance), infections, myocardial ischemia, and emotional stress.

Initial laboratory findings include

- Plasma glucose is very high, usually >300 mg/dL.
- Plasma ph is low, usually <7.3.
- Plasma sodium is low.
- Plasma potassium is normal to high, usually >4.5 mEq/L.
- Plasma bicarbonate is <10 mmol/L.
- Anion gap is high.

- Serum urea nitrogen is high.
- Plasma creatinine is high.
- Plasma acetoacetate is high.
- Plasma β-OH-butyrate is high.
- Plasma free fatty acids are high.
- Plasma osmolarity is high.
- Plasma amylase may be high.
- Leukocytes are high, with or without a left shift.
- Plasma triglycerides are high.

Primary abnormality in DKA is a high serum glucose due to relative insulin deficiency and glucagon excess. The diagnosis is made by first checking the urine for glucose and ketones. In the presence of ketonuria, plasma glucose and ketone levels are checked to rule out ketosis secondary to starvation. Serum ketones are checked using reagent strips that use the nitroprusside test. These strips detect the only true "keto" acid—acetoacetate. β-OH-butyrate, which is initially higher in concentration, is not detected, since it does not have a keto group. The sensitivity for acetone is also very low. High serum osmolarity is simply explained by the presence of elevated glucose and metabolic acids.

Severe hyperglycemia (glucose >1000 mg/dL) can only occur in two situations:

- Severe dehydration
- Chronic renal failure with a low glomerular filtration rate (GFR) and diminished excretion of glucose

Mild-to-moderate hyponatremia is present in DKA. Several factors contribute to this: (1) Hyperosmolar plasma draws intracellular water into the vascular compartment; (2) vomiting leads to volume depletion, and this volume is consequently replaced by the patient drinking water; and (3) pseudohyponatremia in the presence of hypertriglyceridemia/hyperlipidemia.

$$\text{Corrected } Na^+ = 0.016 \text{ (measured glucose} - 100) + \text{measured } Na^+$$

Plasma potassium levels tend to be high on initial laboratory evaluation, despite the fact that there is a total body potassium deficit of several hundred millimoles. Potassium loss occurs because of polyuria and protracted vomiting. Serum levels appear normal or high initially because of cellular shifts as a result of acidosis. These levels tend to fall after a few hours of treatment for acidosis and hence make K^+ replacement mandatory at some stage of treatment. Prerenal azotemia is a reflection of the low intravascular volume secondary to polyuria and vomiting. This is reversible with fluid resuscitation.

Plasma amylase levels may be high. The elevated amylase may be of salivary gland origin. However, an elevated amylase may also indicate the presence of pancreatitis; a lipase- and contrast-enhanced computed tomography scan (after fluid resuscitation) are recommended to diagnose pancreatitis in patients with DKA and an elevated amylase levels. A markedly high white blood cell count with a left shift is usually present in patients with DKA; this does not necessarily indicate an infection. Hypertriglyceridemia is a common finding in DKA and is attributed to impaired activity of lipoprotein lipase, an enzyme that is responsible for lipid disposal and overproduction of very low-density lipoproteins by the liver.

Management (Figure 31-1)

- Strict fluid intake and output
- Nasogastric tube (NGT) if comatose or vomiting
- *No* sedatives or narcotics
- Drug and fluid therapy:
  Insulin replacement
  Fluid replacement
  Potassium replacement
  Phosphate replacement
  Antibiotics in case of suspected infection

Insulin

In the early 1970s, the dose and rate of insulin administration in DKA received much attention. Despite initial skepticism, it subsequently became established that relatively low doses of insulin administered by continuous intravenous infusion or intramuscular injection were appropriate for the vast majority of cases. Most modern protocols now recommend a bolus of 10 U followed by a constant rate of insulin administration (usually 5 U/h) until near normalization of plasma glucose. The insulin for infusion should be added to 0.45% saline (100 U/100 mL) and the container thoroughly mixed before use. If serum potassium is normal or high, start insulin on arrival, otherwise in case of very low serum potassium, hold insulin for an hour or so until 40 to 50 mmol of K^+ are infused. This helps prevent cardiac arrhythmias that may occur with further hypokalemia induced by insulin infusion. The blood glucose concentration should be measured hourly (initially) after starting the infusion, then q2h. If the glucose concentration has not deceased by 100 mg/dL/h, the insulin rate should be doubled. Conversely, if the glucose has fallen by greater than 150 mg/dL/h, the infusion rate should be halved.

Very small doses of insulin suppress hepatic gluconeogenesis and ketogenesis. On the basis of these data, a very-low-dose insulin protocol has been described to avoid the rapid shifts in fluids and electrolytes that are associated with significant morbidity. Using an ~1-U/h infusion to reduce the blood glucose by no more than 50 mg/dL/h.

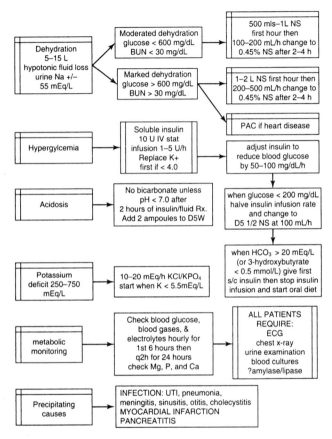

Figure 31-1. Management of diabetic ketoacidosis.

Wagner and colleagues reported this "slow-motion equilibrium" approach to be highly effective and safe.

It is recognized that ketosis and acidosis may persist for many hours after correction of hyperglycemia. There is a broad consensus that further insulin is required after normalization of blood glucose, along with intravenous dextrose (D5% $\frac{1}{2}$ N/S) to avoid hypoglycemia. Most researchers recommend that the rate of insulin be reduced during this phase, perhaps by 50%, or by a variable amount, depending on the blood glucose. It is usually suggested that this second phase of insulin administration should continue until the patient is eating again, and

Table 31-1. Sliding scale for insulin administration (q4–6 h).

Blood Glucose (mg/dL)	Regular Insulin SC (U)
<150	None
150–200	2
201–250	4
251–300	6
>300	8

an overlap with the first subcutaneous insulin injection is advised to avoid hypoinsulinemia. Despite these recommendations, it is not uncommon for relapse of ketoacidosis to occur after correction of hyperglycemia. This may be attributed to either an inadequate rate or a premature cessation of intravenous insulin administration. A subcutaneous sliding scale for the third phase of insulin administration is provided in Table 31-1.

The Extended Insulin Regimen   To prevent relapses of ketoacidosis, an *extended insulin regimen* has been developed. This regimen should be considered in patients with severe ketoacidosis as well as those with significant co-morbidities. In this protocol, the insulin is administered at a constant rate from presentation until normalization of blood 3-hydroxybutyrate concentration and then administered at a reduced rate until oral food intake is reestablished. With this regimen, the insulin infusion is continued at 5 U/h until capillary blood glucose falls to <200 mg/dL. Thereafter, the intravenous insulin is continued at a constant rate of *5 U/h along with 20% glucose* at a variable rate that maintains capillary blood glucose between 90 and 180 mg/dL, until capillary blood 3-hydroxybutyrate falls to <0.5 mmol/L. At this point, the insulin and 20% glucose infusions is stopped, and *500 mL of 5% glucose containing 8 U insulin is infused over 6 hours.* Additional subcutaneous insulin is given at four hourly intervals to maintain blood glucose at <180 mg/dL. At this time, subcutaneous, sliding-scale insulin and oral feeding are started. Where facilities for measuring capillary blood 3-hydroxybutyrate do not exist, a serum HCO_3^- of 20 mEq/L can be substituted for an undetectable hydroxybutyrate level. This regimen has been demonstrated to produce a more rapid resolution of ketosis than the standard regimen.

Fluid Replacement

Patients with DKA are volume depleted; both saline and free water constitute an essential part of treatment. Most patients have a fluid deficit of around 5 to 8 L on presentation. Fluid resuscitation should be started early and continued until after the resolution of the ketoacidosis. Normal saline (NS) or Ringer's lactate given at a rate of 1 to 2 L in the first hour is the initial fluid of choice. Thereafter, depending upon the serum sodium, the fluid should be changed to 0.45% NS; this allows more free water to be delivered, since there is a greater deficit of free water in comparison to sodium. The infusion rate maybe decreased to between 200 and 500 mL/h depending upon urine output and intravascular volume status. This can be safely continued until plasma glucose falls to ~200 mg/dL (see above). At this point, the patient should receive an infusion of dextrose water or D50.456NS and insulin.

Potassium and Phosphate Replacement

Potassium replacement is essential, the serum K^+ levels at presentation determine when it needs to be replaced. Usually, potassium levels are high initially, but after a few hours of treatment with insulin and reversal of acidosis, they drop significantly. Replacement should begin earlier if, however, the K^+ level is normal or low initially. There is also some degree of hypophosphatemia in DKA. However, it does not usually require treatment unless levels fall below 1 mg/dL (0.35 mmol/L). Severe hypophosphatemia may result in damage to skeletal muscles and red blood cells. Repletion is usually achieved in the form of the potassium salt. Replacement should not be too rapid, as it may result in tetany secondary to Ca^{++} precipitation.

Bicarbonate?

Bicarbonate is frequently administered to "correct the acidosis" in patients with DKA. However, paradoxically, bicarbonate has been demonstrated to increase ketone production. Studies have demonstrated an increase in acetoacetate levels during alkali administration, followed by an increase in 3-hydroxybutyrate levels after its completion. In pediatric patients, treatment with bicarbonate has been demonstrated to prolong hospitalization. In addition, bicarbonate may decrease cerebrospinal fluid pH, as increased CO_2 produced by buffering acid crosses the blood–brain barrier, combines H_2O, and regenerates H^+. It is generally believed that adjunctive bicarbonate is unnecessary and potentially disadvantageous in severe DKA. Bicarbonate may be appropriate if the pH remains <7.0 after 2 to 3 hours of fluid and insulin treatment. The bicarbonate should be stopped once the pH is >7.1.

Identification and Management of Precipitating Factors

Infections, particularly urinary tract infections and cellulitis (from diabetic ulcers), are common precipitants in diabetic patients. In addition, it is important to consider craniofacial mucormycosis (examine nose for black exudate) as well as emphysematous pyelonephritis and cholecystitis. Diabetic patients are more predisposed to advanced coronary artery disease, and therefore myocardial ischemia should be excluded.

■ NONKETOTIC HYPEROSMOLAR STATES

Nonketotic hyperosmolar (NKH) states are usually considered to be a disease of elderly patients with noninsulin-dependent diabetes mellitus, but it may occur in younger patients or patients with insulin-dependent diabetes mellitus as well. The pathophysiology that gives rise to NKH requires three interrelated elements to be present: insulin deficiency, renal impairment, and cognitive impairment.

Infection is the most common precipitating factor, being present in 30% to 60% of cases. Pneumonia and urinary tract infections are the most common infections reported in these patients. NKH is common in postoperative patients, particularly those who have undergone orthopedic procedures. NKH does not occur in adequately hydrated patients, and most cases of NKH are associated with restricted access to water. This restriction may be due to impaired cognitive function (dementia, cerebrovascular accident (CVAs), etc.) or the patient's being bedridden or restrained and is exacerbated by the decreased thirst response in the elderly. In addition, some degree of renal impairment accompanies all cases of NKH states. As a result of reduced GFR, they cannot easily excrete a glucose load. When they become hyperglycemic, the glucose is neither metabolized nor excreted. The decline in GFR with dehydration adds further to the hyperglycemia.

The hormonal picture of NKH states is similar to that in DKA. However, although insulin is present, the levels are inadequate to lower glucose and the levels of the counter-regulatory hormones although elevated are not as high as in DKA. In NKH, hyperosmolarity suppresses lipolysis. NKH is characterized by extreme fluid and electrolyte depletion, with intra- and extracellular fluid volumes depleted by as much as 25%. Osmotic diuresis leads to hypotonic fluid loss with electrolyte losses equivalent to roughly one half of water loss. This effect, raising serum sodium, is counterbalanced by pseudohyponatremia secondary to hypertriglyceridemia and hyperglycemia. A mild acidosis may be present (pH > 7.3), owing to accumulation of lactic acid. The characteristic features of NKH are listed in Table 31-2.

The cornerstone of NKH therapy is vigorous, early volume replacement. Hydration alone lowers blood glucose by increasing urinary losses and decreasing levels of counter-regulatory hormones. Initial fluid replacement should be 1 to 2 L in the first 2 hours of treatment,

Table 31-2. Features of nonketotic hyperosmolar states.

Effective osmolarity	≥320 mOsm/L
Blood glucose	≥600 mg/dL
Arterial pH	≥7.3

followed by a total of 7 to 10 L over the next 24 to 48 hours. The choice of initial fluid, isotonic or hypotonic, is controversial. However, normal saline is recommended initially to restore intravascular volume. Once blood pressure, pulse, and urine output have normalized, the fluid should be changed to hypotonic (0.45%) saline to replace the free-water deficit. Potassium replacement is essential and should begin once urine flow is established. Most patients with NKH are more sensitive to insulin than are patients with DKA. In addition, blood glucose concentration can fall precipitously when urine output is reestablished after volume expansion with saline. Treatment with insulin is essential but should be instituted with careful monitoring and only after fluid and electrolyte resuscitation are under way. A bolus dose of insulin is not recommended. An insulin infusion started at a dose of 1 to 5 U/h should be commenced once fluid resuscitation has commenced. The goal in the first 24 hours should be fluid and electrolyte resuscitation rather than normalization of the blood glucose; the blood glucose should be maintained around 250 mg/dL for the first 24 hours. A rapid fall in glucose increases the risk of developing cerebral edema. It is important to identify and treat all precipitating causes.

■ MANAGEMENT OF STRESS-INDUCED HYPERGLYCEMIA

Stress-induced hyperglycemia is a common problem in patients admitted to the ICU, even when glucose homeostasis has previously been normal. Hyperglycemia is a near universal finding in diabetic patients suffering catabolic illnesses, and may worsen prognosis, although this is controversial. The presence of hyperglycemia is associated with an increased risk of infectious complications in surgical patients, and indirect evidence indicates that maintenance of euglycemia can reduce the risk of infection in critically ill patients.

The cause of stress-induced hyperglycemia is multifactorial. Insufficient insulin secretion, insulin resistance, increase in counter-regulatory hormones (i.e., catecholamines, growth hormone, cortisol), age, and cytokine release contribute to the hyperglycemia. Hepatic insulin resistance with increased hepatic output of glucose appears to

Table 31-3. Insulin infusion protocol.

1. If blood glucose (BG) 80–124 mg/dL or if BG falls by
> 50 mg/dL/h

Drip Rate at (U/h)	**DECREASE** by U/h
>2	0.5
2–10	1
10–20	2
>20	4

2. If BG 125 to 200 mg/dL, continue current drip rate.

3. If BG > 200 mg/dL

Drip Rate at (U/h)	**INCREASE** by U/h*
<2	0.5
2–10	1
10–20	2
>20	4

4. For hypoglycemia

BG < 80 mg/dL, STOP insulin infusion and give ½ amp D50.
BG < 60 mg/dL, STOP insulin infusion and give 1 amp D50.

Repeat finger stick in 15 min, and repeat D50 until BG > 100.
When BG > 100, resume insulin infusion at 50% of prior rate.

* Unless BG falls by > 75 mg/dL/h, then decrease by the stated amount.

be more important than impaired glucose uptake. Although much of the clearance of glucose during critical illness is by tissues that do not depend on insulin, insulin-mediated glucose uptake is impaired. Administration of intravenous glucose solutions (particularly total parenteral nutrition) and glucose in dialysis solutions contributes to the hyperglycemia of critical illness. The net result is that many critically ill patients develop hyperglycemia (blood glucose >200 mg/dL).

The postulate that tight control of glycemia may improve the outcome of hospitalized patients is supported by the results of the DIGAMI trial. The DIGAMI trial enrolled patients presenting with acute myocardial infarction who also had diabetes mellitus or hyperglycemia. Patients were randomized either to tight control or usual care. Tight control involved insulin infusions for 24 hours with the goal plasma glucose in the range of 126 to 200 mg/dL, followed by multiple daily insulin injections (continued after discharge from hospital). The mean blood glucose decreased from 277 to 172 mg/dL in the infusion group during the first 24 hours, and from 282 to 210 mg/dL among control patients ($P < 0.0001$). While there was a significant reduction in overall mortality after 1 and 3.4 years of follow-up in the treatment group, in the subgroup of patients in the treatment group without previous insulin use, there was a significant reduction in mortality during the hospital phase (5% vs. 12%; $P < 0.05$).

Patients with stress hyperglycemia are usually managed using subcutaneous insulin injections. These subcutaneous injections prevent large fluctuation in blood glucose level but rarely control blood glucose in the 125- to 200-mg/dL range. I therefore prefer a continuous insulin infusion, which results in much tighter glucose control (supported by the DIGAMI trial).

The following insulin infusion protocol is recommended. The target blood glucose is 125 to 200 mg/dL. Mix 200 U regular insulin in 200 cc normal saline (NS) (= 1 U/cc). Flush tubing with 50 cc of insulin saline infusion before starting drip. Begin IV insulin infusion at a rate of 2 U/h. Check capillary blood every 1 to 2 hours until stable then every 4 to 6 hours. Adjust infusion rate as per Table 31-3.

■ SELECTED REFERENCES

1. Jeeanandam M, Young DH, Schiller WR. Glucose turnover, oxidation, and indices of recycling in severely traumatized patients. *J Trauma*. 1990;30: 582–589.
2. Kannan CR. Bicarbonate therapy in the management of severe diabetic ketoacidosis. *Crit Care Med*. 1999;27:2833–2834.
3. Malmberg K. Prospective randomised study of intensive insulin treatment on long term survival after acute myocardial infarction in patients with diabetes mellitus. DIGAMI (Diabetes Mellitus, Insulin Glucose Infusion in Acute Myocardial Infarction) Study Group. *BMJ*. 1997;314:1512–1515.
4. Malmberg K, Ryden L, Efendic S, et al. Randomized trial of insulin-glucose infusion followed by subcutaneous insulin treatment in diabetic patients with acute myocardial infarction (DIGAMI study): effects on mortality at 1 year. *J Am Coll Cardiol*. 1995;26:57–65.
5. Pomposelli J, Baxter J, Babineau T, et al. Early postoperative glucose control predicts nosocomial infection rate in diabetic patients. *JPEN*. 1998;22: 77–81.
6. Viallon A, Zeni F, Lafond P, et al. Does bicarbonate therapy improve the management of severe diabetic ketoacidosis? *Crit Care Med*. 1999;27: 2690–2693.
7. Wagner A, Risse A, Brill HL, et al. Therapy of severe diabetic ketoacidosis. Zero-mortality under very-low-dose insulin application. *Diabetes Care*. 1999; 22:674–677.
8. Wiggam MI, O'Kane MJ, Harper R, et al. Treatment of diabetic ketoacidosis using normalization of blood 3-hydroxybutyrate concentration as the endpoint of emergency management. A randomized controlled study. *Diabetes Care*. 1997;20:1347–1352.
9. Zerr K, Furary A, Grunkemeier G, et al. Glucose control lowers the risk of wound infection in diabetics after open heart operation. *Ann Thorac Surg*. 1997;63:356–361.

32

Acute Renal Failure

Acute renal failure (ARF) is a common and serious complication in seriously ill hospitalized patients. Indeed, the mortality of ARF in ICU patients has remained in excess of 50% despite improvements in renal-replacement therapy and aggressive supportive care. It is therefore essential that all efforts be made to avoid this complication; i.e., aggressive fluid resuscitation and avoidance of potentially nephro-toxic drugs (especially aminoglycosides and contrast media). The therapeutic intervention of choice in patients with oliguria is fluid resuscitation and *not* furosemide (see Chapter 17). Furthermore, while low-dose dopamine increases renal blood flow and urine output in patients with normal renal function, dopamine *does not* improve renal function, reduce the need for dialysis, or alter the course of ARF in critically ill patients. In addition, studies have demonstrated that furosemide is of no value in modifying azotemia, reducing the need for dialysis, altering the time to recovery of renal function, reducing hospital stay, or impacting survival in established ARF. In patients who remain oliguric/anuric after adequate fluid resuscitation, it is important to exclude urinary tract obstruction (and urinary catheter obstruction), as this is an immediately reversible cause of ARF.

■ PRERENAL AZOTEMIA

Patients with prerenal azotemia (urinary Na < 40mEq/L) and increased serum urea nitrogen (BUN)/creatinine ratio should receive *aggressive fluid resuscitation*. Tables 32-1 and 32-2 highlight the differences between prerenal azotemia and established ARF. Glomerular filtration is highly dependent on renal blood flow and renal

Table 32-1. Laboratory data to differentiate prerenal from renal failure.

Laboratory Test	Prerenal	Renal
Urinalysis	Normal	Proteinuria, casts
Urinary sodium (mEq/L)	<40	>40
Fractional Na excretion	<1	>1
Urinary osmolarity	>600	<300
BUN/Cr ratio	++/+	++/++

Table 32-2. Urinary findings in acute renal failure.

Diagnosis	Urinary Sediment
Prerenal azotemia	Normal (hyaline casts and rare granular casts)
Postrenal azotemia	Can be normal or show hematuria, pyuria, or crystals
Renal: vascular	Often has RBC; eosinophiluria can occur with atheroembolic disease
Renal: glomerulonephritis	RBC, RBC and granular casts
Renal: interstitial nephritis	Pyuria, WBC casts, eosinophils, and eosinophilic casts
Renal: tubular necrosis	Pigmented granular casts, renal tubular epithelial cells, and granular casts

(RBC = red blood cell; WBC = white blood cell.)

perfusion pressure. When both/either fall, the kidney autoregulates to maintain the glomerular filtration rate (GFR). However, when the mean arterial pressure (MAP) falls <60 mm Hg, the filtration pressure drops close to 0. It is therefore essential that all patients with prerenal azotemia be adequately fluid resuscitated to achieve an adequate MAP (>80 mm Hg) and cardiac output (cardiac index >3.0 L/min/m^2). In the elderly and in patients with diseases affecting the integrity of the afferent arterioles, lesser degrees of hypotension may cause a decline in renal function, and oliguria. In patients with compromised renal function, nephrotoxic drugs (particularly aminoglycosides and contract agents) should be avoided.

Other factors that alter the BUN/creatinine ratio

- Dehydration
- Urinary obstruction
- Drugs: corticosteroids, tetracyclines
- Hypercatabolic conditions: sepsis
- Tissue necrosis: gangrene, burns
- Gastrointestinal bleeding

- Reduced muscle bulk
- Increased protein intake
- Urine extravasation in peritoneum

Contrast Agents and the Kidney

It is important to note that intravenous contrast agents are commonly implicated as a cause of renal deterioration in hospitalized patients. The most important risk factor is preexisting renal dysfunction, particularly that caused by diabetic nephropathy. Other risk factors for contrast-induced nephrotoxicity include congestive heart failure, reduced effective arterial volume, multiple myeloma, administration of a high dose of contrast agent, and intracardiac injection. Concomitant use of drugs that impair renal responses, such as angiotensin-converting enzyme (ACE) inhibitors and nonsteroidal anti-inflammatory drugs, may also increase the risk. All attempts should be made to avoid iodinated contrast agents in patients with prerenal azotemia and in patients with acute renal insults. In all patients receiving intravenous contrast agents, vigorous prehydration is required; this is the only measure that has been demonstrated to reduce the incidence of renal compromise following contrast agents. There is evidence that low-osmolality contrast agents lower the risk of nephrotoxicity in patients with elevated serum creatinine concentrations (>1.5 mg/dL). In a meta-analysis of 25 trials, the pooled odds ratio for an increase in serum creatinine of more than 0.5 mg/dL was 0.5 with low-osmolality as compared with high-osmolality contrast agents. No statistically significant benefit could be discerned in patients with normal renal function. Recently, Tepel and colleagues demonstrated that in patients with chronic renal insufficiency who were undergoing computed tomography with a low-osmolality contrast agent, treatment with the antioxidant acetylcysteine (600 mg orally twice daily) and 0.45 percent saline intravenously, before and after administration of the contrast agent, reduced the incidence of decline of renal function compared to patients receiving placebo and saline. Acetylcysteine and vigorous prehydration should be considered in all patients at high risk of contrast induced nephrotoxicity.

In patients with ARF in whom the use of contrast agents is essential, dialysis immediately after the contrast procedure may limit additional renal compromise (contrast agents are dialyzable). However, postprocedure dialysis is not required in patients on chronic hemodialysis who receive an intravenous contrast agent unless they become volume overloaded.

Aminoglycosides and the Kidney

Aminoglycoside antibiotics are reported to be the most common cause of drug-induced nephrotoxicity in hospitalized patients. It is probable that between 5% and 15% of patients treated with an aminoglycoside will develop clinically significant nephrotoxicity. The risk factors for aminoglycoside nephrotoxicity include

- More than 10 days of treatment.
- A second course of aminoglycosides within 3 months of the first course.
- Underlying renal dysfunction/azotemia/renal failure: In patients with renal dysfunction, the half-life of aminoglycosides is increased, resulting in serum levels being elevated for a prolonged period. This enhances the renal uptake of the drug with increased nephrotoxicity. Aminoglycoside antibiotics should therefore be avoided in patients with significant renal dysfunction.
- Advanced age: The increased nephrotoxicity that has been reported in the elderly is probably a consequence of the decreased GFR in this age group.
- Multiple daily dosing schedule.
- Hypokalemia and hypomagnesemia.
- Concurrent administration of nephrotoxic agents, especially vancomycin, amphotericin B, and cyclosporine, will increase the incidence of toxicity.

Strategies to Reduce the Risk of Aminoglycoside Toxicity

- A once-daily (qd) dosing regimen may reduce the risk of nephrotoxicity.
  In patients treated on the qd regimen, therapeutic peak levels will be achieved in almost all patients, and therefore measuring peak levels may not be needed.
  Trough levels should be measured in patients with renal dysfunction and elderly patients (aim for a gentamicin/tobramycin trough <1.0 and preferably <0.5μg/mL).
- Limit duration of course to 7 to 10 days.
- Avoid using aminoglycosides in patients with underlying renal disease.

Common Nephrotoxic Agents

Antibiotics

Aminoglycosides	Acute tubular necrosis (ATN)
Penicillins	Acute interstitial nephritis
Cephalosporins	Acute interstitial nephritis
Sulfamethoxazole	Acute interstitial nephritis, crystals, decreased creatinine secretion
Quinolones	Mechanism unclear
Amphotericin B	ATN, electrolyte wasting, renal tubular acidosis
Pentamidine	ATN

Acyclovir	Crystalluria
Foscarnet	ATN, electrolyte wasting
Rifampicin	Acute interstitial nephritis

Immunosuppressive Agents

Cyclosporine	Intrarenal vasoconstriction
Cisplatin	ATN
Methotrexate	Crystalluria

Antihypertensives

ACE inhibitors	Decreased GFR (especially with renal artery stenosis), acute interstitial nephritis
Contrast agents	Intrarenal vasoconstriction: ATN, acute interstitial nephritis, nephrotic syndrome
Cimetidine	Acute interstitial nephritis, decreased creatinine secretion
Allopurinol	Acute interstitial nephritis
Phenytoin	Acute interstitial nephritis
Lithium	Acute interstitial nephritis

■ MANAGEMENT OF ESTABLISHED ARF

ARF is a reversible process in the majority of cases and often requires only careful fluid and electrolyte management and an adjustment of drug dosage according to the level of the GFR (Table 32-3). Once the patient is in established ARF, no intervention or therapy has been demonstrated to hasten recovery of renal function. However, further kidney insults should be rigorously avoided, as these will delay renal recovery.

There are no hard and fast rules as to when renal replacement therapy (dialysis) should be instituted. However, in critically ill patients with rapid changes in fluid balance and electrolytes, it is usually prudent to start earlier than later. Hemodialysis has been the most frequently used method of renal replacement therapy in the setting of ARF. There are, however, theoretical concerns that dialysis itself may delay the recovery of renal function in patients with ARF. Three factors have been implicated in this regard, namely, (1) decrease in urine output following the start of dialysis, (2) hypotensive episodes, and (3) complement activation due to use of bioincompatible membranes. Recently, a number of studies have demonstrated that, in patients with ARF, dialysis with biocompatible membranes (polymethyl methacrylate membrane) compared with cuprophane membranes results in a higher rate of recovery of renal function, a

Table 32-3. Common drugs used in the ICU that require dosage adjustment in renal failure.

Drug	Dose Based On Estimated Creatinine Clearance		
	>50	10–50%	<10%
Opiates	Unchanged	Unchanged	50–75
Chlordiazepoxide	Unchanged	Unchanged	50
Lorazepam	Unchanged	Unchanged	50
Ceftazidime	Unchanged	50	25
Ceftizoxime	Unchanged	50	25
Cefuroxime	Unchanged	50	25
Other cephalosporins	Unchanged	Unchanged	50
Most penicillins	Unchanged	50–75	25
Ciprofloxacin	Unchanged	50	25
Erythromycin	Unchanged	Unchanged	50–75
Tri/Sulp	Unchanged	75	50
Vancomycin	Monitor levels		
Aminoglycosides	75–50 Monitor levels	AVOID	AVOID
Carbamazepine	Unchanged	Unchanged	75
Amphotericin B	Unchanged	Unchanged	75
Fluconazole	Unchanged	50	25
Acyclovir	Unchanged	50	25
H_2 blockers	Unchanged	75	50
Atenolol	Unchanged	50	25
Allopurinol	Unchanged	50	25
Chlorpropamide	Unchanged	AVOID	AVOID

more rapid rate of recovery of renal function, and improved patient survival. Continuous renal replacement therapy is discussed in Chapter 33.

■ WHEN TO INITIATE RENAL REPLACEMENT THERAPY

The classic criteria for initiating renal replacement therapy (RRT) include

Hyperkalemia (K > 6.5 mmol/L)
Progressive acidosis with pH < 7.20
Fluid overload with pulmonary edema
Pericardial effusion
Uremic symptoms, i.e., nausea, vomiting, altered mental status, asterixis
Increase of serum creatinine >2 mg/dL/day

These recommendations were formulated for patients with chronic renal failure. However, most intensivists (and critical care nephrologists) contend that there is no reason to wait for significant physiological derangements (hyperkalemia, severe acidosis, fluid overload, uremic complication) to develop in the already physiologically fragile, critically ill patient before initiating RRT. The early initiation of RRT facilitates early nutritional support, simplifies fluid management, and may prevent complications. However, no sound data are available to support this strategy. Nevertheless, *earlier may be better.*

■ RHABDOMYOLYSIS AND MYOGLOBINURIA

Rhabdomyolysis with myoglobinuria is commonly encountered in the ICU; causes include

Crush injury
Compartment syndrome
Ischemic limb
Severe sepsis
Cocaine use
Hypothermia
Unconscious patients lying in one position
Alcohol

Rhabdomyolysis should be suspected in a patient with high levels of creatine phosphokinase (CPK) and confirmed by demonstrating myoglobin in the urine. Patients with a CPK >10,000 U/mL are at a high risk of developing ARF. The CPKs should be serially followed, as levels may rise with volume resuscitation (and increased muscle perfusion). All dehydrated patients with elevated CPKs should be rehydrated. Patients with CPKs >3000 to 5000 should be treated to prevent renal failure:

- Maintain a urine output of 100 to 200 mL/h with fluid replacement (NaCl or Ringer's) and the use of a loop diuretic.
- Alkalinize the urine (intravenous sodium bicarbonate).
- Mannitol may also be useful to maintain a high urine output (check osmolarity regularly).
- Monitor fluid balance carefully; do not dehydrate or overload the patient.
- Hypocalcemia is a common complication of rhabdomyolysis. Release of phosphate from injured muscle results in the local precipitation of calcium salts. Hyperphosphatemia also impairs the 1-hydroxylation of vitamin D, thereby decreasing the sensitivity of bone to parathormone. Administration of calcium may result in severe soft tissue calcification. Calcium supplementation should be reserved for patients with clear clinical signs of

hypocalcemia. In patients receiving hemodialysis, the dialysate calcium should be adjusted to prevent a positive calcium balance.

■ SELECTED REFERENCES

1. Barrett BJ, Carlisle EJ. Meta-analysis of the relative nephrotoxicity of high- and low-osmolality iodinated contrast media. *Radiology.* 1993;188:171–178.
2. Chertow G, Sayegh M, Allgren RL. Is the administration of dopamine associated with adverse or favorable outcomes in acute renal failure. *Am J Med.* 1996;101:49–53.
3. Groeneveld ABJ, Tra DD, Van der Meulen J. Acute renal failure in the medical intensive care unit: predisposing, complicating factors and outcome. *Nephron.* 1991;59:602–610.
4. Marik PE, Iglesias J. Low-dose dopamine does not prevent acute renal failure in patients with septic shock and oliguria. NORASEPT II Study investigators. *Am J Med.* 1999;107:387–390.
5. Russo D, Memoli B, Andreucci VE. The place of loop diuretics in the treatment of acute and chronic renal failure. *Clin Nephrol.* 1992;38(suppl 1):S69–S73.
6. Shilliday IR, Quinn KJ, Allison ME. Loop diuretics in the management of acute renal failure: a prospective, double-blind, placebo-controlled, randomized study. *Nephrol Dial Transplant.* 1997;12:2592–2596.
7. Solomon R, Werner C, Mann D, D'Elia J, Silva P. Effects of saline, mannitol, and furosemide to prevent acute decreases in renal function induced by radiocontrast agents. *N Engl J Med.* 1994;331:1416–1420.
8. Tepel M, van der Giet M, Schwarzfeld C, Laufer U, Liermann D, Zidek W. Prevention of radiographic-contrast-agent-induced reductions in renal function by acetylcysteine. *N Eng J Med* 2000;343:80–4.
9. Younathan CM, Kaude JV, Cook MD, Shaw GS, Peterson JC. Dialysis is not indicated immediately after administration of nonionic contrast agents in patients with end-stage renal disease treated by maintenance dialysis. *Am J Roentgenol.* 1994;163:969–971.

33

Continuous Renal Replacement Therapy in Acute Renal Failure

Continuous renal replacement therapies (CRRTs) have been developed to enable the critically ill patient with acute renal failure to be treated more effectively. Acute renal failure in the critically ill patient almost always develops in the setting of shock, sepsis, major surgery, and/or major trauma, and is invariably associated with multiorgan dysfunction and/or failure. In addition, these patients usually have hemodynamic and respiratory abnormalities that make conventional intermittent hemodialysis both technically difficult and fraught with many complications. The patient's fluid, electrolyte, and acid–base status fluctuate widely within a 24-hour period; intermittent dialysis is not suited to these changing circumstances.

Advantages of CRRT include

- Hemodynamically well tolerated
- Minimal change in plasma osmolarity
- Better control of azotemia and electrolytes and acid–base balance
- Very effective in removing fluid
- Technically simple
- Membrane capable of removing cytokines in septic patients
- Better membrane biocompatibility

CRRTs were developed with the aim of providing a more physiological method of renal replacement therapy; i.e., to function more like a normal kidney. Since the early 1980s, CRRT has undergone a remarkable revolution, the major aspects of which include the introduction of countercurrent dialysate flow, the use of double-lumen venous access, and development of modular, portable continuous veno-veno hemodiafiltration (CVVHD) machines.

Continuous arteriovenous hemofiltration (CAVH) was the first continuous renal replacement therapy to be used in ICU patients. Essentially, this was a method of continuously removing a plasma ultrafiltrate and replacing this lost volume with a balanced physiological solution. A hollow-fiber filter (the artificial kidney) was connected at one end to an arterial catheter (usually femoral artery) and to a venous catheter at the other end (usually femoral vein), forming a closed loop system. The patient's own cardiac output perfused the filter (there are no external pumps). The blood flow through the system was dependent upon the cardiac output, mean arterial pressure, and the diameter and length of the connecting tubes. CAVH had serious shortcomings, which included the need for arterial cannulation and the limited solute clearance that could be achieved even under optimal operating conditions (urea clearance of 10 to 12 mL/min). The next development was the addition of a sideport to the hemofilter. Through this port, countercurrent dialysate could be infused to achieve additional diffusive solute clearance; this modified technique was called *continuous arteriovenous hemodiafiltration CAVHD*. Arteriovenous systems are simple because they do not require a peristaltic pump; however, the morbidity associated with arterial cannulation is substantial. Furthermore, blood flow through the filter is limited by the mean arterial pressure and cardiac output. For these reasons, venovenous techniques utilizing a double-lumen central venous catheter have largely replaced arteriovenous methods of CRRT. When venovenous therapy is applied, the blood flow is controlled by a peristaltic pump module with appropriate air bubble traps and pressure monitors. Continuous veno-veno techniques differ according to the membrane used, the mechanism of solute transport, and the presence or absence of dialysis solutions. Specific CRRT machines have been designed that permit the safe and reliable performance of CRRT. These machines have self-loading circuits that include the filter and blood and dialysate lines. These machines have microprocessors that permit different modes of CRRT to be performed while controlling blood and dialysate flow and volume removal.

Although no randomized controlled studies have been *successfully* performed, there are many reasons to postulate that CRRT is superior to standard intermittent hemodialysis (IHD) in critically ill ICU patients. CRRT results in better hemodynamic stability than IHD; this may limit further kidney injury. Uremic control is better with CRRT than with standard IHD, even if the latter is performed daily. This has important implications, as data suggest that in critically ill patients a greater dialysis dose is associated with a better outcome. Furthermore, comparative studies suggest a more rapid improvement of metabolic acidosis and serum phosphate levels. Because volume and uremic control are not a problem with CRRT, patients can receive a protein-rich diet. Because of the rapid shifts of fluid, patients with raised intracranial pressure (IHD can cause surges in intracranial pressure) and patients with limited cardiac reserve tolerate IHD poorly.

■ SELECTED REFERENCES

1. Bellomo R, Ronco C. Acute renal failure in the intensive care unit: adequacy of dialysis and the case for continuous therapies. *Nephrol Dial Transplant.* 1996;11:424–428.
2. Bellomo R, Ronco C. Adequacy of dialysis in the acute renal failure of the critically ill: the case for continuous therapies. *Int J Artif Organs.* 1996;19:129–142.
3. Bellomo R, Ronco C. Continuous versus intermittent renal replacement therapy in the intensive care unit. *Kidney Int.* 1998;53(suppl 66):S125–S128.
4. Clark WR, Mueller BA, Alaka KJ. A comparison of metabolic control by continuous and intermittent therapies in acute renal failure. *J Am Soc Nephrol.* 1994;4:1413–1420.
5. Davenport A, Will EJ, Davidson AM. Improved cardiovascular stability during continuous modes of renal replacement therapy in critically ill patients with acute hepatic and renal failure. *Crit Care Med.* 1993;21:328–338.
6. Misset B, Timset JF, Chevret S, et al. A randomized cross-over comparison of the hemodynamic response to intermittent hemodialysis and continuous hemofiltration in ICU patients with acute renal failure. *Intensive Care Med.* 1996;22:742–746.

34

Adrenal Insufficiency in the Intensive Care Unit

Critical illness can be associated with low concentrations of thyroid hormones—referred to as the *euthyroid sick syndrome*. Depressed levels of gonadotrophins have also been noted in critically ill patients. Depending on the population studied and the diagnostic criteria used, adrenal insufficiency may occur in a substantial number of seriously ill patients. In these patients, adrenal insufficiency may result from both decreased production of adrenocorticotropic hormone (ACTH) as well as decreased responsiveness of the adrenal gland to ACTH.

Cortisol is essential for regulation and control of protein synthesis and therefore cellular function. In addition, cortisol is essential for normal cardiovascular function. Deficiency of cortisol has various clinical manifestations depending on the extent and acuteness of adrenal failure and the clinical setting in which it occurs. Four distinct syndromes of adrenal insufficiency may occur in the ICU setting:

1. Patients may present to hospital with classic Addison's syndrome: nausea, vomiting, malaise, hypotension, hyperpigmentation, etc. (*chronic*).

2. Patients with relative adrenal insufficiency may develop an acute Addisonian crisis due to stress of acute illness; these are patients with intrinsic adrenal disease such as human immunodeficiency virus (HIV), tuberculosis, primary autoimmune adrenalitis, or chronic steroid use who present at the hospital with an acute illness (*acute on chronic*). These patients have an inadequate adrenal reserve, which manifests as an inability to respond adequately (increase cortisol secretion) to a stressor. Patients with acquired immune deficiency syndrome (AIDS) demonstrate both primary and secondary adrenal insufficiency, which may affect 5% to 50% of patients with advanced

disease. HIV infection usually produces primary adrenal insufficiency as a result of opportunistic infection (i.e., cytomegalovirus, mycobacterium, fungus) or due to infection by the HIV virus itself. AIDS is the most common cause of primary adrenal insufficiency seen in medical practice today.

The most common cause of secondary adrenal insufficiency is previous glucocorticoid administration. Adrenal recovery may take 9 to 12 months following discontinuation of chronic steroids. Thus, patients who have received glucocorticoids within the 12 months before ICU admission (for >10 days) should be considered at risk for secondary adrenal insufficiency. Although adrenal suppression from glucocorticoids is clearly dose dependent, it is important to note that even patients receiving as little as 5 mg prednisone daily for many years develop adrenal suppression. In addition, patients receiving inhaled glucocorticoids may develop adrenal suppression.

3. Acute adrenal insufficiency occurs in patients with adrenal hemorrhage (*acute*).

4. Patients with presumably normal premorbid adrenal function may develop adrenal insufficiency in the setting of a severe acute illness (*subacute reversible*). This category of adrenal insufficiency is probably very common in septic ICU patients, yet the diagnosis is frequently missed. Due to differences in diagnostic criteria (see below), the incidence of this condition is uncertain. However, preliminary data suggest that as many as a third of septic ICU patients may suffer from acute reversible adrenal insufficiency. Adrenal insufficiency should be suspected in volume-unresponsive septic patients who are pressor dependent. Adrenal insufficiency should also be considered in patients who cannot be weaned off low-dose dopamine or norepinephrine.

Most signs and symptoms of adrenal insufficiency are nonspecific. Cortisol has a vital role in the maintenance of vascular tone, endothelial integrity, vascular permeability, distribution of body water, and catecholamine synthesis and action. Adrenalectomy predisposes animals to circulatory shock. In humans, chronic adrenal insufficiency is characterized by decreased systemic vascular resistance and decreased myocardial contractility. However, a variety of hemodynamic alterations have been described in patients with acute adrenal insufficiency, including hypovolemic shock (low cardiac output, decreased preload, depressed contractility, elevated systemic vascular resistance) and hyperdynamic shock (high cardiac output, low systemic vascular resistance). Thus, hypotension in patients with acute adrenal insufficiency may mimic hypovolemic or septic shock. Hyponatremia (due to increased vasopressin secretion), hypoglycemia, normocytic anemia, lymphocytosis, and *eosinophilia* are also common. An unexplained eosinophilia in an ICU patient should prompt adrenal testing. Aldosterone deficiency is characterized by hyperkalemia, hyponatremia, metabolic acidosis, and volume depletion secondary to sodium wasting (i.e., with azotemia). In critically ill patients, untreated adrenal insufficiency is usually fatal. Adrenal insufficiency should be suspected in patients with unexplained catecholamine-resistant hypotension, hypotension poorly responsive to fluids and catecholamines, in patients with pressor dependence, and in patients with hyponatremia, hyperkalemia, hypoglycemia, or eosinophilia.

In patients with adequate stress (i.e., hypotension), a random cortisol should be >25 μg/dL. It is incorrect to conclude that the adrenal response to stress is normal when serum cortisol rises to 19 to 20 μg/dL in patients with clinical features of adrenal insufficiency. The short corticotropin (ACTH) stimulation test utilizes 250 μg of cosyntropin to diagnose adrenal insufficiency (primary or secondary). Cosyntropin (250 μg) is administered intravenously, and plasma cortisol is measured before and 30 and 60 minutes after injection. A subnormal response indicates the presence of adrenal insufficiency. Most articles state that adrenal function is considered to be normal if the basal or the postinjection plasma cortisol concentration is >18 μg/dL. Unfortunately, statements such as this are incorrect. The short corticotropin stimulation test was developed to "rule in" adrenal insufficiency at a time when TB was the most common cause of adrenal insufficiency. The test does not rule out adrenal insufficiency, because a normal cortisol response (>20 μg/dL) to 250 μg of corticotropin (a supraphysiologic amount) can be seen in many patients with secondary adrenal insufficiency and corticotropin-resistance syndromes (found in some critically ill patients). Patients have been reported who respond normally to 250 μg of corticotropin but fail to respond to stress (i.e., hypoglycemia, hypotension) or corticotropin-releasing hormone.

Importantly, a plasma level of 100 pg/mL ACTH should produce a maximal cortisol response. Plasma levels of ACTH after 250 μg of cosyntropin are approximately 83,000 pg/mL (830-fold higher than maximal levels). Thus, 250 μg of ACTH is supraphysiologic. I prefer to use a more physiologic dose of 1 μg of ACTH, which produces an ACTH level of approximately 300 pg/mL. Using the 1-μg dose, I have found a number of critically ill patients in shock with basal cortisol levels <12 μg/dL, who fail to respond to the 1-μg dose but increase their cortisol levels >20 μg/dL with 250 μg of ACTH. These patients have improved clinically with hydrocortisone treatment. Thus, I advocate the more physiologic low-dose corticotropin stimulation test.

The precise diagnostic criteria of adrenal insufficiency in critically ill patients remains to be determined. However, a random cortisol level of <25 μg/dL in a critically ill, hypotensive patient should be regarded as being highly suggestive (if not diagnostic) of adrenal insufficiency. The diagnosis can be confirmed by a low-dose corticotropin stimulation test. A 30-minute level of <25 μg/dL (following 1 μg of cosyntropin) should be regarded as diagnostic of adrenal insufficieny. The value of the low-dose ACTH stimulation test is in

Table 34-1. Properties of commonly used corticosteroids.

Agent	Equivalent Dose (mg)	Glucocorticoid Potency	Mineralocorticoid Potency	Duration of Action (hours)
Dexamethasone	0.75	25	0	72
Methylprednisolone	4	5	0.5	36
Prednisolone	5	4	0.8	24
Prednisone	5	4	0.8	24
Hydrocortisone	25	1	1	8

assessing adrenal reserve in an ICU patient in whom the severity of the stressor is uncertain or in patients at moderate-to-high risk of adrenal insufficiency (e.g., HIV patients, those previously using steroids) who are not "adequately" stressed.

Patients should be empirically started on hydrocortisone (or another glucocorticoid), pending results of the low-dose cosyntropin test (Table 34-1). Critically ill patients with life-threatening conditions should receive intravenous hydrocortisone (100-mg bolus followed by 100 mg every 8 hours). If treatment of the patient with glucocorticoids is felt to be indicated before assessing the adrenal axis, the patient should be given dexamethasone (2 to 4 mg) and then testing performed. Dexamethasone does not interfere with the measurement of endogenous cortisol and will not interfere with the response to ACTH. Hydrocortisone should be tapered to maintenance levels once the acute stress has subsided, so as to minimize the immune-suppressive effects of glucocorticoids. Although the sodium-retaining properties of hydrocortisone are often inadequate when administered in maintenance doses, its sodium-retaining properties are sufficient when stress doses are used.

■ SELECTED REFERENCES

1. Beishuizen A, Vermes I, Hylkema BS, Haanen C. Relative eosinophilia and functional adrenal insufficiency in critically ill patients [letter]. *Lancet.* 1999;353:1675–1676.
2. Bollaert PE, Charpentier C, Levy B, et al. Reversal of late septic shock with supraphysiologic doses of hydrocortisone. *Crit Care Med.* 1998;26:645–650.
3. Broide J, Soferman R, Kivity S, et al. Low-dose adrenocorticotropin test reveals impaired adrenal function in patients taking inhaled corticosteroids. *J Clin Endocrinol Metab.* 1995;80:1243–1246.
4. Drucker D, McLaughlin J. Adrenocortical dysfunction in acute medical illness. *Crit Care Med.* 1986;14:789–791.

5. Grinspoon SK, Bilezikian JP. HIV disease and the endocrine system. *N Engl J Med.* 1992;327:1360–1365.
6. Marik PE, Kiminyo K, Olexo S, Zaloga GP. Occult adrenal insufficiency in critically ill patients: an underdiagnosed entity. *Crit Care Med.* 1999; 27(suppl):A141.
7. Richards ML, Caplan RH, Wickus GG, Lambert PJ, Kisken WA. The rapid low-dose (1 microgram) cosyntropin test in the immediate postoperative period: results in elderly subjects after major abdominal surgery. *Surgery.* 1999;125:431–440.
8. Streeten DHP. What test for hypothalamic-pituitary adrenocortical insufficiency? *Lancet.* 1999;354:179–180.

35

Thyroid Diseases in the Critically Ill

■ SICK EUTHYROID SYNDROME/ NONTHYROIDAL ILLNESS SYNDROME

Since the 1960s, it has been known that serum thyroid hormone levels drop during starvation and illness. In mild illness, this involves only a decrease in serum T_3 levels. However, as the severity of the illness increases, there is a drop in both T_3 and T_4. This decrease in thyroid hormone level is seen in starvation, sepsis, surgery, myocardial infarction, transplantation, and in fact, probably any severe illness. Based on the premise that patients with these abnormalities are not hypothyroid despite the low hormone levels in blood, the condition has been called the *sick euthyroid syndrome* (SES). However, some experts in the field believe that some of these patients may in fact have tissue hypothyroidism and prefer the designation of *nonthyroidal illness syndrome*.

Starvation causes a prompt decline in serum T_3 and serum-free T_3. These findings are seen in most severely ill patients. However, it is difficult to differentiate the effects due to the underlying illness from that of short-term starvation, which invariably accompanies any acute illness. Carbohydrate deprivation inhibits the deiodination of T_4 to T_3 by type 1 iodothyronine in the liver, inhibiting the generation of T_3 and preventing the metabolism of rT_3. Consequently, there is a drop in serum T_3 and an elevation of rT_3. Patients who have a drop only in serum T_3, representing the mildest form of SES, do not show clinical signs of hypothyroidism. As the severity of the illness, and often the associated starvation, progresses, there is a gradual development of a more complex syndrome associated with low T_3 and T_4 levels. Generally, thyroid-stimulating hormone (TSH) levels are low despite the low serum hormone levels. The changes in hormone levels with

Table 35-1. Profile of thyroid hormones during acute illness.

Phase of illness	T_3	T_4	FT_4	rT_3	TSH
Mild, early	D	N	N	I	N
Moderate	D	D	D	I	N
Severe	D	D	D	I	D
Early recovery	D	D, N	D, N	I	N, I

(D = decreased; I = increased; N = normal.)

increasing severity of illness are listed in Table 35-1. There is evidence to suggest that hypothalamic function is impaired in patients with SES and that this may, because of low thyrotropin-releasing hormone, result in low TSH and thus low output of thyroid hormones by the thyroid.

A marked decrease in serum T_4 levels is associated with a high probability of death. When serum T_4 levels drop <4μg/dL, the probability of death is about 50%; with serum levels <2μg/dL, the probability of death reaches 80%. Obviously, this raises the question of whether replacement of thyroid hormone would be beneficial in such patients and could increase their chance of survival. There is, however, no clear evidence to date that treatment with T_4 or T_3 is beneficial or disadvantageous in critically ill patients.

■ TOXIC CRISIS: THYROID STORM

Thyroid storm is a life-threatening exacerbation of the hyperthyroid state in which there is evidence of decompensation in one or more organ systems. Thyroid storm is most frequently seen in patients with thyrotoxicosis secondary to Graves's disease, although it can also occur in patients with toxic adenoma or toxic multinodular goiter.

The factors that cause a thyrotoxic patient to develop a thyroid storm are unclear. However, the rapidity with which the thyroid hormone levels rise may be more important than the absolute levels in determining the clinical manifestations. One mechanism for a sudden change in hormone level would be a change in the levels of binding proteins. This has been noted to occur postoperatively and in patients with systemic nonthyroidal illness. In most cases of thyroid storm, a precipitating event can be identified (Table 35-2). Patients generally have all the usual features of thyrotoxicosis (Table 35-3), but these are usually exaggerated and quite severe.

Typical features include fever, profuse sweating, diarrhea, nausea and vomiting, atrial tachyarrhythmia, high output cardiac failure with cardiovascular collapse and shock, angina, as well as altered mental

Table 35-2. Precipitants of thyroid storm.

Infection
Surgery: thyroid and nonthyroidal
Radioidine therapy
Iodinated contrast dyes
Withdrawal of antithyroid drug therapy
Amiodarone
Thyroid hormone ingestion
Diabetic ketoacidosis
Congestive heart failure
Hypoglycemia
Toxemia of pregnancy
Parturition
Severe emotional stress
Pulmonary embolism
Cerebral vascular accident
Bowel infarction
Trauma
Tooth extraction
Vigorous palpation of the thyroid gland

Table 35-3. Symptoms and signs of hyperthyroidism.

Symptoms	Signs
Weakness	Goiter
Fatigue	Hyperkinesis
Heat intolerance	Opthalmopathy
Nervousness	Lid retraction/stare
Increased sweating	Lid lag
Tremor	Tremor
Palpitation	Warm, moist skin
Increased appetite	Muscle weakness
Weight loss	Hyperreflexia
Hyperdefecation	Tachycardia and atrial fibrillation/flutter
Dyspnea	Systolic hypertension
Menstrual abnormalities	Widened pulse pressure
	Fever

status progressing to obtundation and coma. The diagnosis of thyroid storm is a clinical diagnosis in patients with clinical and laboratory features consistent with thyrotoxicosis.

Treatment

There are three components to the therapy of thyroid storm: correcting the hyperthyroidism, normalizing the decompensation of homeostatic mechanisms (e.g., cardiac failure), and treating the precipitating event.

Hyperthyroidism

The first step is to block further synthesis of thyroid hormones. This can be accomplished with the use of propylthiouracil (PTU) and methimazole. PTU is preferred because it has the added benefit of inhibiting the peripheral conversion of T_4 to T_3. It has been recommended that PTU be administered as a loading dose of 600 to 1000 mg followed by 200 to 250 mg every 4 hours to a total dose of 1200 to 1500 mg. Release of the large supply of preformed thyroid hormone within the gland must also be blocked. This can be accompanied with inorganic iodine. These agents should be used, however, only after inhibition of further thyroid hormone synthesis has been achieved with PTU. Iodide may be administered orally or via nasogastric tube as a saturated solution of potassium iodide, 5 drops every 6 hours, or as Lugol's solution, 30 drops each day in three or four divided doses. The radiographic contrast dye ipodate has also been used for this purpose. Ipodate is also a potent inhibitor of the peripheral conversion of T_4 to T_3. A number of techniques that remove excess circulating thyroid hormones from the bloodstream have been employed in patients in thyroid storm. Plasmapheresis, plasma exchange, exchange transfusion, and charcoal plasmaperfusion have all been successful in a limited number of patients. These techniques should be reserved for critically ill patients who have not responded adequately to conventional methods.

Homeostatic Decompensation

Dehydration and electrolyte imbalances need to be aggressively treated with intravenous fluids. Glucose and thiamine should be included in the fluid replacement. Many of the manifestations of hyperthyroidism can be ameliorated with beta-blocking agents. The greatest experience has been with propranolol; the usual starting dose is 20 to 40 mg every 6 hours. Esmolol, a short-acting beta-1-selective agent is a useful alternative. Aggressive treatment of hyperthermia with acetaminophen and cooling blankets should be used. Aspirin can displace thyroid hormones from their binding sites and should therefore be avoided. Shivering should be avoided; if it occurs, it can be blunted with chlorpromazine. Glucocorticoids have traditionally been used for potential relative adrenal insufficiency.

Table 35-4. Clinical features of myxedema coma.

Decreased mental status
Hypoventilation
Hypothermia
Bradycardia
Hyponatremia
Hypoglycemia
Delayed relaxation of tendon reflexes
Sparse body hair
Associated infection

■ MYXEDEMA COMA

Myxedema coma is the most severe expression of hypothyroidism. Patients manifest a marked impairment of central nervous function and cardiovascular decompensation. Recognition of myxedema coma is hampered by its insidious onset. Myxedema coma is usually seen in elderly women in the winter. There is almost always a history of long-standing hypothyroidism. In such patients, a precipitating factor such as a serious infection (usually pneumonia or a urinary tract infection), recent administration of a sedative, or worsening of some preexisting medical condition can usually be identified. Patients are pale and have a characteristic edematous facies with notable periorbital edema. The skin is dry and cold. The major clinical features are summarized in Table 35-4. The diagnosis of hypothyroidism is confirmed by the classic findings of a low T_4 and high TSH.

Treatment

A number of regimens of thyroid hormone replacement have been suggested including large amounts of intravenous T_4, a mixture of intravenous T_4 and oral or intravenous T_3, or T_3 alone. However, most experts recommend intravenous thyroxine alone. Recommendations for intravenous thyroxine are 300 to 500 μg given as a bolus, followed by 50 μg intravenously daily until the patient can take oral medication. In addition, large doses of glucocorticoids are recommended to prevent the precipitation of adrenal crisis in patients with coexisting adrenal insufficiency. Patients frequently require respiratory and hemodynamic support as well as correction of electrolyte disturbances. Precipitating factors should be vigorously identified. The usual signs of infection may be absent (fever, diaphoresis, tachycardia) requiring a careful search for infection sites.

■ SELECTED REFERENCES

1. De Groot LJ. Dangerous dogmas in medicine: the nonthyroidal illness syndrome. *J Clin Endocrinol Metab.* 1999;84:151–164.
2. Smallridge RC. Metabolic and anatomic thyroid emergencies: a review. *Crit Care Med.* 2000;20:276–291.

Part 5

Neurology

36

Acute Cerebrovascular Disease and the Management of Raised Intracranial Pressure

Stroke is the third most common cause of death in the United States, after heart disease and cancer. Over 500,000 Americans suffer a stroke each year, with approximately 175,000 of these patients dying from the acute event. In over 75% of cases, the stroke is ischemic in nature. However, unlike acute myocardial infarction, therapeutic interventions that attempt to limit infarct size have been of limited success. Indeed, apart from thrombolytic therapy in highly select groups of patients (probably <5% of "stroke" patients) and aspirin, no therapeutic intervention has been demonstrated to have an impact on the course of this illness. Considering these data, the rationale for admitting patients to an ICU needs to be evaluated. In addition, aspects of medical care that maximize the potential for recovery and limit complications need to be explored. In most instances, such treatment is best provided by specialized low-technology stroke units.

■ STROKE ICU'S, MEDICAL ICU'S, OR STROKE UNITS

Stroke intensive care units were abandoned in the 1970s after it was demonstrated that such units had very little impact on the outcome of patients following a stroke. The situation is not much different today; for the overwhelming majority of patients suffering a stroke, acute medical interventions in an ICU have not been established to improve outcome, and in fact, certain interventions may be harmful. Admission to and aggressive management in an ICU may only serve to prolong the dying process of a patient who has suffered a catastrophic neurological event. Burtin and colleagues evaluated 199 stroke patients who underwent mechanical ventilation in an ICU. The 1-year survival rate was just 8%. Berrouschot et al. reported a 3-month mortality of 79% in patients admitted to an ICU following a space-occupying (malignant) middle cerebral artery infarction despite aggressive medical care.

A small group of patients who suffer a stroke may benefit from admission to the ICU if they develop a reversible/treatable medical complication. Endotracheal intubation should be reserved for patients with reversible respiratory failure or comatose patients who are likely to have a good prognosis for a functional recovery. Burtin and colleagues have demonstrated that patients with an absent gag reflex on admission to hospital will almost always die from their stroke. Although intubation and hyperventilation are routine, though heroic, measures in patients after severe stroke, their efficacy in reducing mortality and improving functional recovery has never been established. In fact, hyperventilation with induced hypocarbia may reduce perfusion to the penumbral brain regions and increase infarct size. Furthermore, it is arguable that endotracheal intubation and mechanical ventilation will reduce the risk of atelectasis and pneumonia in patients with an impaired level of consciousness, when compared to good nursing and respiratory care without endotracheal intubation.

The failure of specific intervention to improve the outcome of patients suffering a stroke should not imply that physicians should adopt a fatalistic approach when managing these patients. A number of well-conducted clinical trials have demonstrated that the mortality and functional recovery of patients following a stroke is significantly improved when these patients are cared for in a specialized stroke unit as compared to a general medical ward. These units provide specialized nursing care and a well-organized multidisciplinary rehabilitation program. Stroke unit care reduces the medical complications in stroke patients and allows for earlier and more intense rehabilitation. The Stroke Council of the American Heart Association recommends *"rapid transfer of a patient to a hospital that has a specialized stroke care unit."*

■ ACUTE ISCHEMIC STROKES

Ischemic strokes may be conveniently classified as (1) large-vessel, atherosclerotic; (2) cardioembolic; (3) small artery (lacuna); (4) stroke of other identified cause (e.g., vasculitis); and (5) stroke of undetermined cause.

Thrombolytic Therapy for Acute Ischemic Strokes

The National Institute of Neurological Disorders and Stroke (NINDS) recombinant tissue plasminogen activator (rt-PA) stroke trial demonstrated that rt-PA given to patients within 3 hours of the onset of stroke resulted in an 11% to 13% absolute increase in the chance of minimum or no disability at 3 months. Studies with a longer time window for enrollment have demonstrated a higher mortality in the treatment group, largely due to an increased incidence of intracerebral hemorrhage. In the European Cooperative Acute Stroke Study (ECASS), patients with moderate-to-severe acute ischemic strokes were randomized (<6 hours) to placebo or rt-PA. Patients with infarction involving more than one third of the middle cerebral artery territory on computed tomography (CT) scan were excluded. At 30 days, there was a higher mortality in the rt-PA group (17.9% vs. 12.7%). Large parenchymal hemorrhages were increased threefold in the rt-PA group. The lack of benefit in the rt-PA group was ascribed to inappropriate CT scan interpretation in the haste of emergency management of the stroke patients (109 of the 620 randomized patients were not appropriate). In the second European Cooperative Acute Stroke Study (ECASS II), no benefit for rt-PA was demonstrated; furthermore, treatment differences were similar whether patients were treated within 3 hours or 3 to 6 hours. The major complication following rt-PA is intracerebral hemorrhage (ICH). While the risk increases with the size of the infarct and the time delay before initiating therapy, the incidence of symptomatic ICH may be as high as 16% in appropriately selected patients.

As a result of the diverging results between the NINDS and ECASS studies and follow-up cohort studies (Cleveland experience), the role of thrombolysis in acute ischemic stroke remains uncertain. Thrombolytic therapy, however, may have a role in select low-risk patients if treated within 3 hours of the onset of the ictus. The decision to treat an acute ischemic stroke with rt-PA should remain the responsibility of an expert neurologist (and expert neuroradiologist for baseline CT scan assessment), with appropriate access to optimal acute care facilities. In addition, in select cases intra-arterial thrombolytic therapy may have a role in patients with angiographically proven thrombosis.

Antiplatelet Therapy and Anticoagulation

The International Stroke Trial (IST) randomized (using a factorial design) over 19,000 patients within 48 hours of an acute ischemic stroke to 14 days of treatment with placebo, heparin (5000 or 12,500 U q12h), or aspirin 300 mg daily. Aspirin resulted in a 1.1% absolute reduction in recurrent ischemic strokes at 14 days; both heparin regimens had no effect on outcome. Additional studies have demonstrated that heparin, low-molecular-weight heparin (LMWH), and heparinoids do not improve outcome following a stroke. However, treatment with heparin does reduce the incidence of deep venous thrombosis (DVT).

Anticoagulation in Cardioembolic Stroke

Hemorrhage into the infarct occurs in about 30% of cases of all embolic infarcts; it may however, require 3 or 4 days or longer to become apparent on the CT scan. However, magnetic resonance imaging has demonstrated that by 3 weeks hemorrhagic conversion occurs in up to 70% of patients. Hemorrhage ranges from the usual cortical petechiae to confluent hematomas. In nonanticoagulated patients, infarct volume seems to be the only independent predictor of hemorrhagic conversion.

Chronic anticoagulant therapy has been demonstrated to reduce the risk of recurrent embolization in patients who have suffered an embolic stroke. Approximately 80% of patients who have suffered a cerebral embolic stroke will suffer a subsequent embolic stroke without anticoagulation. However, in the "ORG 10172" study, only 2 of 123 patients with cardioembolic strokes treated with placebo (i.e., received no heparin) suffered a recurrent ischemic event during the study period. In the IST trial, recurrent ischemic stroke (during the study period) occurred in 4.9% of patients with cardioembolic stroke randomized to receive placebo compared to 2.8% who received heparin. However, hemorrhagic transformation occurred in 2.1% of patients receiving heparin compared to 0.4% who received placebo. Based on these data, it may be prudent to delay anticoagulation for 10 to 14 days, particularly in patients with large cerebral infarcts and hypertensive patients. The role of transesophageal echocardiography (TEE) in these patients is unclear. However, it may be prudent to perform TEE in patients at high risk of early recurrent embolization, and to commence anticoagulation earlier if clot is visualized within the cardiac chambers and CT scan does not show evidence of hemorrhagic transformation.

The HAEST study compared LMWH and aspirin in 449 patients with an acute ischemic stroke and atrial fibrillation. In this study, the frequency of recurrent ischemic stroke during the first 14 days was 8.5% in the LMWH group and 7.5% in the aspirin group. There was no difference in the rate of ICH between the treatment groups. These data suggest that patients with embolic stroke and atrial fibrillation should receive aspirin during the acute phase of the stroke with the initiation of chronic oral anticoagulation between 10 and 14 days.

Treatment of Hyperglycemia

Both animal and human data suggest that postinfarction hyperglycemia increases neuronal damage with an increase in infarct size. These data suggest that hyperglycemia should be treated, with careful monitoring of the serum glucose (hypoglycemia may also extend an infarct). Results of clinical trials in critically ill patients suggest improved outcome with early enteral nutrition. Prevention of hyperglycemia after initiation of feeding is important (see Chapter 31).

Treatment of Temperature

Experimental studies suggest that hypothermia is neuroprotective after focal brain damage. Furthermore, fever has been shown to worsen the prognosis in acute stroke. It is therefore reasonable to treat fever in stroke patients with antipyretics.

Neuroprotective Strategies

It has been hypothesized that the center of the infarct (which is destined for early cell death) is surrounded by an ischemic penumbra of potentially viable neuronal cells and that medical therapies that can salvage this tissue may limit infarct size. In animal stroke models, extensive reductions of infarct volume occur with many different types of neuroprotective drugs. However, over 150 clinical trials have evaluated different medical therapies in an attempt to limit infarct size; none of these studies have detected a reduction in mortality or disability. These therapies have included calcium channel blockers, N–methyl-D–aspartate (NMDA) receptor blockers, glycine-site NMDA-receptor blockers, gamma-aminobutyric acid agonists, (α-amino-3-hydroxy-5-methyl-4-isoxazole), propionic acid antagonists, choline precursors, basic fibroblast growth factor, corticosteroids, tirilazad (a 21 amino steroid), antileukocyte adhesion molecule therapy (anti-ICAM-1), and isovolemic hemodilution, to name but a few.

■ TREATMENT OF POST-STROKE HYPERTENSION

In health, cerebral autoregulation maintains constant cerebral blood flow between a mean systemic arterial pressure of 60 and 120 mm Hg. However, in patients with chronic hypertension, autoregulation is set at a higher level (approximately 120 to 160), presumably to protect the brain from the effects of persistent hypertension. (See

Figure 18-1, Chapter 18.) After a stroke, the normal mechanisms of cerebral autoregulation are impaired. Perfusion in the ischemic penumbra becomes pressure dependent. A rise in systemic arterial pressure may therefore be an adaptive response to maintain the blood flow to this vulnerable area. In a series of 334 patients hospitalized with acute stroke, Wallace and Levy[17] found that >80% had elevated blood pressure on the day of admission. The blood pressures fell spontaneously and gradually over the next 10 days. By the tenth day post-stroke, only one third of patients remained hypertensive. The mechanisms underlying post-stroke hypertension have not been fully elucidated. Activation of the sympathetic nervous system may be involved as part of a global metabolic response to cerebral infarction, cerebral hemorrhage, or associated edema.

There is no evidence that hypertension has a deleterious effect on the outcome of ischemic strokes during the acute phase. Because lowering the blood pressure in patients with cerebral ischemia may adversely reduce cerebral blood flow—which, because of impaired autoregulation, is particularly dependent upon systemic blood pressure—the practice of "normalizing" blood pressure is potentially dangerous. When a proximal arterial obstruction results in a mild stroke, a fall in blood pressure may result in further infarction involving the entire territory of that artery.

The current recommendations of the American Heart Association are that hypertension in the setting of acute ischemic stroke should be treated only "rarely and cautiously." It is generally recommended that antihypertensive therapy be reserved for patients with a diastolic pressure >120 to 130 mm Hg, aiming to reduce the pressure by no more than an arbitrary figure of 20% in the first 24 hours.

There are no data regarding the comparative effects of different antihypertensive drugs on cerebral blood flow (CBF) in ischemic stroke. To prevent a rapid reduction in blood pressure, short-acting intravenous agents are preferred (see Chapter 20). These agents should be administered in an ICU under close blood pressure monitoring. While nitroprusside is commonly used in this situation, this drug increases intracerebral pressure and has a very narrow therapeutic index, particularly in patients with renal dysfunction (cyanide poisoning). Labetalol (an alpha- and beta-blocker) is currently our drug of choice; however, nicardipine or fenoldopam (a selective DA1 agonist) are suitable alternatives. Intravenous or oral angiotensis-converting enzyme inhibitors, oral or sublingual nifedipine and hydralazine should be avoided due to their unpredictable and poorly titratable antihypertensive effect.

Seizure Prophylaxis

The frequency of seizures during the acute period after stroke is reported to be between 4% and 43%. Recurrent seizures occur in approximately 20% to 80% of cases. There are no data concerning the value of prophylactic administration of anticonvulsants after ischemic stroke. Until such data become available, stroke patients who are seizure-free should not receive anticonvulsant drugs.

Supportive Medical Therapy

General measures are aimed at maintaining an adequate cerebral perfusion pressure and preventing complications.

- Maintain euvolemia; hypovolemia will compromise cardiac output and cerebral perfusion, thereby extending the size of the infarct. Avoid hypotonic solutions, which will increase cerebral edema. Stroke patients may develop the "cerebral salt wasting syndrome," which requires aggressive volume replacement.
- Bed rest with elevation of the head to 20 to 35 degrees.
- Laxatives.
- DVT prophylaxis (stockings/pneumatic boots).
- Mild sedation/anxiolysis for agitated patients. In patients who require deeper sedation/hypnosis (e.g., to facilitate mechanical ventilation), propofol is a useful agent. This drug decreases intracranial pressure (ICP) (and CBF proportionately) and allows frequent neurological assessment due to its short duration of action.
- Regular chest physiotherapy and physical therapy.
- Speech and swallowing assessment. The ability of the patient to swallow should be assessed, as abnormalities of swallowing occur in up to 40% of patients.
- In patients with swallowing dysfunction, enteral feeding should be achieved using a small-bore feeding nasoenteric tube. In the majority of patients, swallowing function will recover in 7 to 10 days. Occasionally, prolonged supportive feeding may be required necessitating placement of a gastrostomy/gastrojejunostomy. Glucose should be maintained <150 to 180 mg/dL.
- Fever should be treated with acetaminophen.
- Give aspirin (if no bleed present and no peptic ulcer disease).
- *Corticosteroids have no role* in the management of cerebral edema and ICP after stroke.

■ INTRACEREBRAL HEMORRHAGES

Approximately 15% of all strokes are hemorrhagic. The mortality rate in the first 30 days after ICH is 35% to 50%, with more than half of the deaths occurring in the first 2 days. Clot volume is the most powerful predictor of outcome. Other important variables are baseline neurologic status and intraventricular hemorrhage volume. Although previously thought to be rare, recurrence or extension of ICH recently has been shown to be a relatively common occurrence affecting as many as one third of patients in the early period after ICH. The principles of management of ICH are similar to those of acute ischemic strokes, with a few exceptions.

A urine toxic screen should be obtained as part of the initial evaluation in ICH patients, particularly the young and the normotensive; substances implicated in the causation of ICH include cocaine, amphetamines, methylphenidate, Talwin-pyribenzamine, phencyclidine, and phenylpropanolamine.

The mainstay of medical therapy is aimed at reducing ICP while maintaining cerebral perfusion pressure in the range of 60 to 70 mm Hg. In patients with intracerebral hematomas, there is almost always a secondary rise in ICP and reflex systemic hypertension. Hypertension may serve to protect CBF, because it preserves cerebral perfusion in the face of high ICP. In patients admitted in the first few hours after ICH, systolic blood pressure and diastolic blood pressure average approximately 190 mm Hg and 100 mm Hg, respectively. The natural history of this hypertensive response is for the blood pressure to decrease toward habitual levels over 7 to 10 days, with the greatest decline occurring in the first 24 hours. There is no good evidence that hypertension provokes further bleeding in patients with intracranial hemorrhage. However, a precipitous fall in systemic blood pressure will compromise cerebral perfusion. This problem is exacerbated in patients with chronic hypertension whose lower limits of autoregulation are set at higher levels than normotensive patients. Furthermore, the hematoma impairs the responsiveness of autoregulation in the surrounding area of marginal ischemia. However, severe hypertension can lead to worsening vasogenic edema. The current recommendation is that cautious lowering of the blood pressure should be instituted when the systolic blood pressure is >200 mm Hg or the diastolic is >110 mm Hg. This recommendation is supported by a recent study that demonstrated that rapid decline in blood pressure within the first 24 hours after presentation was associated with increased mortality in patients with ICH. The rate of decline in blood pressure was independently associated with increased mortality. The effect was independent of other variables known to correlate with outcome after ICH, including hematoma volume, initial Glasgow Coma Score, and presence of ventricular blood.

Those patients with ICH while receiving anticoagulant therapy should have emergent correction of the abnormal coagulation parameters to prevent further enlargement of the hematoma. In patients with ICH and mechanical heart valves, temporary interruption of anticoagulation therapy seems safe in patients without previous evidence of systemic embolization. For most patients at risk of cardioembolic stroke, discontinuation of anticoagulation therapy for 1 to 2 weeks should be sufficient to observe the evolution of a parenchymal hematoma (or to clip or coil a ruptured aneurysm, or to evacuate an acute subdural hematoma). Seizure prophylaxis with anticonvulsants is generally recommended for patients with lobar hematomas. Corticosteroids have no place in the management of patients with ICH, being associated with a higher complication rate.

Surgical Interventions

Routine surgical interventions include placing an ICP monitor in patients who have large hemorrhages or performing a ventriculostomy in patients who display evidence of obstructive hydrocephalus. Urgent surgical decompression is indicated in patients with cerebellar hematomas greater than 3 cm in diameter or with brain stem compression. Open craniotomy and decompression of cortical or lobar hemorrhages has been associated with a higher mortality over medical therapy. The role of stereotactic approaches to clot evacuation has yet to be determined.

■ SUBDURAL HEMATOMA

The collection of fresh blood under the dura mater is referred to as an *acute subdural hematoma.* Data from the traumatic Coma Data Bank indicate that 21% of all severely injured patients have subdural hematomas. Subdural hematoma is usually caused by injury to an artery or vein within or over the brain surface. The clinical presentation includes a wide spectrum of neurological findings secondary to either mass effect or direct brain injury. On CT scan, the lesion is seen as a hyperdense extraaxial collection that is crescent shaped. Patients presenting with acute neurological deficits and a CT scan demonstrating an acute subdural hematoma should undergo emergent surgery. Surgical intervention may not be required for patients with small lesions <3 mm thick on CT scan or those who present neurologically after a significant delay.

■ EPIDURAL HEMATOMA

Like subdural hematoma, epidural hematomas are most commonly associated with head trauma, especially in association with skull fractures. They are rarely seen in adults over the age of 60 years, because after this age, the dura adheres tightly to the inner table of the calvarium. The most common locations are temporal and frontal. When identified, the most common source is the middle meningeal artery. The primary therapy for an acute epidural hematoma is surgery, usually urgently. Mannitol, furosemide, and hyperventilation are used when patients deteriorate clinically from an awake state to one of decreased arousal or agitation.

■ MANAGEMENT OF PATIENTS WITH RAISED ICP

Increased ICP may occur in patients who have cerebral hemorrhage, cerebral infarction with associated edema, primary or metastatic brain tumors, encephalitis, or global anoxic or ischemic brain injury, or following traumatic brain injury.

CBF in human brain tissue averages about 50 mL/100 g/min. Irreversible neuronal damage occurs if CBF drops <18 ml/100 gm/min for a prolonged period of time. CBF is equal to the cerebral perfusion pressure (CPP), which is defined as the difference between the mean arterial blood pressure (MAP) and the ICP, divided by the cerebral vascular resistance. Because the CBF is difficult to measure clinically, the CPP is used as a guide to assessing the adequacy of cerebral perfusion. Both the ICP and MAP need to be measured to determine the CPP. The normal ICP is between 0 and 10 mm Hg. While earlier studies and recommendations centered on the importance of ICP per se, current evidence emphasizes the importance of the CPP. The guidelines proposed by the Brain Trauma Foundation recommend that the CPP should be maintained at a minimum of 70 mm Hg. These guidelines use 20 mm Hg as the threshold for intracranial hypertension.

Aggressive hyperventilation ($Paco_2 \leq 25$ mm Hg) has traditionally been considered a cornerstone in the management of raised ICP. Hyperventilation reduces ICP by causing cerebral vasoconstriction with a subsequent reduction in CBF. Hyperventilation results in a fall in ICP; however, this is associated with a significant fall in jugular venous O_2 saturation. In patients with traumatic head injury, hyperventilation has been associated with a significantly worse neurological outcome when compared to patients who were kept normocapnic. Based on these data, chronic hyperventilation is no longer recommended. Initial target Pco_2 should be 35 to 40 mm Hg with avoidance of hyperventilation. Short-term hyperventilation, however, has a role in reducing ICP in patients who are rapidly deteriorating before other measures can be instituted.

Previous guidelines had advocated moderate-to-severe dehydration as a treatment modality for cerebral edema. This was based on the assumption that such interventions would decrease brain water content and ICP. This reasoning was seriously flawed, as experimental studies demonstrated that cerebral edema was not altered by hydration status and failed to recognize the importance of the cerebral perfusion pressure in preventing secondary brain ischemia. Indeed, acute intracranial disease has been associated with a cerebral salt-wasting syndrome characterized by a negative salt balance and a contracted intravascular volume. Fluid restriction therefore exacerbates the underlying volume depletion, leading to an increased risk of cerebral ischemia. Volume resuscitation with isotonic fluids and restoration of a normal intravascular volume are therefore essential in all patients with acute cerebral insults. Small-volume resuscitation with hypertonic saline has been demonstrated to increase CPP, decrease blood viscosity, and reduce ICP in patients following traumatic head injury. However, this approach to fluid resuscitation has not been demonstrated to improve outcome. The role of small-volume hypertonic saline in the management of patients with elevated ICP has still to be determined.

Osmolar therapy with mannitol is often instituted in patients with elevated ICP. Mannitol is a low molecular weight substance, filtered but not reabsorbed by the kidney, which appears to work via two mechanisms. The acute effect of bolus administration is to expand the intravascular volume, thereby decreasing the hematocrit and blood viscosity and producing an increase intracerebral blood flow. The second mechanism is an osmotic dehydration with its clinical effect varying between 90 minutes to >6 hours. The usual dose of mannitol is 0.25 g/kg body weight to 1.0 g/kg body weight with only a slight variation in duration of action based on doses; therefore, smaller doses that decrease the ICP are preferable. Due to its diuretic effect, mannitol therapy may produce intravascular volume depletion, and this must be prevented; fluid replacement is important when using osmolar therapy. In addition, very rapid bolus administration of mannitol can cause hypotension, apparently due to dilation of skeletal muscle vascular beds. Serum osmolarity must be followed serially as increased doses of mannitol are administered and should not exceed 320 mOsm/L, because renal toxicity significantly increases beyond this level.

Brain tissue shifts secondary to compartmental pressure differentials are the most common cause of neurological deterioration with ischemia-induced cerebral edema rather than ICP elevation-induced hypoperfusion. This may explain in part the lack of effectiveness of medical therapies such as osmotic diuretics and hyperventilation in these patients. Both of these therapies have their main effect on the injured brain and may therefore exacerbate the pressure differentials.

■ SELECTED REFERENCES

1. Berge E, Abelnoor M, Nakstad PH, Sandset PM. Low molecular-weight heparin versus aspirin in patients with acute ischaemic stroke

  and atrial fibrillation: a double-blind randomised study. *Lancet.* 2000;
  355:1205–1210.
2. Berrouschot J, Sterker M, Bettin S, Koster J, Schneider D. Mortality of
  space-occupying ("malignant") middle cerebral artery infarction under
  conservative intensive care. *Intensive Care Med.* 1998;24:620–623.
3. Burtin P, Bollaert PE, Feldmann L, et al. Prognosis of stroke patients undergoing mechanical ventilation. *Intensive Care Med.* 1994;20:32–36.
4. Collaborative systematic review of the randomized trials of organized
  inpatient (stroke unit) care after stroke. *BMJ.* 1997;314:1511–1159.
5. Emergency Cardiac Care Committee and Subcommittees, American Heart
  Association. Guidelines for cardiopulmonary resuscitation and emergency
  cardiac care. Part IV, special resuscitation situations: stroke. *JAMA.* 1992;
  268:2242–2244.
6. Guidelines for the management of patients with acute ischemic stroke.
  A statement for healthcare professionals from a special writing group
  of the Stroke Council, American Heart Association. *Circulation.* 1994;
  90:1588–1601.
7. Hacke W, Kaste M, Fieschi C, et al. Randomised double-blind placebo-controlled trial of thrombolytic therapy with intravenous alteplase in acute
  ischaemic stroke (ECASS II). Second European-Australasian Acute Stroke
  Study Investigators. *Lancet.* 1998;352:1245–1251.
8. Intravenous tissue-type plasminogen activator for treatment of acute stroke.
  The Standard Treatment with Alteplase to Reverse Stroke (STARS) Study.
  JAMA. 2000;283:1145–1150.
9. Katzan IL, Furlan AJ, Lloyd LE, et al. Use of tissue-type plasminogen activator for acute ischemic stroke. The Cleveland area experience. *JAMA.*
  2000;283:1151–1158.
10. Low molecular weight heparinoid, ORG 10172 (Danaparoid), and outcome
  after acute ischemic stroke. A randomized controlled trial. *JAMA.* 1998;
  279:1265–1272.
11. Muizelaar JP, Marmarou A, Ward JD, et al. Adverse effects of prolonged
  hyperventilation in patients with severe head injury: a randomized clinical
  trial. *J Neurosurg.* 1991;75:731–739.
12. NINDS rtPA Stroke Study Group. Tissue plasminogen activator for acute
  ischemic stroke. *N Engl J Med.* 1995;333:1581–1587.
13. O'Connell JE, Gray CS. Treatment of post-stroke hypertension. A practical
  guide. *Drugs & Aging.* 1996;8:408–415.
14. Poungvarin N, Bhoopat W, Viriyavejakul, et al. Effects of dexamethasone
  in primary supratentorial intracerebral hemorrhage. *N Engl J Med.* 1987;
  316:1229–1233.
15. Qureshi AI, Bliwise DL, Bliwise NG, et al. Rate of 24-hour blood pressure
  decline and mortality after spontaneous intracerebral hemorrhage: a retrospective analysis with a random effects regression model. *Crit Care Med.*
  1999;27:480–485.
16. The International Stroke Trial (IST): a randomised trial of aspirin, subcutaneous heparin, both, or neither among 19,435 patients with acute
  ischaemic stroke. *Lancet.* 1997;349:1569–1581.
17. Wallace JD, Levy LL. Blood pressure after stroke. *JAMA.* 1981;246:
  2177–2180.

Aneurysmal Subarachnoid Hemorrhage

Subarachnoid hemorrhage (SAH) is a common and devastating condition. Each year approximately 30,000 Americans suffer from a nontraumatic SAH. Patients who have suffered an SAH are best managed in an ICU or a specialized neurology/neurosurgical unit. Despite improved management, the outcome following SAH remains poor; with an overall mortality of approximately 25% and significant morbidity among the survivors. The most serious complications following the initial bleed are rebleeding and cerebral vasospasm; management of patients with SAH is therefore largely directed to avoiding these complications. The risk of rebleeding (with conservative therapy) is highest in the first month, with a rate of between 20% and 30%. The mortality rate is approximately 70% for patients who rebled. Angiographic vasospasm probably develops to some degree in most patients who suffer a SAH. However, clinically manifest vasospasm occurs in approximately 40% of patients. From 15% to 20% of these patients will suffer a stroke or die despite aggressive management.

■ DIAGNOSIS AND EVALUATION

Computed Tomography Scan and Lumbar Puncture

Noncontrast computed tomography (CT) scanning is the diagnostic test of choice following a suspected SAH. If the scan is performed within 24 hours of the event, clot can be demonstrated in the subarachnoid space in approximately 90% of patients. The diagnostic sensitivity of the CT scan declines after the first day. A diagnostic lumbar puncture should be performed in a patient with a suspected SAH if the initial CT scan is negative. A normal CT scan and a normal spinal fluid examination excludes a SAH and predicts a favorable prognosis in the setting of the sudden onset of a severe headache. The role of magnetic resonance imaging/magnetic resonance angiography in the diagnostic evaluation of SAH remains to be determined.

Clinical Classification

The Hunt and Hess Classification system is the most commonly used grading system to assess the severity of a SAH. The Hunt and Hess grade has important therapeutic and prognostic implications.

Hunt and Hess Classification

  I Asymptomatic or slight headache
 II Moderate-to-severe headache, nuchal rigidity, no neurological deficit other than cranial nerve palsy
III Drowsiness, confusion, or mild focal deficit
 IV Stupor, moderate-to-severe hemiparesis
  V Deep coma, decerebrate rigidity

Cerebral Angiography

Selective catheter angiography is currently the standard for diagnosing cerebral aneurysms as the cause of SAH. Approximately 20% to 25% of cerebral angiograms performed for SAH will not indicate a source of bleeding. It is generally recommended to repeat the angiogram in 2 weeks, because vascular spasm may have obscured the aneurysm. However, only a very small percentage of repeat angiograms will demonstrate an aneurysm. The risk of rebleeding in patients with normal angiograms is low; <4% are reported to rebleed when followed for up to 10 years.

■ INITIAL MANAGEMENT

General measures

- Bed rest with elevation of the head to 20 to 35 degrees
- Mild sedation/anxiolysis for grade I and II patients
- Pain management with morphine sulphate or codeine. Meperidine should be avoided, as it can precipitate seizures.
- Maintain *euvolemia*; dehydration reduces preload, cardiac output, and cerebral perfusion, thereby increasing the risk of cerebral infarction.
- Laxatives.

- Deep venous thrombosis prophylaxis (stockings/pneumatic boots)
- Nimodipine 60 mg q4–6 h, for prevention of cerebral vasospasm
- Ventriculostomy for acute obstructive hydrocephalus
- Although seizure prophylaxis has not been proven to be beneficial, this therapy is generally recommended because of the risk of rebleeding with a seizure. Long-term anticonvulsants are not routinely recommended for patients with no seizure episodes.
- The role of antifibrinolytic agent in preventing rebleeding is unclear. Antifibrinolytic agents, however, have been associated with a higher incidence of cerebral infarction. As a consequence of the trend toward earlier surgery, this form of therapy is no longer recommended.
- Early clinical studies suggest that tirilazad mesylate (a non-glucocorticoid 21-aminosteroid) appears to improve the overall outcome of patients following a SAH. Further studies are required to confirm this observation.

Antihypertensive Agents

The role of antihypertensive agents in preventing rebleeding is controversial. Rebleeding may be related to variations or changes in blood pressure rather than the absolute blood pressure. However, it is generally advised that the systolic pressure be kept <150 mm Hg. Mild sedation and control of pain may adequately control an elevated blood pressure. If antihypertensive agents are used, these should be used with extreme caution. Intravenous agents that can be closely titrated are preferred; an excessive reduction of blood pressure may cause cerebral ischemia. The use of oral or sublingual nifedipine is strongly discouraged. Although nitroprusside is a very short-acting, easily titratable antihypertensive agent, it has been shown to increase intracerebral pressure. Furthermore, doses in excess of 2 mg/min will lead to cyanide accumulation. Intravenous labetalol is the preferred agent; however, intravenous nicardipine can also be used.

Management of Raised Intracranial Pressure

Management of Suspected or Confirmed Intracanial Pressure

(See Chapter 36, "Management of Patients With Raised ICP.")

■ SURGERY

Surgical clipping of the neck of the aneurysm to prevent recurrent bleeding remains the cornerstone of the management of patients with

SAH. Data from many studies strongly suggest that surgical clipping reduces the risk of rebleeding. The timing of surgery is significantly related to the likelihood of preoperative rebleeding. However, the complexity of the aneurysm, the difficulty of the surgical approach, and the clinical grade of the patient influence the timing of surgery. Preliminary studies suggest that intraoperative administration of intracisternal tissue plasminogen activator may reduce the risk of delayed cerebral vasospasm. The risk of rebleeding following incompletely clipped aneurysms is approximately 8%. It is therefore recommended that postoperative angiography be performed in most patients.

■ MANAGEMENT OF CEREBRAL VASOSPASM

Angiographic vasospasm has a typical temporal course, with onset 3 to 5 days after the hemorrhage, maximal narrowing at 5 to 14 days, and gradual resolution over 2 to 4 weeks. Cerebral vasospasm is usually diagnosed by changes in mental status 3 to 10 days after the bleed, not due to another neurological complication and confirmed by angiography or transcranial Doppler imaging.

"Hypervolemic" hemodilution and/or induced arterial hypertension have been shown to be of benefit in uncontrolled reports. However, *hypervolemia* is somewhat of a misnomer. In a patient with normal cardiac and renal function, it is not possible to induce a state of hypervolemia; the excess fluid is just "peed out." In patients with underlying cardiac or renal disease, this approach will lead to pulmonary edema (the intravascular and interstitial compartments are in a dynamic equilibrium). There is no correlation between the central venous pressure (CVP) and intravascular volume; titrating volume replacement to a predetermined CVP is dangerous and is strongly discouraged. Pulmonary artery catheterization is indicated in patients with underlying cardiac disease. The aim of fluid therapy should be to keep the patient well hydrated.

Vasoactive agents are used to increase the cerebral perfusion pressure. Dopamine and/or norepinephrine may achieve this goal. The systolic blood pressure should be kept between 160 and 200 mm Hg (120 to 150 for unclipped aneurysms) and titrated to the patient's neurological state. Dopamine should be used cautiously in patients with cardiac disease. Phenylephrine tends to decrease cardiac output (and therefore cerebral blood flow) and should therefore be avoided. The patient should be closely monitored, and serial transcranial Dopplers performed to monitor the progress of the patient's condition.

Angioplasty of the implicated vessel, high-dose intravenous nicardipine, and intra-arterial papaverine have been reported in patients with vasospasm. The role of these therapeutic interventions remains to be determined.

■ SELECTED REFERENCES

1. Allen G, Ahn H, Preziosi T, et al. Cerebral arterial spasm: a controlled trial of nimodipine in patients with subarachnoid hemorrhage. *N Engl J Med.* 1983;308:619–624.
2. Awad IA, Carter P, Spetzler RF, et al. Clinical vasospasm after subarachnoid hemorrhage: response to hypervolemic hemodilution and arterial hypertension. *Stroke.* 1987;18:365–372.
3. Findlay JM, Kassell NF, Weir BK, et al. A randomized trial of intraoperative, intracisternal tissue plasminogen activator for the prevention of vasospasm. *Neurosurgery.* 1995;37:168–176.
4. Hawkins TD, Sims C, Hanka R. Subarachnoid hemorrhage of unknown cause: a long-term follow-up. *J Neurol Neurosurg Psychiatry.* 1989:52:230–232.
5. Kassell NF, Torner JC, Jane JA, et al. The international cooperative study on the timing of aneurysm surgery, I: overall management results. *J Neurosurg.* 1990;73:18–36.
6. Kassel NF, Haley EC, Apperson-Hansen C, et al. Randomized, double-blind, vehicle-controlled trial of tirilazad mesylate in patients with aneurysmal subarachnoid hemorrhage: a cooperative study in Europe, Australia, and New Zealand. *J Neurosurg.* 1996;84:221–228.
7. Vermeulen M, Lindsay KW, Murray GD, et al. Antifibrinolytic treatment of subarachnoid hemorrhage. *N Engl J Med.* 1984;311:432–437.
8. Wijdicks EFM, Vermeulin M, Hijdra A, van Gijn J. Hyponatremia and cerebral infarction in patients with ruptured intracranial aneurysms: is fluid restriction harmful? *Ann Neurol.* 1985;17:137–140.

38

Neurological and Neuromuscular Complications of Systemic Critical Illness

Neurological complications of acute systemic illnesses involve both central and peripheral parts of the nervous system and contribute to mortality and morbidity. Acute encephalopathy is the most common neurological complication in ICU patients. In addition, a variety of neuromuscular disorders have been described in critically ill patients, including a sensorimotor axonal polyneuropathy (critical illness polyneuropathy), disuse atrophy, steroid-induced myopathy, persistent neuromuscular blockage following the use of neuromuscular blocking agents, and an acute necrotizing myopathy in patients concomitantly receiving a neuromuscular blocking agent and corticosteroids. Some authors have used the term *ICU/critical illness myopathy* to describe the myopathy found in ICU patients. However, as there may be different forms of this condition, I prefer to classify these disorders according to the associated features and inciting factors. It is often extremely difficult to distinguish these disorders from each other on purely clinical grounds, although certain clues may make one more likely. Nerve conduction studies, needle electromyography, and muscle biopsy are often necessary to make a firm diagnosis.

■ SEPTIC ENCEPHALOPATHY

Septic encephalopathy usually is an acute, reversible, generalized disturbance in cerebral function, initially manifested by alteration in attention and alertness, in the presence of sepsis. It is essentially a diagnosis by exclusion, as many factors such as sedative drugs, encephalitis, liver or renal failure, hypoperfusion, fever, adrenal insufficiency, cerebral vascular accidents, and drug fever either alone or in combination may result in disturbed cerebral function.

■ CRITICAL ILLNESS NEUROPATHY

As initially described by Bolton et al. in 1984, critical illness neuropathy is a sensorimotor polyneuropathy that is often a complication of sepsis and multiorgan failure, occurring in 70% of such patients. The severity of the underlying illness, the frequently associated encephalopathy, and the use of nondepolarizing neuromuscular blocking agents and ventilator support make recognition of the onset of the neuropathy difficult. It usually becomes apparent when the patient cannot be weaned from the ventilator. Flaccid weakness of the extremities, often severe, and loss of tendon reflexes are associated findings.

Critical illness polyneuropathy is characterized clinically by reduced ventilatory effort, hyporeflexia, or areflexia. Patients have distal greater than proximal weakness. Creatinine kinase may be normal or slightly elevated, but it is not as high as in a myopathy.

Critical illness polyneuropathy is primarily a distal axonopathy in which distal degeneration of both motor and sensory axons, without inflammation, occurs. The underlying cause of the axonal degeneration may relate to a lack of vascular autoregulation and increased microvascular permeability resulting in endoneurial edema and capillary occlusion. Electrophysiological studies show reduction or absence of both compound muscle and sensory nerve action potentials, fibrillations, and loss of motor unit potentials with a maximal effort. Significant slowing of nerve conduction or nerve conduction blocks are not expected findings and, if present, would implicate other diagnostic possibilities, e.g., Guillain-Barré syndrome. Reduction of diaphragmatic compound muscle action potentials and the presence of fibrillations of chest wall muscles reflect the weaning difficulties.

Multiorgan failure, sepsis, and critical illness polyneuropathy have a mortality rate of 50%. The neuropathy shows spontaneous improvement, with resolution of the underlying illness, but recovery may be limited or absent when the neuropathy is severe. Physical therapy is the only effective rehabilitation therapy available. In general, most of the patients who survive the septic event will recover from the polyneuropathy. However, some patients do not recover; in others the recovery may take years.

■ STEROID MYOPATHY

Steroid myopathy is characterized by a subacute onset of proximal muscle weakness, with atrophy of primarily type 2 fibers on muscle biopsy.

■ NECROTIZING MYOPATHY ASSOCIATED WITH THE USE OF NONDEPOLARIZING BLOCKING AGENTS AND CORTICOSTEROIDS

Neuromuscular junction blocking agents have historically been used in the operating room to augment surgical anesthesia, where they have been found to be remarkably safe. These agents have, however, found their way into ICUs, where they are being used with increasing frequency, and for prolonged periods of time, to facilitate mechanical ventilation. The safety of these drugs has, however, been questioned, due to the increasing number of case reports of prolonged paralysis following their use. In particular, the concomitant use of steroid-based nondepolarizing neuromuscular blocking agents and high-dose corticosteroids has been linked to the syndrome variously known as *acute quadriplegic myopathy*, *acute necrotizing myopathy*, and *thick-filament myopathy*.

The necrotizing myopathy associated with neuromuscular blocking agents is characterized histologically by focal necrosis, degenerative changes, fiber atrophy, and evidence of regeneration, with predominant involvement of the type 1 muscle fiber. Electron microscopy shows extensive myofibribolysis, especially of the thick myofilaments. This syndrome has been reported following the use of vecuronium, pancuronium, and recently atracurium; however, muscle biopsies were not performed in all reported cases. The pathogenetic mechanisms of this neuromuscular disorder are poorly understood. Most of the patients described thus far have received concomitant corticosteroids. However, multiple other factors including electrolyte imbalances (especially hypermagnesemia), acidosis, hypothermia, and aminoglycoside antibiotics may have contributed to the development of this syndrome in these cases. The combination of a neuromuscular blocking agent and corticosteroids should be avoided (see Chapter 48).

■ NEUROMUSCULAR BLOCKADE

Persistent blockade of the neuromuscular junction may occur, particularly in patients with renal and/or hepatic failure, due to the accumulation of the neuromuscular blocking agent and/or its active metabolites.

■ CRITICAL ILLNESS MYOPATHY

A number of authors have described an entity called *critical illness myopathy*. However, it is unclear whether this disorder is a separate clinical entity that can occur in the absence of high-dose intravenous steroids.

39

Management of Traumatic Brain Injury

The annual incidence of traumatic brain injury (TBI) in the United States has been estimated to range from 132 to 367 per 100,000 population per year, with approximately 120,000 severe head injuries (initial Glasgow Coma Score <9) per year. Of the patients with severe head injury, approximately 50% will die before reaching the hospital. Of the estimated 60,000 patients who present to emergency departments, more than 50% of these will have intracranial hypertension at or soon after arrival. Since direct correlations have been reported between increased intracranial pressure (ICP) and adverse outcome, it is important that physicians be able to rapidly identify and treat these patients. It should be emphasized that the management of TBI is complex and will involve early multidisciplinary management.

Cerebral blood flow (CBF) in human brain tissue averages about 50 mL/100 g/min. Irreversible neuronal damage occurs if CBF drops <18 mL/100 g/min for a prolonged period of time. CBF is equal to the cerebral perfusion pressure (CPP), which is defined as the difference between the mean arterial blood pressure (MAP) and the ICP, divided by the cerebral vascular resistance. Because the CBF is difficult to measure clinically, the CPP is used as a guide to assess the adequacy of cerebral perfusion. Both the ICP and MAP need to be measured to determine the CPP. The normal ICP is between 0 and 10 mm Hg. Increased ICP has been defined as a pressure >20 mm Hg persisting for 5 minutes or more. Normal human values for CPP are between 70 and 100 mm Hg.

Since the actual brain damage that occurs at the time of injury cannot be modified, the maximization of neurological recovery depends upon minimizing secondary insults to the brain. As a result of metabolic and molecular derangements and diminished autoregulation, the traumatized brain is particularly vulnerable to ischemia. In patients who have died from head injury, post-traumatic ischemic lesions have been reported in up to 80% of patients at postmortem. The prevention of cerebral ischemia is considered the most important goal in the management of the patients following TBI.

■ ENDOTRACHEAL INTUBATION

The main objective of management is to maintain adequate cerebral perfusion and oxygenation. Patients with TBI who are unable to protect their airway should be intubated early. Precautions in intubation need to be taken in the patient with an uncleared cervical spine, because the incidence of concomitant spine injury in head injury patients ranges from 6% to 8%. Patients with suspected or confirmed cervical spine injuries should be intubated with extreme caution, with every effort taken to avoid hyperextension of the neck. Intubation may be performed by either the oral or nasal route, preferably by an experienced intubator. It has been taught that patients with a suspected or proven basal skull fracture should not be intubated nasally, due to the possibility of intracranial placement of the endotracheal tube. However, recent studies indicate that this complication is exceedingly rare and probably related to poor technique.

The only way to effectively prevent the increases in ICP associated with gagging and coughing during intubation is to chemically paralyze the patient. This, however, precludes nasotracheal intubation. When the orotracheal route is used, the intubator's assistant must provide in-line traction to prevent excessive extension of the neck. Intubation can also be achieved using a flexible bronchoscope/laryngoscope (by those experienced with the technique). Although these patients' mental status may be depressed, they are not anesthetized. Significant increases in ICP may occur with airway stimulation associated with laryngoscopy and intubation. Rapid-sequence induction anesthesia is therefore always required. Hypnotic agents that reduce vascular tone may result in profound postintubation hypotension, particularly in patients who have received inadequate volume resuscitation. Extreme care must be taken to avoid these profound fluctuations in blood pressure and ICP during endotracheal intubation.

The use of induction agents and muscle relaxants to optimize airway management has been found to be safe and effective in patients with TBI. Traditionally, this has been accomplished with sodium thiopental (3 to 5 mg/kg) and succinylcholine (1 to 2 mg/kg), though newer alternatives such as etomidate (0.2 to 0.4 mg/kg) and rocuronium (0.6 to 1.2 mg/kg) may have added benefits. Etomidate is a carboxylated imidazole hypnotic agent that has a rapid and predictable onset of action with a short duration of action. Like sodium thiopental, etomidate reduces ICP by decreasing the cerebral meta-

bolic rate for oxygen and CBF. The most distinctive property of etomidate as compared with other rapid-acting agents is its minimal
effect on cardiovascular parameters. Succinylcholine has a number of
potential disadvantages in head-injured patients including increased
ICP, increased CBF, and abnormal potassium release. Rocuronium is
a steroidal nondepolarizing muscle relaxant, which in a dose of 0.9 to
1.2 mg/kg has a duration of onset similar to succinylcholine. Rocuronium is devoid of significant hemodynamic effects and exhibits no
untoward effects on intracranial dynamics. Esmolol (a short-acting
beta-blocker) and fentanyl (50 to 100 μg) are used during rapid-
sequence intubation to attenuate the sympathetic response.

■ INITIAL MANAGEMENT (SEE ALSO CHAPTER 36, "MANAGEMENT OF PATIENTS WITH RAISED ICP")

Once the patient is intubated, the patient should be placed on 100%
oxygen, with the inspired fraction of oxygen only titrated down once
the patient has been transferred to the ICU and invasive monitoring
initiated. Aggressive hyperventilation ($Paco_2 \leq 25$ mm Hg) has traditionally been considered a cornerstone in the management of severe
TBI because it causes a rapid reduction in ICP. Hyperventilation
reduces ICP by causing cerebral vasoconstriction with a subsequent
reduction in CBF. This, however, is associated with a significant fall in
jugular venous O_2 saturation. In 1991, Muizelaar and colleagues published the results of a prospective randomized clinical study in which
they demonstrated that hyperventilation post head injury was associated with a significantly worse neurological outcome when compared
to patients who were kept normocapnic. Based on these data, chronic
hyperventilation is no longer recommended. Initial target Pco_2 should
be 35 to 40 mm Hg with avoidance of hyperventilation. Short-term
hyperventilation, however, has a role in reducing ICP in patients who
are rapidly deteriorating before other measures can be instituted.

While earlier studies and recommendations centered on the importance of ICP per se, current evidence emphasizes the importance of
the CPP. The guidelines proposed by the Brain Trauma Foundation
recommend that the CPP should be maintained at a minimum of
70 mm Hg. After the establishment of an airway and ventilation, the
restoration of blood pressure and normal circulating volume is of
utmost importance. According to the Brain Trauma Foundation guidelines for the management of severe head injury, a MAP of ≥90 mm Hg
should be targeted; this was chosen based on attaining cerebral perfusion pressures >70 mm Hg. These guidelines use 20 mm Hg as the
threshold for intracranial hypertension.

Previous guidelines had advocated moderate-to-severe dehydration as a treatment modality for cerebral edema. This was based on the assumption that such interventions would decrease brain water content and ICP. This reasoning was seriously flawed, as experimental studies demonstrated that cerebral edema was not altered by hydration status and failed to recognize the importance of the cerebral perfusion pressure in preventing secondary brain ischemia. Indeed, acute intracranial disease has been associated with a cerebral salt wasting syndrome characterized by a negative salt balance and a contracted intravascular volume. Fluid restriction therefore exacerbates the underlying volume depletion, leading to an increased risk of cerebral ischemia. Volume resuscitation with restoration of a normal intravascular volume is therefore essential in all patients with acute cerebral insults.

As for the type of fluid (crystalloid vs. colloid) with which to resuscitate, controversy continues to exist. Hypotonic solutions should not be administered due to the increased permeability of the blood–brain barrier after head trauma. Hypertonic saline (7.5% saline) has been shown to be beneficial in a subset of head injury patients due to improved hemodynamic parameters. Hypertonic salt solutions restore blood pressure and cardiac output by having a positive inotropic effect and by extracting water from the intracellular space to restore intravascular losses. However, the indications as well as optimal timing and volume of hypertonic saline need to be determined in prospective clinical studies.

Due to the extreme sensitivity of the brain to even transient episodes of hypotension, the initiation of vasopressors is recommended as temporizing or supplementary measures to fluid resuscitation. Dopamine or norepinephrine may be used in this situation. While phenylephrine will increase blood pressure, it will usually lower cardiac output and hence CBF. Disadvantages of pressor therapy include difficulty in determining adequacy of intravascular volume resuscitation due to the increased systemic vascular resistance. While the data suggest that a decline in blood pressure should be avoided in the head-injured patient, even when the baseline blood pressure is high, induced hypertension may either increase or decrease ICP, depending on the cerebral circulation's ability to autoregulate. Induced hypertension with vasopressor agents should, therefore, be used with extreme caution and only with very close monitoring.

After adequate resuscitation, the initial therapy for increased ICP is sedation and analgesia. Even though patients may appear comatose, they still respond to painful and noxious stimuli, often with an increase in ICP and blood pressure. Most frequently, narcotics (morphine or fentanyl) should be considered first-line therapy, since they provide both analgesia and depression of airway reflexes, which are required in the intubated patient. Fentanyl has the advantage of having minimal hemodynamic effects. Propofol is the hypnotic agent of choice in patients with an acute neurological insult, as it is easily titratable and rapidly reversible once discontinued. These properties permit predictable sedation yet also permit periodic neurological examination.

Muscle relaxation (paralysis) with various agents, commonly vecuronium or rocuronium, will avoid patient asynchrony with the ventilator. The major drawback of muscle relaxation is the difficulty in assessing the neurologic examination and following the clinical progression, limiting it to pupillary changes and radiologic imaging studies such as computed tomography (CT) and magnetic resonance imaging (MRI) scans. The benefit of neuromuscular-blocking drugs in patients with TBI has recently been challenged. However, as it may take up to 30 minutes to carefully load a patient with sufficient sedation and analgesia to control airway reflexes in response to mechanical ventilation, early paralysis is important in preventing ventilator dyssynchrony with gagging and coughing, which produce ICP surges. Once the patient has been stabilized and adequate sedation and analgesia achieved, the neuromuscular blocker may be stopped. The use of a propofol infusion (titrated to deep sedation), together with fentanyl may obviate the need for paralysis.

Other general principles in the management of intracranial hypertension that should never be overlooked include lowering the body temperature of patients with fever, elevation of the head of the bed up to 30 degrees, prevention of jugular venous outflow obstruction (keeping the patient's head midline, avoiding extrinsic compression of the jugular veins by hematomas, masses), adequate arterial oxygenation, and seizure prophylaxis. While some studies have suggested that patients be nursed flat, Feldman and colleagues have demonstrated that head elevation to 30 degrees significantly reduced ICP in the majority of patients without reducing CPP or CBF.

Seizure prophylaxis is frequently overlooked in the head-injured patient. The cerebral metabolic rate of oxygen increases by 200% to 300% with seizure activity, and in the presence of TBI, this increased metabolic rate will not be met with sufficient increase in blood flow to prevent ischemia. Seizure prophylaxis is currently recommended for 7 days following the injury in patients with severe TBI. The agent most commonly recommended is phenytoin; loading dose of 18 mg/kg and usual maintenance dose of 5 mg/kg/day following serum drug levels to a goal of 10 to 20 mg/L. However, in contrast to short-term prophylaxis of seizures, there is no evidence that long-term prophylaxis is effective.

If, despite adequate resuscitation and sedation, the patient continues to have evidence of increased ICP, osmolar therapy with mannitol should be initiated. Mannitol therapy may be instituted before ICP monitoring if signs of transtentorial herniation are present or neurological deterioration not attributable to systemic pathology is evident. Mannitol is a low-molecular-weight substance, filtered but not reabsorbed by the kidney, which appears to work via two mechanisms. The acute effect of bolus administration is to expand the intravascular volume, thereby decreasing the hematocrit and blood viscosity and producing an increase in CBF. The second mechanism is an osmotic dehydration, with its clinical effect varying between 90 minutes to >6 hours. The usual dose of mannitol is 0.25 g/kg body weight to 1.0 g/kg body weight, with only a slight variation in duration of action based on doses; therefore, smaller doses that decrease the ICP are preferable. Due to its diuretic effect, mannitol therapy may produce dehydration, and this must be prevented; fluid replacement is important when using osmolar therapy. In addition, very rapid bolus administration of mannitol can cause hypotension, apparently due to dilation of skeletal muscle vascular beds. Serum osmolarity must be followed serially as increased doses of mannitol are administered and should not exceed 320 mOsm/L, because renal toxicity significantly increases beyond this level. The use of loop diuretics, such as furosemide, along with mannitol has been advocated by some due to its synergistic effect. The combination may reduce the ICP to a greater extent as well as for greater duration, though little data support this. This combination may, however, result in severe intravascular depletion.

The use of corticosteroids for increased ICP has only been efficacious in cerebral edema associated with tumors. In head injuries, steroids have been shown to lack efficacy and carry the risks of potential side effects (i.e., hyperglycemia, increased risk of infections), and their use must be avoided. Multiple other modalities are currently under investigation for the treatment of intracranial hypertension including oxygen radical scavengers, calcium channel blockers, and excitatory amino acid receptor blockade. None of the above therapies are currently recommended.

■ FURTHER MANAGEMENT IN THE INTENSIVE CARE UNIT

Once the patient is stabilized and has been transferred to the ICU, the establishment of physiologic monitoring (arterial line, pulmonary artery catheter, ICP monitoring) facilitates and directs the further management of these patients. The role of ICP monitoring in patients with TBI is, however, controversial. No randomized controlled studies have been performed (or are likely to be performed) demonstrating that ICP monitoring improves outcome. However, ICP monitoring has become an integral part of the management of patients with severe TBI in virtually all trauma centers in the United States. The improved outcome of patients with severe TBI in the United States has been ascribed to intensive management protocols that include ICP monitoring. Furthermore, several studies have shown that under conditions of aggressive ICP management, the probability of a good outcome is inversely proportional to the maximum ICP and the percentage of the time spent at levels of >20 mm Hg.

Invasive ICP-monitoring devices provide the most accurate, reliable information for clinical determination of ICP. ICP monitoring should be instituted in patients with Glasgow Coma Score <8, since intracranial hypertension in this population >60%. Currently available methods include extradural, subdural, intraparenchymal, and intraventricular catheters. Extradural measurement of ICP is frequently unreliable and should not be used; ICP measurements from subdural, intraparenchymal, or ventricular sites within a compartment are essentially equivalent. A general principle that must be remembered when inserting ICP monitors is that of compartmentalization. This occurs due to blockage of cerebrospinal fluid by mass lesions with resultant pressure gradients. Once compartmentalization occurs, ICP measured in another nonfluid coupled compartment may not reflect the one with the mass lesion, often underestimating the ICP. Therefore, ICP monitoring should be performed, whenever possible, within the compartment of interest on the ipsilateral side of the lesion, if a supratentorial mass is present. Among current techniques, the ventricular catheter and fiberoptic pressure devices are preferable. Ventricular catheterization remains the most invasive method of determining ICP and carries the highest incidence of serious risk (e.g., hemorrhage, infection), ranging between 5% and 10% total complication rate in university teaching hospitals. Advantages of the ventricular catheter include the ability to externally drain cerebrospinal fluid as a therapeutic maneuver. The role of continuous monitoring of jugular venous oxygen (JVo_2) saturation in the head-injured patient is unclear. Episodes of JVo_2 desaturation may reflect cerebral ischemia. However, Cruz has demonstrated that early JVo_2 desaturation may represent high cerebral extraction of oxygen and indicate cerebral viability rather than cerebral ischemia.

Throughout the course of therapy for intracranial hypertension, suspicion must be maintained for a surgical mass or intracranial lesion. If intractable ICP occurs or the ICP becomes unresponsive to escalating therapy, repeat imaging (CT or MRI) should be considered immediately. Signs of brain swelling appear in 70% of patients within 1 hour post injury with an increase at 2 hours to 87% of patients; the severity of swelling decreases after 48 hours. Especially early in the course of head injury, any neurological deterioration or worsening mental status should warrant the consideration of repeat CT imaging. Once sustained elevations of ICP are noted and no localized intracranial lesions (i.e., epidural, subdural, contusion) are found, generalized brain edema should be suspected.

For intracranial hypertension refractory to therapy, second-tier therapies should be considered, including barbiturate coma, hypothermia, and hypertensive therapy. In animal models, hypothermia has been shown to reduce neuronal loss in ischemic head injury and improve behavioral outcome. Recently, Marion and colleagues have demonstrated that moderate hypothermia (33°C) for 24 hours in patients with severe TBI hastened neurological recovery and may have improved outcome. Barbiturate coma should be consideration in hemodynamically stable, salvageable patients with severe head injury with intracranial hypertension refractory to maximal medical and surgical ICP-lowering therapy. Barbiturates have been shown to lower ICP when other treatments have failed and have improved outcomes. On the other hand, the prophylactic use of barbiturates has not been demonstrated to be of benefit, and such therapy increases the incidence of hypotension. A variety of dosage regimens have been proposed, ranging from 3 to 10 mg/kg pentobarbital given over 0.5 to 3 hours. Maintenance infusions of 0.5 to 3 mg/kg/h have been suggested. Monitoring of serum pentobarbital levels is recommended; therapeutic levels are between 2.5 and 4 mg/dL, though electroencephalographic evidence of "burst suppression" is the goal of therapy. When burst suppression is seen on electroencephalogram, near-maximal CBF and metabolism reduction have occurred. Patients in barbiturate coma usually have small reactive pupils with cessation of all motor function, requiring full ventilatory support. Consequently, barbiturate coma requires vigilant monitoring for cardiovascular complications. The incidence of ventilator-associated pneumonia is increased, possibly due to suppression of ciliary action.

■ SELECTED REFERENCES

1. Bullock R, Chestnut R, Clifton G, Ghajar J, Marion DW, Narayan RK. *Guidelines for the Management of Severe Head Injury*. New York: Brain Trauma Foundation; 1996.
2. Cruz J. Relationship between early patterns of cerebral extraction of oxygen and outcome from severe acute traumatic brain swelling: cerebral ischemia or cerebral viability? *Crit Care Med*. 1996;24:953–956.
3. Feldman Z, Kanter MJ, Robertson CS, et al. Effect of head elevation on intracranial pressure, cerebral perfusion pressure, and cerebral blood flow in head-injured patients. *J Neurosurg*. 1992;76:207–211.
4. Harrigan MR. Cerebral salt wasting syndrome: A review. *Neurosurgery*. 1996;38:152–160.
5. Marion DW, Penrod LE, Kelsey SF, et al. Treatment of traumatic brain injury with moderate hypothermia. *N Engl J Med*. 1997;336:540–546.
6. Marmarou A, Anderson RL, Ward JD. Impact of ICP instability and hypotension on outcome in patients with severe head trauma. *J Neurosurg*. 1991; 75:S59–S66.

7. Muizelaar JP, Marmarou A, Ward JD, et al. Adverse effects of prolonged hyperventilation in patients with severe head injury: a randomized clinical trial. *J Neurosurg*. 1991;75:731–739.

8. Temkin NR, Dikmen SS, Wilensky AJ, et al. A randomized, double-blind study of phenytoin for the prevention of post-traumatic seizures. *N Engl J Med*. 1990;323:497–502.

40

Seizures and Status Epilepticus

Status epilepticus (SE) is a term used to describe continuous seizures lasting at least 5 minutes or two or more discrete seizures between which there is incomplete recovery of consciousness. Some patients have no observable, repetitive motor activity, and the detection of ongoing seizures requires electroencephalography. Convulsive SE has many complications including hypertension, cardiac arrhythmias, hyperthermia, vomiting with aspiration, hyperglycemia, metabolic acidosis, injuries including vertebral and other fractures, and rhabdomyolysis with renal failure. Mortality caused by SE itself is approximately 2%; however, the overall mortality is approximately 30%, owing to the illness causing SE.

■ THE EMERGENCY EVALUATION OF PATIENTS WITH A SEIZURE

Is the patient experiencing a seizure?

Differential Diagnosis

- Syncope
- Transient ischemic attack
- Migraine with aura
- Movement disorder

Is there an acute condition precipitating the seizure?

- Central nervous system infection; bacterial meningitis, abscess, viral encephalitis

- Head trauma
- Alcohol withdrawal
- Anticonvulsant withdrawal
- Drugs including tricyclic antidepressants overdose (OD), penicillins, isoniazid (INH), metronidazole, acyclovir, methylxanthines, phenothiazines, meperidine, cocaine, amphetamines
- Cerebrovascular event
- Metabolic abnormality; hypoglycemia, hyponatremia, hypocalcemia
- Special considerations: human immunodeficiency virus, renal failure, pregnancy

If no acute precipitant, is there a chronic or remote precipitant?

- Previous head injury, cerebrovascular accident, central nervous system infection

Initial Management of Patients With SE

- History and focused examination
- Chemistry panel, glucose, urine toxicology screen, anticonvulsant drug levels
- Computed tomography of the head followed by lumbar puncture

■ GUIDELINES FOR THE TREATMENT OF SE

(Figure 40-1)

- Establish an intravenous line with saline, and give 100mg thiamine and glucose (50mL of 50%).
- Give supplemental oxygen by nasal cannula or mask.
- The VA Cooperative SE trial established that lorazepam is the agent of choice for terminating SE. An initial dose of 0.1mg/kg in adults, repeated as necessary is recommended.
- Treat hyperthermia with passive cooling.
- Screen patient for presence of rhabdomyolysis, i.e., myoglobinuria and creatine phosphokinase (CPK). If CPK > 3000, consider instituting saline diuresis and urinary alkalinization (see Chapter 32).
- Once the seizure activity is controlled, endotracheal intubation is often required for airway protection. Do not try to intubate a patient actively seizing. A muscle relaxant may be required to optimize airway management in patients with ongoing seizures. Succinylcholine has a number of potential disadvantages including abnormal potassium release. Rocuronium is a steroidal non-

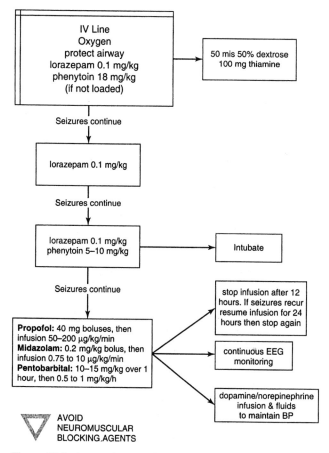

Figure 40-1. Approach to treating status epilepticus.

depolarizing muscle relaxant, which in a dose of 0.9 to 1.2 mg/kg, has a duration of onset similar to succinylcholine. Rocuronium is devoid of significant hemodynamic effects and exhibits no untoward effects on intracranial dynamics. Vecuronium, in a dose of 0.1 mg/kg, is a useful alternative.

Table 40-1. Anticonvulsants dosing and therapeutic levels.

Drug	Serum Level (µg/mL)	Daily Dose (mg)
Phenytoin	10–20 total	4 mg/kg/day
	1–2 free fraction	200–500
Carbamazepine	4–12	600–2400
Phenobarbital	15–45	60–300
Ethosuximide	40–100	500–1500
Valproic acid	50–100	750–3000

- A long-acting anticonvulsant is required (Table 40-1).
    Phenytoin is the most commonly used maintenance mediation, given in a dose of **15 to 20 mg/kg** (not standard dose of 1000 mg). Phenytoin is given in saline (insoluble in D5W) at a rate not to exceed 50 mg/min with continuous electrocardiograph (ECG) monitoring. Phosphenytoin (a water-soluble prodrug) can be given at a rate of 100 to 150 mg. Phenytoin equivalents (PE)/min, to a dose of 15 to 20 PE/kg.
    An additional dose of 5 to 10 mg/kg phenytoin should be given if seizures continue.
- Patients who continue in SE after treatment with lorazepam and phenytoin traditionally have been treated with phenobarbital (20 mg/kg IV), but the results of the VA study suggest that this is unlikely to result in the rapid termination of SE. At this point, SE should be considered refractory SE, and treatment should progress to one of the agents used for the treatment of refractory SE.
- The following agents have been used for the control of refractory SE. Endotracheal intubation and mechanical ventilation are essential. Continuous electroencephalogram (EEG) monitoring is suggested.
    Propofol is an intravenous anesthetic agent with potent anti-convulsant properties. The drug is extremely lipid soluble, has a rapid onset of action, and has been used successfully in refractory SE. A dose of 40 mg every 10 seconds until control of seizures (2 to 2.5 mg/kg) is suggested, followed by an infusion of 50 to 200 µg/kg/min.
    Midazolam: Bolus of 0.2 mg/kg followed by an infusion at 0.75 to 10 µg/kg/min.
    Pentobarbital: 10 to 15 mg/kg followed by a maintenance dose of 0.5 to 1 mg/kg/h to control seizures and attain the desired EEG.
    Propofol is more likely than midazolam to provide rapid control of refractory SE, exhibits less tachyphylaxis than midazolam, and produces less hypotension than pentobarbi-

tal for an equivalent degree of seizure control. The infusion should be stopped after 12 hours. If seizures recur, resume infusion for 24 hours then stop again.

- Patients who reach the stage of refractory SE should undergo continuous EEG monitoring. The goal regarding the activity on the EEG remains a matter of debate. Many patients can achieve complete seizure control with a background of continuous slow activity and do not incur the greater risks associated with the higher dose of medication required to achieve burst-suppression pattern. Conversely, few patients will continue to have frequent seizures that emerge out of a burst-suppression background. These patients will presumably need even higher doses of medication, which may result in very long periods of suppression or even a "flat" EEG. Treating a patient with SE without continuous EEG monitoring is akin to treating patients with ventricular tachycardia without continuous ECG monitoring. Without continuous EEG monitoring, one must rely on occasional samples of the EEG, which are therefore associated with risks for under- and overtreatment. It is very important to note that between 20% and 30% of patients treated for SE will continue to have EEG evidence of seizures without clinical evidence of seizures, so-called *aconvulsive seizures*.

Electroencephalographic Monitoring

EEG monitoring is an underutilized tool in patients with SE. EEG monitoring is essential in patients who have received a long-acting paralytic agent, in patients who remain unconscious after the initial seizure, and in patients who require prolonged therapy for refractory SE. Relatively simple EEG-monitoring devices are available for continuous monitoring in the ICU.

Phenytoin

Phenytoin is the most commonly used anticonvulsant in the ICU, and therefore an understanding of the pharmacokinetics and pharmacodynamics of this drug is important.

Phenytoin is metabolized by the liver and follows zero-order kinetics; i.e., the metabolic process is saturable and therefore doubling the dose *does not* double the serum concentration (the serum concentration increases exponentially). A small increase in the dose may result in a large increase in serum levels (into the toxic range).

Phenytoin is 90% protein bound. Only the free fraction is pharmacologically active. Critically ill patients frequently have a decreased serum albumin concentration, which increases the free phenytoin fraction (may cause toxicity). The therapeutic concentration (10 to 20µg/mL) reflects both the bound and unbound fractions. Therefore, in hypoalbuminemic patients, the free-phenytoin concentration should be monitored (1 to 2µg/mL).

Drugs that cause autoinduction of hepatic enzymes increase phenytoin clearance, whereas drugs that inhibit hepatic enzymes cause phenytoin clearance to decline.

Drugs That Increase Phenytoin Metabolism
(Decreased Phenytoin Levels)

- Barbiturates
- Ethanol
- Folic acid
- Rifampin

Drugs That Decrease Phenytoin Metabolism
(Increased Phenytoin Levels)

- Omeprazole
- Cimetidine
- Amiodarone
- Oral antiocoagulants
- Sulfonamides and trimethoprim
- Chloramphenicol
- Disulfiram
- Isoniazid
- Phenylbutazone

Other Drug Interactions

- Steroids (decreased levels)
- *Cyclosporin* (decreased levels)
- Digoxin (decreased levels)
- Amiodarone (increased phenytoin, decreased amiodarone)
- Anticoagulants (increased phenytoin, increased International Normalized Ratio (INR) with bleeding)

Toxicity

- May cause hypotension, bradycardia, heart block, arrhythmias, and asystole (particularly if infused too rapidly).
- Contraindicated in patients with second- or third-degree heart block. An external pacemaker should be available in patients with conduction defects.
- Ataxia, nausea, vomiting, nystagmus, involuntary movements, confusion, hallucinations.

- Hypersensitivity reactions, including *skin rashes*, *hepatitis*, *fever*, Stevens-Johnson syndrome and the Dilantin (phenytoin) hypersensitivity syndrome.

■ SELECTED REFERENCES

1. Lowenstein DH, Alldredge BK. Status epilepticus. *N Engl J Med.* 1998; 338:970–976.
2. Treiman DM, Meyers PD, Walton NY. A comparison of four treatments for generalized convulsive status epilepticus. Veterans Affairs Status Epilepticus Cooperative Study Group. *N Engl J Med.* 1998;339:792–798.

41

Guillain-Barré Syndrome and Myasthenia Gravis

■ GUILLAIN-BARRÉ SYNDROME

Diagnosis

Clinical Features

- Ascending symmetrical muscle weakness that evolves over several days to a week.
- Nadir of neurologic deficit occurs by 28 days in 95% of cases.
- Full recovery in 80% of patients.
- Pain and aching discomfort in muscles.
- Paraesthesias.
- Hypotonia with absent reflexes.
- Facial diplegia is common.
- Autonomic dysfunction with fluctuating blood pressure and pulse, facial flushing, profuse diaphoresis.
- Fisher syndrome: ophthalmoplegia, ataxia, areflexia.

Cerebrospinal Fluid

- Normal pressure.
- Acellular (but occasionally 10 to 50 cells are found).
- Protein is normal initially but rises to reach a peak in 4 to 6 weeks.

Electromyogram
- May be normal early in disease
- Then reduction in conduction velocity or conduction block
- Prolonged distal latencies

Differential Diagnosis

- Subacute polyradiculopathies: infectious mononucleosis, hepatitis, diphtheria, human immunodeficiency virus, Lyme disease
- Cervical myelopathy
- Early pontine infarction
- Porphyric polyneuropathy
- Botulism
- Toxic polyneuropathies: triorthocresyl phosphate, thallium
- Lupus polyneuropathy
- Acute myasthenia gravis
- Polymyositis
- Tick paralysis

Management

The most common reason for admitting patients with Guillain-Barré syndrome (GBS) to the ICU is for respiratory monitoring and impending ventilatory failure. Adequate ventilation in any individual relies on the triad of adequate inspiratory effort, effective expiratory forces, and the ability to cough and protect the airway. Any or all of these components may be affected to some degree in patients with GBS. Frequent clinical assessments of patients with GBS are essential. Respiratory rate, cough, the ability to count to 20 on one breath, evaluation of bulbar function, strength of the shoulder shrug, and the presence or absence of paradoxic inward movement of the abdominal wall muscles with inspiration need to be evaluated every 4 hours while the patient is awake. Respiratory muscle function should also be evaluated quantitatively by measuring the vital capacity and forced expiratory pressures every 2 to 4 hours.

It is essential that all patients with GBS have baseline pulmonary function tests upon hospital admission. This information allows appropriate triage of patients: either close monitoring on a ward service or respiratory monitoring in an ICU. If the vital capacity is ≤20mL/kg, then the patient should be admitted to the ICU. A vital capacity of ≤15mL/kg requires intubation and mechanical ventilation. Specific indications for intubation are indicated below. However, no patient should have mechanical ventilation withheld because he/she does not meet specific guidelines for measures of respiratory function. It is always better to intubate patients electively before a crisis ensues. A rising $Paco_2$ is a late sign of respiratory distress. A falling Pao_2 or arterial saturation is a very late sign of respiratory distress.

Criteria for Mechanical Ventilation

Clinical

> Restlessness, anxiety
> Tachycardia
> Tachypnea
> Staccato speech
> Inability to count to 20 on one breath
> Use of accessory muscles

Respiratory Function

> Vital capacity (VC) ≤15 mL/kg
> Maximal inspiratory pressure (PiMax) <20 mm Hg

Treatment

Supportive

- Prophylaxis to prevent deep venous thromboses. Pulmonary embolism is the most common cause of death. Compression boots and/or subcutanous heparin are recommended. In patients who require long-term ventilation, anticoagulation with coumadin to achieve an international normalized ratio (INR) between 1.5 and 2.5 is a practical approach.
- Consider early tracheostomy in patients with severe disease.
- Early enteral tube feeding.
- Pulmonary toilet and chest physiotherapy to prevent atelectasis and pneumonia.
- Physical therapy to prevent flexion contractures.
- Regular turning to prevent decubitus ulcers.
- Early diagnosis and treatment of pulmonary and urinary tract infections.

Specific Treatment

- Plasmapheresis: A number of large randomized trials have clearly established the usefulness of plasma exchange in the rapidly evolving phase of GBS. Plasmapheresis instituted within 2 weeks of the onset of the disease shortens the course of the illness.

- Intravenous administration of immune globulin (0.4 g/kg/day for 5 consecutive days) has been reported to be as effective as plasma exchange. This therapy, however, is generally considered second line and reserved for patients who cannot tolerate plasmapheresis or when plasmapheresis is not available.
- *Corticosteroids have no beneficial effects in patients with GBS.*

Autonomic Dysfunction

Significant autonomic dysfunction occurs most often in patients with severe motor weakness and respiratory failure. Features include

- Cardiac arrhythmias: tachyarrhythmias, bradycardia, asystole
- Labile blood pressure
- Electrocardiographic (EKG) changes
- Pupillary abnormalities
- Sweating abnormalities
- Urinary retention
- Gastrointestinal tract dysfunction: gastroparesis, ileus, diarrhea, constipation

Weaning From Mechanical Ventilation

The time to wean patients from mechanical ventilation is when clinical and respiratory function criteria for mechanical ventilation no longer exist. Weaning patients with neuromuscular disorders differs from that of patients with pulmonary disease, who can be liberated from the ventilator once the underlying lung disease process has resolved without an extended weaning process. The process of weaning in patients with neuromuscular disorders should be thought of as a respiratory muscle conditioning program. Short intervals of conditioning should be interspersed with generous rest periods, with patients resting at night. This process may be accomplished by either intermittent mandatory ventilation or pressure-support weaning. Rapid weaning with T-piece trials may be tolerated by patients with less severe disease.

■ MYASTHENIA GRAVIS

Patients with myasthenia gravis may be admitted to the ICU for respiratory support or postoperatively following a thymectomy.

Diagnosis

- Myasthenic facies: drooping eyelids, immobile mouth, snarling smile, hanging jaw in classic case.
- Other signs include ptosis, diplopia, difficulty in speaking or swallowing, limb weakness.
- Marked limb weakness and respiratory difficulty are seen in patients with severe disease (monitor and treat as for GBS).
- Electromyogram (EMG) and single-fiber EMG: reduction of the amplitude of compound action potentials during repetitive stimulation and blocking of single muscle fiber transmission.
- Edrophonium test: Increase in muscle strength after 10-mg dose (give 1-mg test dose first).
- Antibodies against the acetylcholine receptor can be demonstrated in 85% to 90% of patients.
- Exclude concomitant autoimmune diseases, such as Grave's disease and pernicious anemia.
- Exclude botulism, which presents with diplopia, ptosis, and opthalmoparesis, with pupils that are usually large and dilated.

Management

- Anticholinesterase drugs: pyridostigmine (Mestinon) is the drug preferred by most clinicians, the dose is 15 to 90 mg q6h. *A cholinergic crisis* occurs due to overdosing with anticholinesterase drugs and is manifested by muscarinic effects (nausea, vomiting, pallor, sweating, salivation, diarrhea, bradycardia, etc.) with increasing weakness. If the muscarinic effects are not present and weakness from pyridostigmine is suspected, the tensilon test should be done. The weakness of a cholinergic crisis is unaffected (or worsened) by tensilon. If the weakness improves, the patient is not receiving enough anticholinergic drug.
- Avoidance of drugs that increase weakness (Table 41-1)
- Indications for thymectomy
    - All cases of thymoma
    - All patients <50 years old who have responded poorly to anticholinesterase drugs
- A trial of steroids is indicated in patients who have responded poorly to thymectomy and anticholinesterase drugs. An initial worsening during the first 7 to 10 days may occur, necessitating close observation.
- Plasmapheresis: Striking temporary remissions may be obtained by the use of plasmapheresis. This form of treatment may be life-saving during a crisis.

Table 41-1. Drugs that increase weakness in myasthenics.

Anesthetics, general
  Curare, decamethonium, gallamine, halothane, methoxyflurane

Anesthetics, local
  Lidocaine (xylocaine)

Antibiotics
  Aminoglycoside antibiotics, bacitracin, clindamycin, fluoroquinolones,
    tetracyclines

Antiarrhythmics
  Lidocaine, procainamide, quinidine

Antihypertensives
  Beta-blockers, verapamil, diuretics that deplete potassium

Antirheumatics
  Chloroquine, D-penicillamine

Antiseizure drugs
  Diazipam, phenytoin, trimethadione

Hormones
  Corticosteroids and adrenocorticotropic hormone, oral contraceptives,
    thyroid hormone

Sedatives
  Barbiturates, narcotics, benzodiazepines, chlorpromazine, promazine,
    phenezine

■ SELECTED REFERENCE

1. Randomised trial of plasma exchange, intravenous immunoglobulin, and combined treatments in Guillain-Barré syndrome. Plasma Exchange/Sandoglobulin Guillain-Barré Syndrome Trial Group. *Lancet.* 1997;349: 225–230.

Part 6

Infection

42

Management of Septic Patients

The American College of Chest Physicians/Society of Critical Care Medicine developed a set of terms and definitions to define sepsis in a more precise manner. The term *systemic inflammatory response syndrome (SIRS)* was coined to describe the systemic response to a wide variety of insults and characterized by two or more of the following clinical manifestations:

1. A body temperature of >38°C or <36°C

2. A heart rate of >90 beats/min

3. Tachypnea, as manifested by a respiratory rate of >20 breaths/min

4. A WBC count of >12,000 cells/mm^3, or <4000 cells/mm^3 or the presence of >10% immature neutrophils

When SIRS is the result of a confirmed infectious process, it is termed *sepsis*. Severe sepsis is defined as sepsis plus either organ dysfunction, evidence of hypoperfusion, or hypotension. Septic shock is a subset of severe sepsis and is defined as sepsis-induced hypotension, persisting despite adequate fluid resuscitation, along with the presence of hypoperfusion abnormalities or organ dysfunction.

The most common primary focus of infection and the spectrum of implicated pathogens in patients with sepsis are listed in Tables 42-1 and 42-2.

■ CARDIOVASCULAR CHANGES IN SEPSIS

Sepsis and septic shock result in a severe decrease in systemic vascular resistance and generalized blood flow maldistribution. In >90% of

Table 42-1. The most common primary focus of infection in patients with sepsis.

Respiratory tract	25%
Intra-abdominal/pelvis	25%
Bacteremia	15%
Urinary tract	10%
Skin	5%
Intravascular catheter	5%
Unknown/other	15%

Table 42-2. The microbiology of sepsis in the nonimmunocompromised host.

Categories	
Gram-negative	25%
Gram-positive	25%
Mixed gram-negative/positive	20%
Fungal (*Candida*) only	3%
Anaerobes	2%
Unknown	25%
Gram-negative bacteria	
Escherichia coli	25%
Klebsiella/Citrobacter	20%
Pseudomonas aeruginosa	15%
Enterobacter spp.	10%
Proteus spp.	5%
Other gram-negative bacteria	25%
Gram-positive bacteria	
Staphylococcus aureus	35%
Enterococcus spp.	20%
Coagulase-negative staphylococcus	15%
Streptococcus pneumoniae	10%
Other gram-positive bacteria	20%

patients with septic shock who have been aggressively volume loaded to ensure the absence of hypovolemia, cardiac output is normal or elevated. Despite the high cardiac output, clinical and experimental studies have demonstrated that sepsis is characterized by biventricular systolic (depressed ejection fraction) and diastolic dysfunction (decreased chamber compliance), with an increase in both end-diastolic and end-systolic volume. This characteristic pattern occurs within the first 24 hours of the onset of sepsis. The decreased systolic function is most easily identified clinically by a low left ventricular stroke work index (LVSWI). The cardiac output and indices of ventricular function normalize as patients recover from the septic insult, while ventricular function remains depressed (despite inotropic agents) in the nonsurvivors.

The effective intravascular volume is reduced in patients with sepsis and is a major factor leading to circulatory instability and collapse. In patients who have been inadequately fluid resuscitated, septic shock may present as a hypodynamic state with a low cardiac output. Multiple factors are responsible for the decreased intravascular volume, including an increase in venous capacitance and venous pooling, a generalized increase in microvascular permeability, increased insensible losses, and poor fluid intake.

Although the cardiac output is increased in sepsis, this flow is not evenly distributed; a reduction in blood flow to the myocardium and skeletal muscle, but most notably to the stomach, duodenum, small bowel, and pancreas is characteristic, while blood flow to the brain and kidneys is preserved. A reduction in splanchnic blood flow with a reduction in gastric and ileal mucosal flow appears to be a consistent finding in sepsis. The gut is highly susceptible to diminished tissue perfusion and oxygenation, as it has a higher critical oxygen delivery (Do_2) than the whole body and other vital organs, and the mucosal countercurrent microcirculation renders the villi particularly vulnerable to ischemia. The decreased mucosal blood flow to the gut may be particularly important, and circumstantial evidence has linked this phenomenon to the development of progressive organ dysfunction. Experimental and clinical studies have demonstrated that mesenteric hypoperfusion following sepsis results in mucosal hypoxia, intramucosal acidosis, and increased intestinal mucosal permeability leading to bacterial translocation.

■ MANAGEMENT PRINCIPLES

The management of patients with severe sepsis is based largely on treating or eliminating the source of infection, the use of appropriate antimicrobial agents, and hemodynamic and other physiological supportive measures. Immunomodulation therapy remains of unproven value at this time. The remainder of this chapter evaluates therapeutic strategies for the management of patients with severe sepsis. These recommendations apply to the management of the immunocompetent patient; however, many of the principles apply to the immunocompromised host.

Identification and Eradication of the Source of Infection

One of the most challenging features of the sepsis syndrome is that of identifying and eradicating, as early as possible, the source of infection. The majority of patients presenting with severe sepsis usually have a pulmonary, genitourinary, primary bloodstream, intra-abdominal, or intravenous catheter as a source of infection. Recent studies have demonstrated that in approximately 75% of patients with presumed sepsis an etiological agent can be isolated, these being equally divided among gram-positive and gram-negative organisms (see Table 42-2).

It has been known for centuries that, unless the source of the infection is controlled, the patient cannot be cured of his/her infective process and that death will eventually ensue. Surgical control or percutaneous drainage of the infective process is, therefore, essential; in most patients with severe intra-abdominal infections, recovery will not occur without them. Infected central venous catheters must be removed from patients with catheter-related sepsis.

Antimicrobial Agents

Antimicrobial therapy remains the cornerstone of treatment in patients with sepsis. The choice of antibiotics is largely determined by the source or focus of infection, the patient's immunological status, and whether the infection is nosocomial or community-acquired. Although antimicrobial therapy should be targeted against specific microorganisms, in the vast majority of cases, empiric therapy is started as soon as the diagnosis of sepsis is contemplated. Initial empiric management often requires more than one antibiotic to cover the most likely potential pathogens. Once a pathogen is isolated, monotherapy is adequate for most infections. The indications for double-antimicrobial therapy include suspected or proven *Pseudomonas aeruginosa* infections, enterococcal infections, the treatment of febrile-neutropenic patients, and severe intra-abdominal infections. In patients with culture-negative sepsis, continuation of the initial empiric combination is warranted. Additional antibiotics or a change in antibiotics may be required in patients with culture-negative sepsis who do not appear to be responding to the initial empiric regimen.

To rapidly achieve adequate blood and tissue concentrations, antibiotics should be given intravenously, at least initially. Dosing regimens should take into account whether the antibiotic "kills" by time-dependent kinetics (e.g., beta-lactam antibiotics, vancomycin) or concentration-dependent kinetics (e.g., aminoglycoside). Recent data suggest that the clinical effectiveness of beta-lactam antibiotics and vancomycin is optimal when the concentration of the antimicrobial agent at the site of infection exceeds the minimum inhibitory concentration (MIC) of the infecting organism for a prolonged period of time. In addition, antibiotic dosing should also take into account the patient's hepatic and renal function. Antibiotics are continued until clinical improvement is noted and ordinarily are not continued for more than 2 weeks, except in cases of osteomyelitis and endocarditis.

Hemodynamic Support

As mentioned earlier in this chapter, peripheral vasodilation with hypotension and abnormal distribution of blood flow is characteristic in patients with sepsis. Several studies have demonstrated that indices of inadequate tissue perfusion and oxygenation are strong predictors of multiorgan dysfunction and death in septic patients. Aggressive volume resuscitation is considered the best initial therapy for the cardiovascular instability of sepsis. Hypotension can often be reversed with fluid administration alone. Fluid requirements for the initial resuscitation of patients with septic shock are frequently large, with up to 10 L of crystalloid or 4 L of colloid being required in the first 24 hours.

The choice of crystalloid or colloid (or both) for resuscitation of septic patients remains a controversial issue (see Chapter 17). Crystalloids have generally been recommended as the volume expander of first choice. It has, however, been suggested that in patients with sepsis, colloidal replacement fluids may limit the degree of "third-space" loss. Hydroxyethyl starch solutions have a number of theoretical advantages in patients with sepsis. In septic and trauma patients, hydroxyethyl starch solutions have been demonstrated to inhibit endothelial activation and endothelial-associated coagulation. Furthermore, in both clinical and experimental studies in sepsis and trauma, resuscitation with hydroxyethyl starch solutions has been demonstrated to result in less tissue edema and better preserved microcapillary integrity than resuscitation with crystalloid solutions. Despite the theoretical advantages of hydroxyethyl starch solutions, there are no conclusive data that the type of resuscitation fluid has a major impact on outcome. However, albumin is not recommended as a volume expander, even in hypoalbuminemic patients with sepsis.

Patients with sepsis have a markedly abnormal ventricular response to volume infusion, with a significantly smaller increase in LVSWI than controls in response to fluid challenges. Furthermore, due to the massively reduced systemic vascular resistance, patients may remain hypotensive despite adequate fluid resuscitation. Should hypotension or signs of inadequate organ perfusion persist after adequate fluid resuscitation, invasive hemodynamic monitoring should be considered. Although the benefit of pulmonary artery catheterization in this setting remains unproven, this procedure allows for the rational titration of fluid and vasoactive drug therapy. A volumetric pulmonary artery catheter may provide additional useful information to guide volume replacement (see Chapter 18).

Those patients who remain hypotensive and/or display evidence of end-organ dysfunction despite adequate fluid resuscitation are likely to benefit from the use of vasoactive agents. The failure to improve tissue perfusion may lead to progressive multiorgan failure and death. However, the true risk/benefit ratio and the optimal choice of inotropic agents in this setting have yet to be determined in well-controlled clinical studies. Reluctance to optimize hemodynamics with vasopressors may stem from the traditional belief that vasopressors produce adverse vasoconstrictive effects peripherally that outweigh their positive effects on the central circulation. Furthermore, high doses of vasopressors are frequently required as septic patients demonstrate hyporesponsiveness to these agents.

Dopamine has traditionally been the vasoactive drug of choice in patients with sepsis. The Third European Consensus Conference in Intensive Care Medicine recommended dopamine as the "most appropriate first choice" in septic patients requiring vasoactive support. Furthermore, many authorities advocate the use of other pressor agents only in patients who prove to be "dopamine-resistant." However, dopamine may not be the ideal drug for a number of reasons. In sepsis, chronotropic sensitivity to beta-adrenergic stimulation is increased. In addition, it has been demonstrated that the beta-adrenergic properties of dopamine predominate in patients with sepsis. The increase in blood pressure with dopamine is predominantly due to an increase in cardiac output, mainly due to an increase in heart rate. Tachycardia and tachydysrhythmias may become the rate-limiting factor in its use. The positive chronotropic and inotropic effects of dopamine will elevate myocardial oxygen requirements, which may not be adequately met by increased coronary flow. In addition, dopamine has been demonstrated to cause an uncompensated increase in oxygen requirements together with a maldistribution of blood flow in vital tissue beds. Furthermore, recent studies suggest that dopamine suppresses the circulating concentrations of all the anterior pituitary-dependent hormones (except cortisol). This latter action may have a deleterious effect on the metabolic and immune status of the patient with sepsis.

Norepinephrine improves the hemodynamic parameters in the majority of patients with sepsis, and it may improve tissue oxygen utilization. In spite of many practitioners' concerns, no data indicate that this agent has a deleterious renal effect. Dobutamine has been demonstrated to increase oxygen delivery and reverse both systemic and local indices of tissue hypoxia in patients with sepsis. However, the use of dobutamine in isolation may cause or potentiate hypotension due to beta-2-mediated vasodilation. The coexistence of a decreased ejection fraction and widespread vasodilation implies that it is may be advantageous to use two drugs with different receptor profiles to attain the desired effect. The *combination of dobutamine and norepinephrine* has been demonstrated to increase both the cardiac output and peripheral vascular resistance and to improve indices of tissue oxygenation in patients with severe sepsis.

There are concerns about the use of epinephrine in patients with sepsis, as this agent has been shown to cause a significant increase in the serum lactate concentration with an associated fall in the serum pH. This rise in lactate has not been demonstrated with the use of the other commonly used inotropic agents. The increased lactate production may be due to increased glycogenolysis and/or a maldistribution of blood flow. Data on the hemodynamic effect of phenylephrine in patients with sepsis are limited. While this agent will increase blood pressure and systemic vascular resistance, it will usually lower cardiac output. Dopexamine is an analogue of dopamine that produces systemic vasodilation through stimulation of β_2-adrenoceptors and dopamine receptors. Dopexamine has been demonstrated to increase splanchnic blood flow in septic patients; however, the role of this agent, particularly in hypotensive septic patients, is unclear.

When the patient with sepsis remains hypotensive in spite of exogenous catecholamines, phosphodiesterase inhibitors and vasopressin can be considered. There is, however, limited experience with the use of these agents in sepsis. Vasopressin effectively reverses the hypotension that accompanies sepsis, but the significant peripheral and intestinal vasoconstriction that this agent produces may limit its use.

Adrenal insufficiency should always be suspected in patients who fail to respond to catecholamines, who require high doses of catecholamines, and who remain pressor dependent. The incidence of adrenal insufficiency in patients with septic shock is unclear; however, the incidence may be as high as 30%. A low-dose adrenocorticotropic hormone test and stress doses of glucocorticoids are suggested when this disorder is suspected (see Chapter 34). A rapid and dramatic improvement in hemodynamics may occur within a few hours of the administration of exogenous corticosteroids.

Goals of Hemodynamic Support and the Evidence of a Systemic Oxygen-Debt Sepsis

Following the studies of Shoemaker et al. in surgical patients, it has become a common practice to increase systemic Do_2 in patients with sepsis on the assumption that these patients had an overt or occult oxygen debt. Furthermore, an elevated arterial lactate concentration in septic patients was presumed to be a marker of cellular oxygen deficiency and was used to identify patients who would respond to maneuvers that increase systemic Do_2. Recent evidence suggests that both of these postulates may be incorrect. Experimental and clinical data suggest that the increased lactate levels in sepsis are due to hypermetabolism rather than a systemic oxygen debt. These data, therefore, seriously question the scientific validity of driving up Do_2 to "supranormal" levels in patients with sepsis. This is supported by recent clinical trials that have failed to demonstrate an improvement in outcome with this strategy.

The primary aim of the initial phase of resuscitation is to restore an adequate tissue perfusion pressure; a mean arterial pressure of 75 to 80 mm Hg and a cardiac index of least 2.8 L/min/m^2 would be reasonable initial goals. A number of studies have demonstrated that in septic patients, gastric intramucosal acidosis is a better predictor of outcome than the hemodynamic and oxygen-derived variables obtained by invasive hemodynamic monitoring. Preliminary data suggest that therapy directed at preventing intramucosal hypercarbia may reduce morbidity and mortality in critically ill patients. However, well-conducted, randomized controlled trials are needed to confirm this observation.

■ OTHER SUPPORTIVE THERAPIES

Red blood cell transfusions are commonly used to augment systemic oxygen delivery in patients with sepsis. However, clinical studies have not consistently demonstrated that this maneuver increases oxygen utilization at either the whole-body level or within individual organs. Furthermore, the transfusion of poorly deformable red blood cells in patients with sepsis may cause microcapillary occlusion and tissue ischemia. Blood transfusions have also been shown to be immunosuppressive and to increase the risk of postoperative infections and organ failure in surgical patients. The results of a large randomized trial failed to demonstrate any benefit of increasing the transfusion threshold from 7 g/dL to 10 g/dL in critically ill ICU patients.

Recent data suggest that early enteral nutrition, particularly with the use of immune-enhancing diets, improves the hormonal, metabolic, and immunological derangements that occur in critically ill patients with sepsis. Postpyloric feeding should be considered in those patients who tolerate gastric tube feedings poorly.

■ ADJUNCTIVE THERAPIES FOR SEPSIS

Corticosteroids are potent anti-inflammatory agents whose use in sepsis has been suggested for decades. Ten randomized, placebo-controlled studies have investigated the utility of pharmacologic doses of corticosteroids in patients with severe sepsis. Meta-analyses of these studies have been unable to demonstrate a beneficial effect of corticosteroids and suggest that in some patients their use may be harmful. Similarly, attempts at modulating the immune response with anti-endotoxin and anti-cytokine therapy, as well as inhibitors of platelet-activating factor, bradykinin, and prostaglandin synthesis have similarly failed to demonstrate a survival benefit in patients with sepsis.

Recently, a number of studies have suggested a survival advantage in patients with sepsis who were treated with stress doses of corticosteroids. The hypothalamic-pituitary-adrenal axis was incompletely studied in these reports; it is therefore possible that the improved survival was due to the treatment of patients with adrenal insufficiency. Further data are required before "stress doses" of steroids can be routinely recommended in septic patients.

■ COMPLICATIONS OF SEPSIS

1. Acute respiratory distress (see Chapter 12)
2. Acute renal failure (see Chapter 32)
3. Disseminated intravascular coagulation (see Chapter 50)
4. Multiorgan dysfunction syndrome (see Chapter 51)

■ SELECTED REFERENCES

1. Bone RC. The sepsis syndrome: definition and general approach to management. *Clin Chest Med.* 1996;17:175–182.
2. Bollaert PE, Bauer P, Audibert G, Lambert H, Larcan A. Effects of epinephrine on hemodynamics and oxygen metabolism in dopamine-resistant septic shock. *Chest.* 1990;98:949–953.
3. Briegel J, Forst H, Haller M, et al. Stress doses of hydrocortisone reverse hyperdynamic septic shock: a prospective, randomized, double-blind, single-center study. *Crit Care Med.* 1999;27:723–732.
4. Gattinoni L, Brazzi L, Pelosi P, et al. A trial of goal-oriented hemodynamic therapy in critically ill patients. *N Engl J Med.* 1995;333:1025–1032.
5. Hayes MA, Timmins AC, Yau E, et al. Elevation of systemic oxygen delivery in the treatment of critically ill patients. *N Engl J Med.* 1994;330: 1717–1722.
6. Marik PE, Varon J. The hemodynamic derangements in sepsis: implications for treatment strategies. *Chest.* 1998;114:854–860.
7. Shoemaker WC, Appel PL, Kram HB, Waxman K, Lee TS. Prospective trial of supranormal values of survivors as therapeutic goals in high risk surgical patients. *Chest.* 1988;94:1176–1186.
8. Society of Critical Care Medicine Consensus Conference Committee. American College of Chest Physicians/Society of Critical Care Medicine Consensus Conference: definitions for sepsis and organ failure and guidelines for the use of innovative therapies in sepsis. *Crit Care Med.* 1992;20: 864–874.
9. Third European Consensus Conference in Intensive Care Medicine. Tissue hypoxia: how to detect, how to correct, how to prevent? *Am J Respir Crit Care Med.* 1996;154:1573–1578.
10. Van den Berghe G, de Zegher F. Anterior pituitary function during critical illness and dopamine treatment. *Crit Care Med.* 1996;24:1580–1590.

43

Assessment of New Fever in the Non-neutropenic Intensive Care Unit Patient

Fever is a common problem in ICU patients. The presence of a fever frequently results in the performance of diagnostic tests and procedures that significantly increase medical costs and expose the patient to unnecessary invasive diagnostic procedures and the inappropriate use of antibiotics. The main diagnostic dilemma is to exclude noninfectious causes of fever and then to determine the site and likely pathogens of those with infections. It should be recalled that *antibiotics are not antipyretic agents* and that antibiotics should be used only in patients likely to have *a bacterial infection*. Furthermore, it is important to appreciate that not all patients with infections are febrile. Approximately 10% of septic patients are hypothermic and 35% are normothermic at presentation. Septic patients who fail to develop a temperature have a significantly higher mortality than febrile septic patients.

Temperature is most accurately measured by an intravascular thermistor, but measurement by an electronic probe in the mouth, rectum, or external auditory canal is an acceptable alternative. The Society of Critical Care Medicine practice parameters define fever in the ICU as a temperature >38.3°C (≥101°F). Unless the patient has other features of an infectious process, only a temperature >38.3°C (≥101°F) warrants further investigation. Furthermore, unless the patient is clinically deteriorating (low blood pressure, decreased urine output, increased confusion, worsening coagulopathy) or the temperature is ≥39°C (102°F), it may be prudent to perform blood cultures and then observe the patient before embarking on the *"fever diagnostic workup."* *All neutropenic patients* with a fever should be started on antimicrobial therapy immediately after cultures are obtained. In patients with an obvious focus of infections (e.g., purulent nasal discharge, abdominal tenderness, profuse green diarrhea) and chest x-ray changes, only a focused diagnostic workup is required.

■ CAUSES OF FEVER

For reasons that are not entirely clear, most noninfectious disorders usually do not lead to a fever >38.9°C (102°F); therefore, if the temperature increases above this threshold, the patient should be considered to have an infectious cause of the fever. However, patients with drug fever may have a temperature >102°F. Similarly, fever secondary to blood transfusion may exceed 102°F. The following noninfectious causes of a fever should be excluded in ICU patients:

- Alcohol/drug withdrawal (see Chapter 52)
- Postoperative fever (48 hours postoperative)
- Post-transfusion fever
- Cerebral infarction/hemorrhage
- Myocardial infarction
- Pancreatitis
- Acalculous cholecystitis (see Chapter 44)
- Ischemic bowel
- Aspiration pneumonitis
- Acute respiratory distress syndrome
- Subarachnoid hemorrhage
- Fat emboli
- Transplant rejection
- Deep venous thrombosis/pulmonary emboli (see Chapter 13)
- Gout/pseudogout
- Hematoma
- Cirrhosis (without primary peritonitis)
- Gastrointestinal bleeding
- Phlebitis/thrombophlebitis
- Adrenal insufficiency (see Chapter 34)
- Intravenous contrast reaction
- Neoplastic fevers
- Decubitus ulcers

Most of those clinical conditions listed above are clinically obvious and do not require additional diagnostic tests to confirm their presence. However, a few of these disorders require special consideration. Although drug-induced fever is commonly cited as a cause of fever, fewer than 300 cases of this condition have been reported in the literature. Furthermore, only a single case of drug fever has been reported in an ICU patient population. However, on the basis of the number of medications administered to patients in the ICU, one would expect drug fever to be a relatively common event. Although the true incidence of this disorder is unknown, drug fever should be considered in patients with an otherwise unexplained fever, particularly if they are receiving beta-lactam antibiotics, procainamide, or diphenylhydantoin. Drug fever is usually characterized by high spiking temperatures and shaking chills. It may be associated with leukocytosis and eosinophilia. Relative bradycardia, although commonly cited, is uncommon.

Atelectasis is commonly implicated as a cause of fever. Standard ICU texts list atelectasis as a cause of fever, although they provide no primary source. Engoren studied 100 postoperative cardiac surgery patients and was unable to demonstrate a relationship between atelectasis and fever. Furthermore, when atelectasis is induced in experimental animals by ligation of a main stem bronchus, fever does not occur. The role of atelectasis as a cause of fever is unclear; however, atelectasis probably does not cause fever in the absence of pulmonary infection.

Febrile reactions complicate about 0.5% of blood transfusions but may be more common following platelet transfusion. Febrile reactions usually begin within 30 minutes to 2 hours after a blood product transfusion is begun. The fever generally lasts between 2 and 24 hours and may be preceded by chills. An acute leukocytosis lasting up to 12 hours commonly occurs following a blood transfusion.

While fever may occur in patients with deep venous thrombosis, in patients suspected of deep venous thrombosis, the predictive value of fever is poor. Furthermore, in critically ill ICU patients, fever without other features of ileofemoral thrombosis is uncommon and does not warrant routine venography as part of the initial diagnostic workup of pyrexia in ICU patients.

The common infectious causes of fever in the ICU include (see Chapters 10 and 44):

- Ventilator-associated pneumonia
- Catheter-related sepsis
- Sinusitis
- *Clostridium difficile* infection
- Abdominal sepsis
- Primary gram-negative septicemia
- Complicated wound infections

Urinary tract infections (UTIs) have been reported to be common in ICU patients, among whom they are reported to account for between 25% and 50% of all infections. However, it is likely that most of these patients had "asymptomatic bacteriuria" rather than true infections of the urinary tract. The treatment of patients with "asymptomatic bacteriuria" is based on a single study performed in the early 1980s that is not applicable today. Platt and colleagues demonstrated that in hospitalized patients bacteriuria with <10^5 colony-forming units (CFU) of bacteria per milliliter of urine during bladder catheterization was associated with a 2.8-fold increase in mortality. Based on this study, thousands of ICU patients with urinary tract colonization have been treated with antibiotics.

Most ICU patients require an indwelling urinary catheter for monitoring fluid balance and renal function. Colonic flora rapidly colonize the urinary tract in these patients. Bacteriuria defined as a quantitative culture of ≥10^5 CFU/mL has been reported in up to 30% of catheterized hospitalized patients. The terms *bacteriuria* and *UTI* are generally although incorrectly used as synonyms. Bacteriuria implies colonization of the urinary tract without bacterial invasion and an acute inflammatory response. UTI implies an infection of the urinary tract. Criteria have not been developed for differentiating asymptomatic colonization of the urinary tract from symptomatic infection. Furthermore, the presence of white cells in the urine is not useful for differentiating colonization from infection, as most catheter-associated bacteriurias have accompanying pyuria.

While catheter-associated bacteruria is common in ICU patients, data from the early 1980s indicate that <3% of catheter-associated bacteriuric patients will develop bacteremia caused by organisms in the urine. This finding is supported by the recent publications of Maki and colleagues. These authors reviewed 1497 catheterized patients and were unable to demonstrate a clinical difference (symptoms and signs of infection) between those patients who had ≥10^5 CFU/mL and those with sterile urine or <10^5 CFU/mL. Furthermore, only 1 patient with ≥10^5 CFU/mL developed bloodstream infection. These data imply that the surveillance for and treatment of isolated bacteruria in most ICU patients is incorrect. Bacteriuria should, however, be treated following urinary tract manipulation or surgery, in patients with kidney stones, and in patients with urinary tract obstruction.

Nosocomial meningitis is exceedingly uncommon in hospitalized patients who have not undergone a neurosurgical procedure. Lumbar puncture, therefore, need not be performed routinely in patients (non-neurosurgical) who develop a fever in the ICU unless they have meningeal signs or contiguous infection.

■ BLOOD CULTURES

Bacteremia and candidemia have been documented in up to 10% of ICU patients and are an important cause of morbidity and mortality in the ICU. Blood cultures are therefore indicated in *all* febrile patients. Surveillance blood cultures, however, are expensive and add very little to the management of patients in the ICU.

Blood cultures are ideally drawn before the onset of a temperature spike. In reality this is not possible, and therefore spreading out the collection of blood cultures increases the likelihood of blood collection during bacteremia. It is therefore recommended that at least two and no more than three sets of blood cultures should be obtained by separate needle sticks from different venipuncture sites. Colonization of the lumen of central venous catheters occurs within a short period of time after placement. Therefore, blood cultures should not be obtained through intravascular catheters unless the catheter has been recently placed. The volume of blood drawn in adult patients is the single most important factor governing the sensitivity of blood cultures. Therefore, it is recommended that a minimum of 10 mL and preferably 20 mL of blood be removed per draw divided among the minimum number of blood culture containers as recommended by the manufacturer. Resin-containing medium offers little clinical benefit to the majority of ICU patients. Once bloodstream infection is identified, repeated or follow-up cultures are not necessary in most cases.

■ SCINTIGRAPHY, COMPUTED TOMOGRAPHY SCANNING, AND ULTRASOUND EXAMINATIONS

Scintigraphic scanning techniques have a low sensitivity and specificity in ICU patients and are therefore not recommended. The advantages of computed tomography (CT) scanning and/or ultrasound over scintigraphy is that the results of the test can be obtained immediately with superior anatomic resolution, which can be used to guide drainage procedures.

■ FEVER DIAGNOSTIC WORKUP

The following approach is suggested in ICU patients who develop a fever (Figure 43-1). Due to the frequency and excess morbidity and mortality associated with bacteremia, blood cultures are recommended in all ICU patients who develop a fever. A comprehensive physical examination and review of the chest radiograph are essential. Noninfectious causes of fever should be excluded. In patients with an "obvious" focus of infections (e.g., purulent nasal discharge, abdominal tenderness, profuse green diarrhea, pulmonary infiltrate, erythema at catheter insertion site), a focused diagnostic workup is

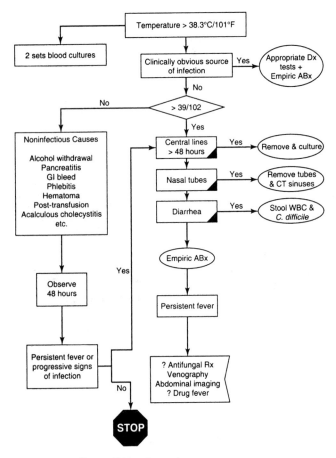

Figure 43-1. Fever diagnostic workup.

required. If there is no clinically obvious source of infection and unless the patient is clinically deteriorating (falling blood pressure, decreased urine output, increasing confusion, rising serum lactate concentration, falling platelet count, or worsening coagulopathy) or the temperature is >39°C (102°F), it may be prudent to perform blood cultures and then observe the patient before embarking on the further diagnostic tests and commencing empiric antibiotics. Urine culture is indicated only in patients with abnormalities of the renal system or following urinary tract manipulation. In patients with a temperature ≥39°C and no obvious source of infection, central venous catheters that have been in situ for over 4 days should be removed and cultured (see Chapter 44). *All neutropenic* patients with fever and patients with severe (as outlined above) or progressive signs of sepsis should be started on broad-spectrum antimicrobial therapy immediately after obtaining appropriate cultures.

Clinical signs that should prompt the institution of empiric antimicrobial therapy include

- Hypotension requiring volume resuscitation or inotropic support
- Falling urine output
- Falling platelet count
- Rising serum lactate concentration
- Progressive hyperglycemia
- Development of a coagulopathy, i.e., prolonged prothrombin time or partial thromboplastin time

Re-evaluation of the patient's status after 48 hours—using all available results and the evolution of the patient's clinical condition—is essential. In patients whose clinical picture is consistent with infection and in whom no clinically obvious source has been documented, removal of all central lines (>48 hours old, with semiquantitative or quantitative culture) is recommended as well as stool analysis for white blood cells and *C. difficile* toxin in those patients with loose stools, and CT scan of sinuses with removal of all nasal tubes. Empiric broad-spectrum antibiotics should be started at this point in patients with persistent fever and signs of infection. Additional diagnostic tests may be appropriate at this time including venography, a differential blood count for eosinophils (diagnosis of drug fever), and abdominal imaging. If fever persists despite empiric antibiotics and no source of infection has yet been identified, empiric antifungal therapy may be indicated if the patient has risk factors for candidal infection (see Chapter 44).

■ EMPIRIC ANTIBIOTICS

In patients with a persistent temperature, patients with a clinical picture strongly suggestive of infection, and patients with a temperature >39°C (102°F), empiric antibiotics should be commenced. The most appropriate empiric regimen will depend upon the most likely sites of infection, *the resident ICU bacteria and their sensitivity pattern.* The following are "generic" recommendations, which should be modified according to the factors listed above:

- *Vancomycin* in patients at risk of central venous catheter infection; must be stopped if culture of catheter (semiquantitative) and blood are negative.
- *Metronidazole* (oral) if *C. difficile* enterocolitis is suspected.
- *Vancomycin or oxacillin* (or equivalent) **AND** *gram-negative coverage* (double cover if pseudomonas is endemic in the ICU) for suspected ventilator associated pneumonia (VAP). Specific anaerobic cover is not required. Change/stop antibiotics once culture data are available.
- *Gram-negative coverage* and *anaerobic coverage* for suspected abdominal infection.
- *Vancomycin **AND** gram-negative coverage* for a clinical picture strongly suggestive of infection and no obvious site/source infection until culture data are available.

48 Hours Later

- If the patient has improved and the organism has been isolated, antibiotics **must** be changed according to the narrowest adequate spectrum coverage.
- If the patient has improved and no organism has been isolated, *stop vancomycin* and continue other antibiotics.
- If the patient has not improved and no organism has been isolated, stop *vancomycin*, continue other antibiotics, and add *fluconazole* (if the patient is at risk for *Candida* infection, see Chapter 44).
- If *C. difficile* toxin is negative and *C. difficile* enterocolitis is likely (see Chapter 44), perform flexible sigmoidoscopy *and* biopsy or abdominal CT scan (increased colonic wall thickness).
- If fever persists, *and* there is no obvious source of infection, *and* no organism has been isolated, *and* the patient is hemodynamically stable, perform differential count for eosinophils and consider *drug fever*; stop antibiotics and repeat cultures.

■ TREATMENT OF FEVER IN THE ICU

Almost all febrile ICU patients are treated with acetaminophen and external cooling methods to render the patients afebrile. However, fever is a basic evolutionary response to infection and may be an important host defense mechanism. The preponderance of evidence suggests that temperature in the range of the usual fever renders host defenses more active and many pathogens more susceptible to these defenses. Therefore, it seems illogical to treat fever per se. In addition, temperature is an important physical sign allowing the physician to monitor the response to treatment. Furthermore, acute hepatitis may occur in ICU patients with reduced glutathione reserves (alcoholics, malnourished persons, etc.) who have received regular therapeutic doses of acetaminophen. Based on these data, it is recommended that febrile episodes not be routinely treated with antipyretic therapy; an evaluation of the relative benefits and risks of antipyretic treatment should be evaluated in each individual case. Fever should, however, be treated in patients with acute brain insults, patients with limited cardiorespiratory reserve (i.e., ischemic heart disease), and patients in whom the temperature increases above 40°C (104°F).

Hypothermia blankets are frequently used in ICU patients with febrile episodes. However, studies have demonstrated that hypothermia blankets are no more effective in cooling patients than are antipyretic agents. Furthermore, the use of hypothermia blankets is associated with large temperature fluctuations and rebound hyperthermia. In addition, there is a fundamental illogic to the use of external application of cold to lower temperature in a patient with true fever. Because of the altered hypothalamic set point, the patient is already responding as if to a cold environment. External cooling may result in augmented hypermetabolism and a persistent fever. Indeed, Lenhardt and colleagues demonstrated that active external cooling in volunteers with induced fever increased oxygen consumption by 35% to 40% and was associated with a significant increase in epinephrine and norepinephrine levels.

■ SELECTED REFERENCES

1. Adelson-Mitty J, Fink MP, Lisbon A. The value of lumbar puncture in the evaluation of critically ill, non-immunosuppressed, surgical patients: a retrospective analysis of 70 cases. *Intensive Care Med.* 1997;23:749–752.
2. Chandrasekar PH, Brown WJ. Clinical issues of blood cultures. *Arch Intern Med.* 1994;154:841–849.
3. Cunha BA. Fever in the critical care unit. *Crit Care Clin.* 1998;14:1–14.
4. de Kleijn EM, Oyen WJ, Claessens RA, Corstens FH, van der Meer JW. Utility of scintigraphic methods in patients with fever of unknown origin. *Arch Intern Med.* 1995;155:1989–1994.
5. Engoren M. Lack of association between atelectasis and fever. *Chest.* 1995; 107:81–84.
6. Krieger JN, Kaiser DL, Wenzel RP. Urinary tract etiology of bloodstream infections in hospitalized patients. *J Infect Dis.* 1983;148:57–62.
7. Lenhardt R, Negishi C, Sessler DI, et al. The effects of physical treatment on induced fever in humans. *Am J Med.* 1999;106:550–555.
8. Mackowiak PA, LeMaistre CF. Drug fever: a critical appraisal of conventional concepts. An analysis of 51 episodes in two Dallas hospitals and 97 episodes reported in the English literature. *Ann Intern Med.* 1987;106: 728–733.

9. Meduri GU, Mauldin GL, Wunderink RG et al. Causes of fever and pulmonary densities in patients with clinical manifestations of ventilator-associated pneumonia. *Chest*. 1994;106:221–235.

10. Metersky ML, Williams A, Rafanan AL. Retrospective analysis: are fever and mental status indications for lumbar puncture in a hospitalized patient who has not undergone neurosurgery. *Clin Infect Dis*. 1997;25:285–288.

11. O'Donnel J, Axelrod P, Fisher C, Lorber B. Use of and effectiveness of hypothermia blankets for febrile patients in the intensive care unit. *Clin Infect Dis*. 1997;24:1208–1213.

12. O'Grady NP, Barie PS, Bartlett J, et al. Practice parameters for evaluating new fever in critically ill adult patients. *Crit Care Med*. 1998;26:392–408.

13. Platt R, Polk BF, Murdock B, Rosner B. Mortality associated with nosocomial urinary tract infection. *N Engl J Med*. 1982;307:637–642.

14. Styrt B, Sugarman B. Antipyresis and fever. *Arch Intern Med*. 1990;150:1589–1597.

15. Tambyah PA, Maki DG. Catheter-associated urinary tract infection is rarely symptomatic: a prospective study of 1497 catheterized patients. *Arch Intern Med*. 2000;160:678–82.

16. Tambyah PA, Maki DG. The relationship between pyuria and infection in patients with indwelling urinary catheters: a prospective study of 761 patients. *Arch Intern Med*. 2000;160:673–677.

44

Nosocomial Infections in the Intensive Care Unit

■ CATHETER-ASSOCIATED SEPSIS

Catheter-associated sepsis is defined as bloodstream infection due to an organism that has colonized a vascular catheter. Approximately 5% of patients with indwelling vascular catheters (uncoated) will develop bloodstream infection ($\approx$10 infections per 1000 catheter days). The incidence of catheter-associated sepsis increases with the length of time the catheter is in situ, the number of ports, and the number of manipulations. Approximately 25% of catheters become colonized (>15 colony-forming units, CFU) and approximately 20% to 30% of colonized catheters will result in catheter sepsis. *Staphylococcus aureus* and coagulase-negative staphylococci are the most common infecting (and colonizing) organisms, followed by enterococci, gram-negative bacteria, and *Candida* species. Antibiotic-coated catheters significantly reduce catheter colonization and catheter-associated bloodstream infection. Femoral catheters *are not associated* with a higher infection rate. Similarly, neither the type of occlusive dressing nor the frequency of dressing change affects the incidence of catheter-associated sepsis.

Replacement of a colonized catheter over a guidewire is associated with rapid colonization of the replacement catheter. If catheter sepsis is strongly suspected, the catheter must be changed to a *new* site, with withdrawal blood cultures and culture of the catheter tip. In patients with limited venous access or in patients in whom catheter sepsis is less likely, the catheter can be changed over a guidewire; however, withdrawal blood cultures and culture of the catheter tip must be performed and the catheter removed if the cultures are positive.

The *routine* replacement of central venous catheters is no longer recommended. Central venous catheters should remain in situ until

- Purulent discharge, cellulitis, or erythema develops at the puncture site
- Catheter malfunction
- Any positive blood cultures since the line was inserted
- Septic clinical pattern with no other obvious source of infection

However, it may be prudent to replace a *multilumen catheter* after 10 to 14 days even if the above criteria are not met. All lines that are inserted in emergent situations under conditions that are not strictly aseptic should be removed within 24 hours and replaced at a new site. Patients with colonized catheters (>15 CFU), with negative blood cultures, and no signs of infection should not be treated with antibiotics. All catheters removed from potentially septic patients should be cultured (tip and intracutaneous segment).

■ NOSOCOMIAL SINUSITIS

Nosocomial sinusitis is a common problem in ICU patients. Risk factors include nasotracheal tubes, nasogastric tubes, and patients nursed in a supine position. Almost all patients with nasotracheal tubes will develop opacification of their maxillary sinuses within 3 to 5 days of intubation. Approximately a third of these cases will prove to have infectious sinusitis. It is therefore desirable that patients in whom the length of nasotracheal intubation is expected to exceed 3 days should have all nasal tubes removed and reinserted through the mouth.

Diagnostic Approach

- Computed tomography CT scan of the paranasal sinuses should be performed in patients with a purulent nasal discharge or an offensive nasal discharge, and in patients who have an undiagnosed fever with risk factors for developing sinusitis.
- Plain x-rays are of *no value* in diagnosing nosocomial sinusitis.
- Not all patients with radiological sinusitis, i.e., opacification of the sinuses, have infectious sinusitis. Patients who have opacification of the maxillary sinuses should undergo transnasal puncture and aspiration (the nasal mucosa must be thoroughly cleaned before culture, to limit contamination). Only about 30% to 40% of patients with opacification of their maxillary sinuses will have positive cultures with purulent aspirates.

Microbiology of Nosocomial Sinusitis

- Similar spectrum to that of nosocomial pneumonia
- Often polymicrobial
- *Pseudomonas* spp.
- *Acinetobacter* spp.
- *S. aureus*
- *Candida* spp.
- *Hemophilus influenzae*
- Anaerobes

Treatment of Infectious Sinusitis

- Remove all nasal tubes.
- Treat with broad-spectrum antibiotics, tailored to the sinus aspirate Gram stain and culture.
- Local vasoconstrictors and nasal toilet.

■ CANDIDA INFECTIONS IN THE ICU

Candida species are important opportunistic pathogens in the ICU. The Centers for Disease Control National Nosocomial Infection Study reported that 7% of all nosocomial infections were due to candidal species. Patients with candidal infection have been shown to have a longer hospital stay and higher mortality compared to case-matched controls.

It is important to realize that *Candida* species are constituents of the normal flora in about 30% of all healthy people. Antibiotic therapy increases the incidence of enteric colonization by up to 70%. It is probable that *most ICU patients become colonized with* Candida *species soon after admission. Not all patients colonized with* Candida *will become infected with* Candida. Non-neutropenic patients with isolation of *Candida* species from pulmonary samples (tracheal aspirates, bronchoscopic, or blind sampling methods), even in high concentrations, are unlikely to have invasive candidiasis. Indication for initiation of antifungal therapy in these patients should be based on histologic evidence or identification from sterile specimens. Similarly, isolation of *Candida* species from the urine in ICU patients with indwelling catheters usually represents colonization rather than infection. Although candiduria may be observed in up to 80% of patients with systemic candidiasis, most patients with candiduria do not have disseminated infection or upper urinary tract infection. The initial treatment for candiduria consists of the elimination of factors contributing to its occurrence, such as indwelling catheters, immunosuppression, or broad-spectrum antibiotics. These options are clearly not possible in most ICU patients. The indwelling catheter should be changed with close observation of the patient. The role of amphotericin B bladder irrigations in these patients is unclear. In patients with pyuria, worsening renal function, and/or systemic signs of infection, it may be prudent to perform blood cultures as well as renal imaging.

The factors predisposing to systemic *Candida* infection include the following:

- Broad-spectrum antibiotics are the single most important risk factor.
- Indwelling intravenous and urinary catheters.
- Parenteral alimentation.
- ICU stay >7 days.
- Perforated viscus.

Clinical features and diagnosis of systemic fungal infections:

- The clinical diagnosis of systemic candidal infection is particularly difficult in the ICU patient. On the one hand, the clinical picture may be indistinguishable from that of a bacteremia with an acute onset of high fever, rigors, tachycardia, and hypotension. Conversely, a low-grade fever or hypothermia may be the only manifestation.
- *Candida* may infect the eyes, causing an endophthalmitis. Funduscopy should therefore be part of the daily examination of the ICU patient.
- Although the respiratory tract is frequently colonized, invasive pulmonary candidiasis is uncommon.
- Approximately 10% of patients will present with a macular rash or discrete skin nodules.
- Other features of systemic candidiasis may include a myocarditis, meningitis, cerebral microabscesses, myositis, endocarditis, osteomyelitis, and arthritis.
- The ante mortem diagnosis of systemic candidiasis is exceedingly difficult, and therefore this diagnosis requires a high index of suspicion (an ante mortem diagnosis of candidal infection is made in only 15% to 40% of patients with systemic candidiasis proven at autopsy).
- Only about 50% of patients with systemic candidiasis at postmortem have ante mortem positive blood cultures.
- Serology has been shown to be of little value in the diagnosis of systemic candidiasis, as have assays for the detection of circulating candidal antigens.

- An association has been demonstrated between the number of sites colonized with *Candida* and the occurrence of invasive candidiasis in high-risk patients.
- A single positive blood culture is highly predictive of candidal infection and should never be considered a contaminant.

Management

- The initial treatment of candidal infections should include removal of all possible foci of infection, including removal of intravascular lines and urinary catheters.
- Candidemia may resolve spontaneously after removal of an intravascular catheter. There is, however, increasing evidence that metastatic foci of infection may develop in patients who do not receive systemic antifungal therapy.
- Drainage is an integral part of the management of patients with intra-abdominal suppuration in whom *Candida* is isolated from a peritoneal culture.
- Amphotericin B has long been the standard treatment for candidemia. However, recent data suggest that fluconazole and amphotericin B may be equally efficacious in the treatment of non-neutropenic patients with candidemia. C. *krusei*, however, is intrinsically resistant to fluconazole.

Drug Therapy

Amphotericin B

- A total dose of 6 to 8 mg/kg is recommended, although some authors have recommended a total dose as high as 2 g. After a 1-mg test dose, amphotericin B is usually given in a daily dose of 0.5 mg/kg over a 2-week period. A daily dose of 1 mg/kg may be given, which is usually well tolerated. Amphotericin B should be given as an infusion in 5% dextrose in water over 8 hours.
- Amphotericin B is associated with reversible nephrotoxicity. Fluid and sodium loading may reduce incidence of nephrotoxicity. The dosage should not be reduced in patients with pre-existing renal dysfunction, as only a small fraction of the drug is excreted by the kidney.
- Amphotericin B is associated with a proximal renal tubular acidosis and a profound loss of Na^+, K^+, and Mg^{++} in the urine. These electrolytes must be aggressively replaced.
- Fever, chills, and headaches commonly occur at the initiation of therapy and are probably mediated by the release of tumor necrosis factor and interleukin-1. These side effects can be mini-

mized by infusing the drug slowly and by premedication with antihistamines and nonsteroidal anti-inflammatory agents.

- Liposomal amphotericin B has been demonstrated to be at least as effective as conventional amphotericin B. However, with the liposomal preparation, significantly fewer patients experience infusion-related fever (17% vs. 44%), chills or rigors (18% vs. 54%), and other reactions, including hypotension. Nephrotoxic effects are significantly less frequent among patients treated with liposomal amphotericin B than among those treated with conventional amphotericin B (19% vs. 34%).

Fluconazole

- Loading dose: 800 mg.
- Maintenance dose: 400 mg as a single daily dose. The dose must be adjusted according to the calculated creatinine clearance.

Prophylaxis

- Delaying or preventing oropharyngeal, gut, and skin colonization with *Candida* species may prevent systemic infection.
- Ketoconazole has been shown to reduce the incidence of candidal infections in high-risk surgical patients.
- It is likely that fluconazole may prove to be effective in preventing infection with *Candida* species in high-risk ICU patients. The role of such prophylaxis has yet to be determined.

■ *CLOSTRIDIA DIFFICILE* COLITIS

Clostridia difficile is the agent that causes pseudomembranous colitis and antibiotic-associated diarrhea and has become a common nosocomial pathogen. Approximately 20% of all hospitalized patients become "infected" with *C. difficile*, of whom only about a third develop diarrhea. *Clostridia difficile* is responsible for virtually all cases of pseudomembranous colitis and for up to 20% of cases of antibiotic-associated diarrhea without colitis. The spores of *C. difficile* are easily transmitted by the oral–fecal route from one patient to the next and may become widely disseminated throughout a hospital. Although reported in the preantibiotic era, antibiotics are the most important risk factor leading to colonization and colitis. The normal colonic flora resists colonization by *C. difficile*; however, broad-spectrum antibiotics with activity against enteric bacteria disrupt the normal flora, allowing colonization. Approximately 25% of hospitalized adults recently treated with antibiotics will become colonized with *C. difficile*. Once established in the colon, pathogenetic strains of *C. difficile* produce two exotoxins (toxin A and B) that cause diarrhea and colitis.

Antimicrobial Agents That Induce *C. difficile*

Frequent Induction

- Ampicillin and amoxicillin
- Cephalosporins
- Clindamycin

Infrequent Induction

- Tetracyclines
- Sulphanomides
- Erythromycin
- Chloramphenicol
- Trimethoprim
- Quinolones

Rare or no Induction

- Parenteral aminoglycosides
- Metronidazole
- Vancomycin

The majority of hospital patients infected with *C. difficile* are asymptomatic. *Clostridia difficile* infection commonly presents as diarrhea that is mild to moderate, sometimes accompanied by lower abdominal cramping. Symptoms usually begin during or shortly after antibiotic therapy but are occasionally delayed for several weeks. Severe colitis without pseudomembrane formation may occur with profuse, debilitating diarrhea, abdominal pain, and distention. Common systemic manifestations include fever, nausea, anorexia, and malaise. A marked neutrophilia and increased numbers of fecal leukocytes are common. Pseudomembranous colitis is the most dramatic manifestation of *C. difficile* infection; these patients have marked abdominal and systemic signs and symptoms and may develop a fulminant and life-threatening colitis.

Stool assay for toxins A or B are the main clinical tests used to diagnose *C. difficile* infection. The gold standard test is the tissue culture cytotoxicity assay. This test has a high sensitivity (94% to 100%) and specificity (99%). The major disadvantages of this test are its high expense and the time needed to complete the assay (2 to 3 days). Therefore, this test is no longer routinely performed. Toxin enzyme-linked immunosorbentassay (ELISA) tests are less sensitive (70% to 90%) than the cytotoxicity test but demonstrate excellent specificity (99%) and can be rapidly processed, and they have largely replaced the cytotoxicity assay. It is suggested that two stool specimens be examined for leukocytes and toxin (ELISA test). Should the ELISA be negative and a high index of suspicion for *C. difficile* exist, the following are recommended: (1) sigmoidoscopy, and/or (2) cytotoxicity assay, and/or (3) CT scan of the abdomen looking for thickened colonic wall.

Management

Treatment of asymptomatic carriers is not recommended. Antidiarrheal agents that reduce intestinal peristaltic activity may delay clearance of the organism and are therefore not recommended. The first step in managing patients is to discontinue antibiotic therapy, if possible. Patients with mild diarrhea may not require any other treatment. However, in the ICU, this is often not possible, and therefore specific therapy aimed at eradicating *C. difficile* is necessary. The treatment options for *C. difficile* infection remain limited, although promising agents are currently being assessed. Metronidazole is the first-line drug of choice for those patients requiring specific *anti-C. difficile* treatment; oral metronidazole (250 mg, q6h). Much of the interest in alternative therapies has centered on the difficult management issues posed by patients with multiple symptomatic recurrences of *C. difficile* infection. However, it is now clear that the majority of these episodes are due to reinfections with new *C. difficile* strains and not relapses caused by the original bacterium. Hence, the true efficacy of the alternative regimens remains unclear. Individuals susceptible to *C. difficile* reinfections need to be protected from exposure to *C. difficile* until their bowel flora recovers. While several biotherapeutic approaches to the treatment and prevention of *C. difficile* infection have been described, few controlled data are available. Oral vancomycin (125 mg, q6h) is reserved for patients who cannot tolerate or who do not have a response to metronidazole. Patients who cannot tolerate oral medication can be treated with intravenous metronidazole. In general, sigmoidoscopy should be avoided in severe colitis because of the risk of perforation.

■ ACALCULOUS CHOLECYSTITIS

Acalculous cholecystis, while relatively uncommon, is an important "infection" in critically ill patients. It is often unrecognized and is therefore potentially life threatening. Only about 10% of cases of acute cholecystitis in the ICU are associated with gallstones, which are usually considered an incidental finding rather than the cause. Critically ill patients have multiple factors that increase their risk for developing this complication.

The diagnosis of acalculous cholecystitis is often exceedingly difficult and requires a high index of suspicion. Pain in the right upper quadrant is the finding that most often leads the clinician to the correct diagnosis, but it may frequently be absent. Nausea, vomiting, and fever are other associated clinical features. The clinical findings and laboratory workup in patients with acalculous cholecystitis are, however, often nonspecific. The most difficult patients are those recovering from abdominal sepsis who deteriorate again, misleadingly suggesting a flare-up of the original infection.

Radiological investigations are required for a presumptive diagnosis. Ultrasound is the most common radiologic investigation used in the diagnosis of acalculous cholecystitis, with a sensitivity and specificity of greater than 80% and 90%, respectively (features include increased wall thickness, intramural lucencies, gallbladder distention, pericholecystic fluid, and intramural sludge). Wall thickness of ≥3 mm is reported to be the most important diagnostic feature on ultrasound examination, with a specificity of 90% and a sensitivity of 100%. In ICU patients, hepatobiliary scintigraphy has a high false-positive rate (>50%), limiting the value of this test. However, a normal scan virtually excludes acalculous cholecystitis. CT scanning has been reported to have a high sensitivity and specificity; however, no prospective studies have been performed comparing ultrasonography with CT scanning in the diagnosis of acalculous cholecystitis.

Management

Once the presumptive diagnosis has been made, the management consists of both medical and interventional therapies. The gallbladder either needs to be drained or removed surgically. Percutaneous cholecystomy is usually the initial procedure of choice, with interval cholecystomy performed when (and if) the patient is considered a suitable surgical candidate. It should be noted that acalculous cholecystitis is primarily a "noninfectious" disease, with bacterial invasion a secondary event (at least a third of patients have sterile bile). However, antibiotics with adequate gram-negative coverage are usually prescribed.

■ VENTILATOR-ASSOCIATED PNEUMONIA (SEE CHAPTER 10)

■ URINARY TRACT INFECTION (SEE CHAPTER 43)

■ NOSOCOMIAL CYTOMEGALOVIRUS (AND HERPESVIRUS) INFECTION IN "NONIMMUNOCOMPROMISED" ICU PATIENTS

Primary cytomegalovirus (CMV) infection usually takes place in childhood, after which the virus remains latent. Depending on the country of residence and social status, between 50% and 100% of the population harbor CMV and are CMV seropositive (immunoglobulin G). In immunocompromised patients, such as those with acquired immune deficiency syndrome and immunosuppressed transplant recipients, the virus becomes reactivated; CMV infections in these patients are an important cause of morbidity and death. CMV may, however, become reactivated during other immunosuppressive illnesses. It is well known that critical illness, particularly sepsis and the systemic inflammatory response, results in perturbations of the immune system. Of particular significance, it has been suggested that tumor necrosis factor may play a role in activating CMV. However, these patients are not classically considered immunocompromised, and CMV infection is not considered a pathogen in these patients. This postulate appears to be incorrect. A number of studies have documented active CMV infections in nonimmunocompromised ICU patients. While the presence of viral antigen and DNA may merely represent carriage of the virus, histologic documentation of CMV pneumonitis has been reported in a number of these patients. CMV pneumonitis should therefore be considered a cause of ventilator-associated pneumonia. Papazian and co-workers reported 18 cases of CMV pneumonitis in 36 (48%) nonimmunocompromised ICU patients with acute respiratory distress syndrome (ARDS) who underwent open lung biopsy. CMV pneumonitis should therefore be considered in patients with nonresolving ARDS and in septic ICU patients who develop ventilator-associated pneumonia. Kutza and colleagues have elegantly demonstrated that the number of CMV-positive peripheral leukocytes increases after about the fifth day of critical illness, peaks at the height of the illness and then declines with recovery. These data suggest that CMV reactivation and CMV infection should be considered in chronic critically ill (~7 to 10 days) ICU patients. It is likely that other herpesviruses may become reactivated in critical illness. Tuxen and colleagues reported the presence of herpes simplex tracheobronchitis in 14 of 46 (30%) patients with ARDS.

■ SELECTED REFERENCES

Catheter-Associated Sepsis

1. Cobb DK, High KP, Sawyer WT, et al. A controlled trial of scheduled replacement of central venous and pulmonary artery catheters. *N Engl J Med.* 1992;327:1062–1068.
2. Darouiche R, Raad I, Heard SO, et al. A comparison of two antimicrobial-impregnated central venous catheters. *N Engl J Med.* 1999;340: 1–8.
3. Pearson ML. Guidelines for the prevention of intravascular device related infections. *Infect Control Hosp Epidemiol.* 1996;17:438–473.

Nosocomial Sinusitis

4. Holzapfel L, Chastang C, Demingeon G, et al. Randomized study assessing the systematic search for maxillary sinusitis in nasotracheally mechanically ventilated patients. *Am J Respir Crit Care Med.* 1999;159:695–701.
5. Rouby JJ, Laurent P, Gosnach M, Cambau E, Lamas G, Zouaoui A, et al. Risk factors and clinical relevance of nosocomial maxillary sinusitis in the critically ill. *Am J Respir Crit Care Med.* 1994;150:776–783.

Candida

6. el Ebiary M, Torres A, Fabregas N, et al. Significance of the isolation of *Candida* species from respiratory samples in critically ill, non-neutropenic patients. An immediate postmortem histologic study. *Am J Respir Crit Care Med.* 1997;156:583–590.
7. Nolla-Salas J, Sitges-Serra A, Leon-Gil C, et al. Candidemia in non-neutropenic critically ill patients: analysis of prognostic factors and assessment of systemic antifungal therapy. Study Group of Fungal Infection in the ICU. *Intensive Care Med.* 1997;23:23–30.
8. Rello J, Esandi ME, Diaz E, et al. The role of *Candida* sp isolated from bronchoscopic samples in nonneutropenic patients. *Chest.* 1998;114: 146–149.
9. Rex JH, Bennett JE, Sugar AM, et al. A randomized trial comparing fluconazole with amphotericin B for the treatment of candidemia in patients without neutropenia. Candidemia Study Group and the National Institute. *N Engl J Med.* 1994;331:1325–1330.
10. Voss A, le Noble JL, Verduyn Lunel FM, Foudraine NA, Meis JF. Candidemia in intensive care unit patients: risk factors for mortality. *Infection.* 1997;25:8–11.

C. difficile Infection

11. Manabe YC, Vinetz JM, Moore RD, et al. *Clostridium difficile* colitis; an efficient clinical approach to diagnosis. *Ann Intern Med.* 1995;123:835–840.

Acalculous cholecystitis

12. Deitch EA, Engel JM. Acute acalculous cholecystitis. Ultrasonic diagnosis. *Am J Surg.* 1981;142:290–292.
13. Kiviniemi H, Makela JT, Autio R, et al. Percutaneous cholecystostomy in acute cholecystitis in high-risk patients: an analysis of 69 patients. *Int Surg.* 1998;83:299–302.
14. van Overhagen H, Meyers H, Tilanus HW, Jeekel J, Lameris JS. Percutaneous cholecystectomy for patients with acute cholecystitis and an increased surgical risk. *Cardiovasc Intervent Radiol.* 1996;19:72–76.

CMV (+ Herpes) Infection

15. Docke WD, Prosch S, Fietze E, et al. Cytomegalovirus reactivation and tumour necrosis factor. *Lancet.* 1994;343:268–269.
16. Kutza AS, Muhl E, Hackstein H, Kirchner H, Bein G. High incidence of active cytomegalovirus infection among septic patients. *Clin Infect Dis.* 1998;26:1076–1082.
17. Papazian L, Thomas P, Bregeon F, et al. Open-lung biopsy in patients with acute respiratory distress syndrome. *Anesthesiology.* 1998;88:935–944.
18. Papazian L, Fraisse A, Garbe L, et al. Cytomegalovirus. An unexpected cause of ventilator-associated pneumonia. *Anesthesiology.* 1996;84:280–287.
19. Tuxen DV, Cade FF, McDonald MI, et al. Herpes simplex virus from the lower respiratory tract in adult respiratory distress syndrome. *Am Rev Respir Dis.* 1982;126:416–419.

45

Infections in the Immunocompromised Host

With advances in the management of patients with hematological malignancies, solid tumors, and organ transplantation, a large population of immunocompromised patients has emerged at risk of developing serious infections. The implicated pathogens are largely dependent on the degree and type of immune suppression. In general, the most common definable sites of infection in the immunocompromised host are bloodstream, lung, and mucosal surfaces.

The organisms most commonly associated with infection in the compromised host are listed in Table 45-1. Although virtually any organism can cause infection in severely immunocompromised patients, the predominant organisms are gram-negative bacilli such as *Pseudomonas aeruginosa*, *Escherichia coli*, and *Enterobacter* spp. followed by *Staphylococcus aureus*, and coagulase-negative staphylococci. Fungal infections develop with increasing severity and duration of granulocytopenia. Infections caused by *Pneumocystis carinii* and cytomegalovirus (CMV) are seen predominantly in patients with defects in cell-mediated immunity (e.g., lymphoma, corticosteroids, transplant patients). Pneumococcus and hemophils cause severe infections in splenectomized patients.

Patients with profound neutropenia (i.e., an absolute neutrophil count of less than 500/mm^3) are at high risk of severe life-threatening infections. The risk increases with the duration and severity of the neutropenia as well as with concurrent breaches of mucosal integrity. Because of the blunted inflammatory response in patients with neutropenia, the signs and symptoms of infection can be minimal, so a heightened index of suspicion for infection is essential. Patients who have had neutropenia for >10 days are vulnerable not only to acute bacterial infections but also to second or even multiple infectious complications from bacteria, fungi, viruses, or parasites.

Table 45-1. Pathogens in immunocompromised patients.

Granulocytopenic
  Bacteria
    Gram-negative bacteria
      • *Escherichia coli*
      • *Pseudomonas aeruginosa*
      • *Enterobacter* spp.
      • *Klebsiella pneumoniae*
      • *Acinetobacter* spp.
    Gram positive
      • *Staphylococcus aureus*
      • Coagulase-negative staphylococci
      • Group D streptococci
      • *Corynebacterium* spp., especially *C. jeikeium*
  Fungi
    • *Candida* spp.
    • Aspergillus

T Cell dysfunction
  Bacteria
    • *Streptococci* spp., including *S. pneumoniae*
    • *Listeria monocytogenes* (including meningitis)
    • *Legionella* spp.
    • *Mycobacterium* spp.
    • *Salmonella* spp.
  Viruses
    • Cytomegalovirus
    • Varicella-zoster virus
    • Herpes simplex virus
  Fungi
    • *Pneumocystis carinii*
    • *Candida* spp. (especially of mucosal surfaces)
    • *Cryptococcus neoformans*
    • *Histoplasma capsulatum*
  Protozoa
    • *Toxoplasma gondii*
    • *Cryptosporidium*

Patients who are functionally asplenic (e.g., from sickle cell disease) or who have had a splenectomy, especially those in whom a splenectomy was performed because of a malignant disorder (e.g., Hodgkin's disease), have increased vulnerability to life-threatening infections with encapsulated bacteria (e.g., *Streptococcus pneumoniae, Neisseria meningitidis,* and *Hemophilus influenzae*), particularly if they have not been immunized. Such patients require prompt antimicrobial treatment.

In addition to neutropenia, severe alterations in either humoral or cellular immunity can lead to life-threatening infections. Patients with substantial depressions of CD4 cell counts (to <200/mm³) are at risk for life-threatening infections with *P. carinii* and acute infections with other organisms that might have serious consequences if not promptly evaluated and treated (e.g., *Toxoplasma gondii* encephalitis and CMV retinitis). The risk of these infections is also heightened by certain immunosuppressive agents (e.g., cyclosporine) that are given after solid-organ transplantation or for the treatment of serious autoimmune diseases. Although bacterial infections with gram-negative or gram-positive organisms are the most common infectious complications immediately after transplantation, the profound alterations in cellular immunity also heighten the risk of serious opportunistic infections (such as *P. carinii*, CMV, and aspergillus infection).

■ THE FEBRILE NEUTROPENIC PATIENT

Since the 1980s, the dominant organisms responsible for infection in immunocompromised hosts with neutropenia have changed. Gram-positive organisms, especially the coagulase-negative staphylococci, have emerged as the leading cause of acute bacterial infections associated with fever and neutropenia in patients in the United States and western Europe. The increased prevalence of these organisms may be partly due to the increased use of indwelling intravenous-access devices, although this trend began before the routine use of these devices.

In the patients without an obvious site of infection, empiric therapy directed against enteric gram-negative therapy is warranted. Traditionally, a beta-lactam/aminoglycoside combination together with vancomycin has been advocated; however, recent studies indicate that monotherapy with agents such as imipenem or ceftazidime may be adequate. Most authorities recommend that vancomycin should *not* be added empirically because of the increased frequency of gram-positive infections in this patient population (due to the increasing emergence of vancomycin-resistant enterococci). A number of randomized clinical trials have demonstrated that there is no survival advantage to including vancomycin in the initial management of febrile neutropenic patients (including those with indwelling catheters). Vancomycin should be reserved for patients who are infected with methicillin-resistant staphylococcus aureus (MRSA) and vancomycin-susceptible enterococci or patients who have clinical evidence of catheter-associated infection (local infection at catheter site).

Antibiotic therapy should then be adjusted according the isolates recovered and their sensitivities. However, a broad-spectrum regimen should be maintained for the duration of neutropenia. In patients who have defervesced on broad-spectrum antibiotics, therapy should continue until *all* of the following conditions have been met: (1) >3 days without fever, (2) >10 days total duration of antibiotic therapy, (3) resolution of clinical and laboratory signs of infection, and (4) reversal of neutropenia with a total neutrophil count of a least 500/mm^3.

If the fever has not resolved by the third day and no specific pathogens isolated, vancomycin (and in some instances an aminoglycoside, if not already being administered) should be added. Should fevers persist for 7 days of neutropenia, it is customary to begin empiric antifungal therapy with amphotericin B. Fluconazole may be an effective alternative.

■ PNEUMONIA IN THE COMPROMISED HOST

The lung is one of the most common sites of infection in immunocompromised hosts. A wide variety of pathogens are implicated. The differential diagnosis is complicated by the fact that noninfectious pulmonary complications are common in the immunocompromised host. Neutropenic patients are most prone to gram-negative bacillary pneumonia; those with prolonged or profound neutropenia are susceptible to *Aspergillus* infection. Patients with depressed cell-mediated immunity are susceptible to infection with CMV, herpes simplex virus (HSV), pneumocystis, as well as cryptococcus, histoplasma, and *Nocardia* species.

Focal or multifocal infiltrates suggest infection with bacteria or *Aspergillus*. Diffuse disease is more characteristic of HSV, CMV, and *P. carinii* pneumonia (PCP) as well as noninfectious processes (drug toxicity, lymphangitic carcinomatosis). Bronchoscopic protected specimen brush sampling and bronchoalveolar lavage (BAL) are recommended as part of the initial diagnostic workup. The BAL specimen should be sent for (1) cytology and PCP staining; (2) detection of viral antigens and DNA by polymerase chain reaction (PCR) (CMV, HSV, influenzae, adenovirus, parainfluenza, respiratory syncytial virus); and (3) fungal culture. Sputum/lavage fluid culture for *Aspergillus* has a significant false-negative and false-positive rate; definitive diagnosis can be made with certainty only by open lung biopsy. High-resolution computed tomography scanning may be helpful in patients with suspected *Aspergillus* or lymphangitis. Segmental areas of consolidation with ground-glass attenuation or nodules with the "halo sign" are seen in patients with invasive aspergillosis. Spiral computed tomography is sensitive for identifying pulmonary emboli, metastatic pulmonary nodules, lymphangitic carcinomatosis, endobronchial tumors, and pleural involvement.

Part 7

Miscellaneous Intensive Care Unit Topics

46

Intensive Care Unit Admission and Discharge Criteria

The advanced life support technology that can be provided in the ICU is intended to provide temporary physiologic support for patients with potentially reversible organ failure or dysfunction. In general, only patients who have a reasonable prospect of recovery should be treated in the ICU. The merits of each potential ICU admission should be assessed on an individual basis, taking the following factors into account:

1. The patient's wishes or advance directives regarding life-support treatment
2. The patient's underlying disease(s) and physiologic function
3. The severity and reversibility of the patient's acute condition

When the reversibility and prognosis of a patient's condition are uncertain, a *time-limited therapeutic trial* in the ICU may be justified. A do not resuscitate (DNR) order does not preclude a patient from being admitted to the ICU; this is a specific instruction not to perform advanced cardiac life support once the patient's heart has stopped (i.e., the patient has died). The patient with advanced chronic disease, the patient with terminal illnesses, and the patient who has suffered a catastrophic insult should only be admitted to the ICU if there is a reasonable chance that the patient may benefit from aggressive management in the ICU *and* if the patient or surrogate is prepared to accept the burden (i.e., pain, suffering) that such therapy may incur. It should be appreciated that death is the only certainty of life, and that the ICU is not a halfway station between life on earth and the hereafter; this implies that not all dying patients need to (or will benefit from) admission to an ICU.

Once a patient is admitted to the ICU, the appropriateness of continuing care in the ICU should be evaluated on an ongoing fashion;

the fact that aggressive life supportive therapy has been provided to a patient does not imply that it cannot be withdrawn. Patients should only remain in the ICU as long as they continue to derive benefit from the physiological support provided in the ICU. When all the ICU beds are filled, the ICU/Critical Care Director or his/her designee will have the responsibility to admit/discharge patients from these units. Triage decisions should be made explicitly, fairly, and justly. Ethnic origin, race, sex, social status, sexual preference, or financial status should not be considered in triage decisions. Triage decisions may be made without patient, surrogate, or attending physician consent.

In evaluating the appropriateness of an admission to the ICU, the priority of the admission should be determined as well as the disease-specific or physiologic indications for admission (as outlined below).

■ PRIORITIZATION OF POTENTIAL ICU ADMISSIONS

This system defines a range of patients, from those who will benefit most (Priority 1) to those who will not benefit at all (Priority 4) from admission to an ICU.

Priority 1

Priority 1 patients are critically ill, unstable patients in need of *intensive treatments and monitoring* that usually cannot be provided outside of the ICU. Examples of such treatments include ventilator support, continuous titration of vasoactive drug infusion, etc. These patients have no limits placed on the extent of therapy they are to receive. Illustrative case types include postoperative patients or those with acute respiratory failure requiring mechanical ventilatory support, and shock or hemodynamic instability requiring invasive monitoring and/or titrated vasoactive drugs.

Priority 2

Priority 2 patients are those who require the *intensive monitoring* services of an ICU and are at risk to require immediate intensive treatment. No limits are placed on the extent of therapy these patients are to receive. Examples of these patients include patients with underlying heart, lung, renal, or central nervous system disease who have an acute severe medical illness or have undergone major surgery, or those patients requiring invasive hemodynamic monitoring.

Priority 3

Priority 3 are critically ill, unstable patients whose previous state of health, underlying disease, or acute illness reduces the likelihood of recovery and therefore benefit from ICU treatment. These patients may receive intensive treatment to relieve acute illness, but therapeutic efforts may stop short of measures such as intubation or cardiopulmonary resuscitation. Examples include patients with metastatic malignancy complicated by infection, pericardial tamponade, or airway obstruction, or patients with end-stage heart or lung disease complicated by a severe acute illness.

Priority 4

Priority 4 are patients who generally are not appropriate for ICU admission. Admission of these patients should be on an individual basis, under unusual circumstances, and at the discretion of the ICU attending/ICU director. These patients can be placed in the following categories:

1. Little or no additional benefit from ICU care (compared to non-ICU care) based on low risk of active intervention that could not safely be administered in a non-ICU setting (i.e., too well to benefit from ICU care). These include patients with peripheral vascular surgery, hemodynamically stable diabetic ketoacidosis, conscious drug overdose, mild congestive heart failure, etc.

2. Patients with terminal, irreversible illness who face imminent death (i.e., too sick to benefit from ICU care). These include patients with severe irreversible brain damage, irreversible multiorgan system failure, metastatic cancer unresponsive to chemotherapy and/or radiation therapy (unless the patient is on a specific treatment protocol), brain-dead nonorgan donors, patients in a persistent vegetative state, patients who are permanently unconscious, etc.

This group *includes* patients with decision-making capacity who decline intensive care and/or invasive monitoring and who elect to receive comfort care only. This group *excludes* brain-dead patients who are organ donors or potential organ donors (these patients require intensive monitoring and/or treatment in an ICU).

Transfer from Another Hospital: Variable Priority

The priority of transfers from other hospitals should be based on the current ICU census as well as the nature of the patient's acute condition and the risks of interhospital transfer. Consent for transfer must be obtained from the patient or his/her surrogate by the transferring attending physician before transfer.

■ DISEASE-SPECIFIC INDICATIONS FOR ICU ADMISSION

1. **Cardiovascular System**
   a. Acute myocardial infarction (AMI) complicated by ongoing pain, arrhythmias, congestive heart failure (CHF), or hemodynamic instability
   b. Patients suffering an AMI who are candidates for, or have received, reperfusion therapy
   c. Unstable angina
   d. Cardiogenic shock
   e. Acute CHF with respiratory failure and/or requiring hemodynamic support
   f. Hypertensive emergencies, i.e., accelerated hypertension with encephalopathy, chest pain, pulmonary edema, aortic dissection, or eclampsia

2. **Pulmonary System**
   a. Acute respiratory failure requiring emergent ventilatory support, including noninvasive positive-pressure ventilation
   b. Severe asthma, with forced expiratory volume in 1 second (FEV_1) or peak flow <40% predicted, pulsus paradoxus >18 mm Hg, pneumothorax or pneumomediastinum, $Paco_2$ > 40 mm Hg, or an "exhausted" patient
   c. Hemodynamically unstable patients with pulmonary emboli and/or patients who are candidates for thrombolytic therapy

3. **Neurological Disorders**
   a. Patients suffering a cerebrovascular accident (CVA) who are candidates for, or have received, thrombolytic therapy (i.e., within a 3-hour window following the onset of the CVA) and patients with cerebellar or brain stem CVAs
   b. Central nervous system or neuromuscular disorders with deteriorating neurologic or ventilatory function
   c. Patients with subarachnoid hemorrhage (Hunt & Hess Grades I–IV)

4. **Drug Ingestion and Drug Overdose**
   a. Hemodynamically unstable drug ingestion
   b. Drug ingestion with significantly altered mental status with inadequate airway protection

    c. Seizures following drug ingestion
    d. Drug ingestion requiring mechanical ventilation
    e. Drug ingestion requiring acute hemodialysis/hemoperfusion

5. Gastrointestinal Disorders
    a. Gastrointestinal bleeding from any source with
        i. Hemodynamic instability: systolic arterial pressure <100 mm Hg, or pulse rate >120/min, or postural hypotension after 1000 mL of fluid resuscitation (but excluding postural hypotension on presentation alone)
        ii. Hypotension requiring pressors
        iii. Ongoing bleeding (bright red blood on nasogastric aspirate; red or maroon blood per rectum)
        iv. Rebleeding
        v. Erratic mental status
        vi. Unstable co-morbid disease
        vii. Coagulopathy (international normalized ratio (INR) >1.4 and/or partial thromboplastin time >40 seconds)
    b. Fulminant hepatic failure
    c. Acute hemorrhagic pancreatitis (three or more Ranson criteria)

6. Endocrine
    a. Diabetic ketoacidosis with severe acidosis, hemodynamic instability, or altered mental status
    b. Hyperosmolar state with coma and/or hemodynamic instability
    c. Thyroid storm or myxedema coma
    d. Severe hyponatremia, hypernatremia, or hypercalcemia with altered mental status
    e. Hyperkalemia, severe and acute
    f. Adrenal crisis

7. Postoperative Care
    a. Postoperative patients requiring hemodynamic monitoring, ventilatory support, treatment of hemodynamic instability or airway monitoring
    b. Neurosurgical patients requiring hemodynamic monitoring or aggressive, titrated treatment of intracranial hypertension and vasospasm, etc.

8. Miscellaneous
Septic shock or sepsis syndrome requiring hemodynamic monitoring or hemodynamic or respiratory support.

■ PHYSIOLOGIC INDICATIONS FOR ICU ADMISSION

1. Apical pulse <40 or >150 beats/min (>130 beats/min if age >60 years)
2. Mean arterial pressure (MAP) <60 mm Hg after adequate fluid resuscitation (1500 mL) or the need for vasoactive agents to maintain a MAP >60 mm Hg
3. Diastolic blood pressure >110 mm Hg **and** one of the following:
   a. Pulmonary edema
   b. Encephalopathy
   c. Myocardial ischemia
   d. Dissecting aortic aneurysm
   e. Eclampsia or preeclampsia (diastolic >100 mm Hg)
   f. Subarachnoid hemorrhage (diastolic >100 mm Hg)
4. Respiratory rate >35/min (sustained) and respiratory distress
5. Pao_2 <55 mm Hg with Fio_2 ≥0.4 (acute)
6. Serum potassium >6.5 mEq/L (acute)
7. pHa <7.2 or >7.6 (diabetic ketoacidosis pHa <7.0)
8. Serum glucose >800 mg/dL
9. Serum calcium >15 mg/dL
10. Temperature (core) <32°C

■ DISCHARGE CRITERIA

To maximize the efficient use of ICU resources, the discharge process should be ongoing and continuous. Once admitted, it may be possible to determine that a patient is too well to benefit or too sick to benefit from continued intensive care. Patients should be discharged from the ICU when it can be determined that the patient is no longer benefitting from being in the ICU. The discharge process should be a collaborative one between the intensivist, the primary care physician or surgeon, and the nursing staff to ensure that the needs of the patients can be met by the receiving unit. General criteria for ICU discharge have been met when the need for intensive care is no longer present because

1. The indication for initial or continued treatment has reverted spontaneously or with therapy.

2. Therapy provided has not reversed the reason for admission and little benefit will be attained from continued intensive therapy.

3. The need for intensive monitoring is no longer present.

4. The patient has responded to treatment, but the long-term prognosis is such that continuing further care is unacceptable to the patient or his/her surrogate.

■ SELECTED REFERENCES

1. Adelman M. An intensivists view: Who should be admitted to the intensive care unit? *New Jersey Med.* 1993;80:617–618.

2. Bone RC, McElwee NE, Eubanks DH, Gluck EH. Analysis of indications for intensive care unit admission. Clinical efficacy assessment project: American College of Physicians. *Chest.* 1993;104:1806–1811.

3. Bone RC, McElwee NE, Eubanks DH, Gluck EH. Analysis of indications for early discharge from the intensive care unit. Clinical efficacy assessment project: American College of Physicians. *Chest.* 1993;104:1812–1817.

4. Mulley AG. The allocation of resources for medical intensive care. In: Presidents Commission for the Study of Ethical Problems in Medicine and Biomedical Research, *Securing Access to Health Care*. Washington, DC: Government Printing Office; 1983:285–311.

5. Task Force on Guidelines—Society of Critical Care Medicine. Recommendations for intensive care unit admission and discharge criteria. *Crit Care Med.* 1988;16:807–808.

47

Severity of Illness Scoring Systems

The degree of illness of patients admitted to ICUs varies enormously. The severity of illness affects resource and manpower utilization, length of stay, complication rate, and outcome. To adequately compare and contrast critically ill patients, it is useful to quantitate the severity of their illness. To achieve this goal, a number of severity of illness scoring systems have been developed. Most of these scoring systems are based on the premise that the severity of a patient's illness is related to the degree of physiological derangement of the major organ systems. Points are assigned according to the degree of derangement of readily available physiological variables, and a total score is then computed (Table 47-1; APACHE II scoring system). It is then assumed that for patients with similar disease processes the risk of death is related to the severity of illness score.

Severity of illness scoring systems are commonly used as an indicator of the quality of care delivered, as they allow the computation of the ratio between actual and predicted outcome (standardized mortality ratio). However, the main value of these scoring systems is to describe the severity of illness of patients within an ICU, as well as to compare groups of patients within an ICU. Severity of illness scoring systems are also extremely valuable in ensuring equal randomization of patients in clinical trials.

APACHE II

The APACHE II (Acute Physiology and Chronic Health Evaluation), APACHE III, SAPS II (Simplified Acute Physiology Score), and MPM II (Mortality Probability Model) scoring systems are the principal severity of illness scoring systems used in ICU patients. Of these, the APACHE II scoring system is the most well known, the most

Table 47-1. APACHE II scoring system.

Physiologic Variable	+4	+3	+2	+1	0	+1	+2	+3	+4
Temperature	≥41	39–40.9		38.5–38.9	36–38.4	34–35.9	32–33.9	30–31.9	≤29.9
Mean arterial pressure	≥160	130–159	110–129		70–109		50–69		≤49
Heart rate	≥180	140–179	110–139		70–109		55–69	40–54	≤39
Respiratory rate	≥50	35–49		25–34	12–24	10–11	6–9		≤5
FiO_2 >0.5 A-aDO_2	≥500	350–499	200–349		<200				
FiO_2 <0.5 PaO_2					>70	61–70		55–60	<55
Arterial pH	≥7.7	7.6–7.69		7.5–7.59	7.33–7.49		7.25–7.32	7.15–7.24	<7.15
Serum sodium	≥180	160–179	155–159	150–154	130–149		120–129	111–119	≤110
Serum potassium	≥7	6–6.9		5.5–5.9	3.5–5.4	3–3.4	2.5–2.9		<2.5
Serum creatinine	≥3.5	2–3.4	1.5–1.9		0.6–1.4		<0.6		
Hematocrit	≥60		50–59.9	46–49.9	30–45.9		20–29.9		<20
White blood cell count	≥40		20–39.9	15–19.9	3–14.9		1–2.9		<1
GCS: score = 15-GCS									

APACHE II Score = APS Points + Age points + Chronic health points (0/2/5)

Age	Points
≤44	0
45–54	2
55–64	3
65–74	5
≥75	6

widely used and the most frequently cited. This model was developed by Knaus and colleagues at George Washington University Hospital in Washington, D.C., and was published in 1985. The developers of this model selected those variables that they thought to be relevant to patient outcome and then arbitrarily weighted each variable. The APACHE II score includes 12 physiological variables, an age score and a chronic health score. The worst values (greatest deviation from normal) for each of the 12 physiological variables are collected during the first 24 hours after admission to the ICU. Each physiological variable is assigned a score that can range from 0 to 4 depending on the degree of deviation from normal. The final APACHE II score is the sum of the points assigned to the 12 physiological variables as well as points for age and chronic health status. The final APACHE II score can range from 0 to 71. Most ICU patients have an APACHE II score between 10 and 20. Patients with an admission APACHE II score >20 are severely ill with a high predicted mortality, while those with a score of <10 are unlikely to have a life-threatening illness. In some ICUs, the APACHE II score is calculated daily as a means of tracking the patient's illness severity over time. However, the APACHE II score calculated from variables collected within the first 24 hours of ICU admission is the most useful and frequently cited score. The APACHE II predictive model assigns disease-specific coefficients to 42 diseases that represent the majority of ICU diagnoses. The patient's probability of dying is then calculated using a logistic equation that takes into account the APACHE II score and the disease coefficient.

APACHE III

APACHE III is the most recent version of the scoring system developed by Knaus and colleagues. This commercially available model includes 17 physiological variables that were determined to contribute independently to outcome. The weighting of these variables was determined statistically to increase the explanatory power of the APACHE III score. The final APACHE III score is determined by the sum of the physiological points together with age and chronic health points. The final APACHE III score can vary between 0 and 300. The disease-specific coefficients and the formula to calculate the predicted mortality are not in the public domain.

SAPS II

SAPS II was described in 1993 by Le Gall and colleagues and is based on a European/North American multicenter database. It was developed and validated in a cohort of 12,997 patients from 110 hospitals in Europe and 27 in North America. This model includes 17 variables, including 12 physiology variables (weighted according to their degree of deviation from normal ranges), age, type of admission, and three underlying diagnoses (acquired immune deficiency syndrome, metastatic cancer, hematologic malignancies). The worst values for all variables are collected during the first 24 hours after admission to the ICU, their weights are summed, and the final result is the SAPS II score. A logistic regression equation enables the conversion of the score into a probability of hospital death. This model does not use disease-specific coefficients in the calculation of the predicted mortality.

Mortality Probability Model

The second version of the Mortality Probability Model (MPM II) was described in 1993 by Lemeshow and co-workers and is based on the same database as SAPS II. In this model, the choice of variables and their weights were done by logistic regression, and the final result is expressed as a probability of mortality (and not as a score). The MPM II contains 15 variables, including age, three physiologic variables, three chronic diseases, five acute diagnoses, type of admission, mechanical ventilation, and cardiopulmonary resuscitation before admission.

Performance of Predictive Models

The performance of these predictive models has been tested in a spectrum of ICU populations by determining their discrimination and calibration. Discrimination is the ability of a model to distinguish between a patient who will live and one who will die. Calibration compares the observed mortality with that predicted by the model within severity strata. In general, APACHE II and III, SAPS II, and MPM II show good discrimination. However, in most studies the calibration was poor. These scoring systems, particularly APACHE II, have been tested in patients within specific diagnostic categories. These studies have demonstrated the scoring systems to perform equally well for groups of patients with specific diseases as compared to heterogeneous ICU patients. However, APACHE II has consistently performed poorly in patients with trauma with or without head injury. Consequently, a number of trauma severity scoring systems have been developed, including the Revised Trauma Score (RTS), the Injury Severity Score (ISS), and the Trauma-Injury Severity Score (TRISS). In patients with acute head injury, the Glasgow Coma Scale remains the best severity scoring system.

APACHE II remains the most widely used and recognized severity scoring system. The score is relatively easy to calculate with the probability equation being in the public domain. SAPS II and MPM II do not seem to offer any particular advantages over APACHE II. While the operating characteristics of APACHE III are slightly better than that of APACHE II, it is debatable whether this justifies the large financial investment.

Severity scoring systems allow us to scientifically describe ICU patients. This information is useful in clinical research, where one of the most important controls is the ability to define the severity of illness of the individual patients being studied. Severity scoring systems cannot accurately predict individual patient outcome and should never be used for this purpose. The allocation of resources and admission and discharge criteria should be based on sound clinical criteria and not on severity scores. Mortality ratios are commonly used in the evaluation of the quality of care provided in different ICUs. It should, however, be appreciated that the outcome of patients is influenced by many factors including the type of hospital and referral base, source of patients, patient case mix, and discharge patterns. Many of these factors are "unmeasured" by the current scoring systems and therefore make comparison between hospitals based on standardized mortality ratios extremely unreliable. While the mean severity score and mortality ratio are useful in tracking trends within a particular ICU, they should be used with extreme caution as an indicator of quality of care.

■ SELECTED REFERENCES

1. Baker SP, O'Neil B, Haddon W. The injury severity score: a method for describing patients with multiple injuries and evaluating emergency care. *J Trauma*. 1974;14:187–196.
2. Boyd CR, Tolson MA, Copes WS. Evaluating trauma care: The TRISS method. *J Trauma*. 1987;27:370–378.
3. Champion HR, Copes WS, Sacco WJ. A revision of the trauma score. *J Trauma*. 1989;29:623–629.
4. Knaus WA, Draper EA, Wagner DP, Zimmerman JE. APACHE II: A severity of disease classification system. *Crit Care Med*. 1985;13:818–828.
5. Knaus WA, Wagner DP, Draper EA, Zimmerman JE, Bregner M, Bastos PG. The APACHE III prognostic system. Risk prediction of hospital mortality for critically ill hospitalized adults. *Chest*. 1991;100:1619–1636.
6. Le Gall JR, Lemeshow S, Saulnier F. A new simplified acute physiology score (SAPS II) based on a European/North American multicenter study. *JAMA*. 1993;270:2957–2963.
7. Lemeshow S, Teres D, Klar J, Avrunin JS, Gehlbach SH, Rapoport J. Mortality prediction models (MPM II) based on an international cohort of intensive care unit patients. *JAMA*. 1993;270:2478–2486.
8. Marik PE, Varon J. Severity scoring and outcome assessment: computerized predictive models and scoring systems. *Crit Care Clin*. 1999;15:633–646.

48

Sedation, Analgesia, and Paralysis in the Intensive Care Unit

Anxiety is an almost universal feature of ICU patients. Clinically significant anxiety has been reported in up to 70% of ICU patients. Severe anxiety is not limited to mechanically ventilated patients; indeed, Treggiari-Venzi and colleagues demonstrated that up to 30% of nonintubated surgical ICU patients had severe anxiety. Consequently, sedation is an integral component of the management of the ICU patient. The primary objective of sedation is to allay anxiety, enhance patient comfort, promote sleep, and facilitate mechanical ventilation. The desirable level of sedation/hypnosis will depend in large part upon the patient's acute disease process as well as the need for mechanical ventilation. However, the ideal level of sedation is one from which the patient can be easily aroused with maintenance of the normal sleep–wake cycle. Assessing the degree of sedation and titrating the drug regimen to predetermined end points are essential, as both oversedation and inadequate sedation are associated with significant complications.

Complications of undersedation include severe anxiety with delusional behavior, interference with medical and nursing care, sympathetic overactivity with increased myocardial oxygen consumption, self-injury, and self-extubation. Severe anxiety with inadequate sedation has been reported to be the most important factor leading to unplanned extubations. Oversedation is associated with significant morbidity including prolonged intubation with an increased risk of pulmonary complications and disorientation and "ICU-psychosis" following emergence. In addition, oversedation may mask significant neurological and neuromuscular complications.

In anxious patients, it is important to exclude treatable causes of anxiety and not just increase the amount of sedative drugs being used. Treatable causes of anxiety include

- Uncontrolled pain
- Ventilator settings inappropriate (especially, inadequate flow rate)—respiratory incoordination
- Drug or alcohol withdrawal syndrome
- Increased work breathing, e.g., pneumothorax, kinked/blocked tube
- Pulmonary edema
- Loud ventilator alarms and monitors
- Poor communication with patient as regards diagnosis, therapy, etc.

The use of continuous vs. intermittent sedation in the ICU is controversial. It has been assumed that because of its smoother pharmacokinetic and pharmacodynamic profile a continuous infusion would result in smoother sedation without periods of agitation and deep sedation. Furthermore, a continuous infusion requires a smaller cumulative dose. However, Kollef and colleagues in a prospective observational study have suggested that a continuous infusion of sedation is associated with prolonged mechanical ventilation. This observation, however, needs to be confirmed by other studies. Kress and colleagues demonstrated that the daily interruption of sedative-drug infusions (midazolam or propofol) in patients receiving mechanical ventilation decreased the duration of mechanical ventilation and the length of ICU stay. This approach is highly recommended for the following reasons:

- It allows daily assessment of neurological function that would otherwise not be possible (see Chapters 2 and 38).
- It prevents oversedation and reduction of total sedative dosages.

■ ASSESSING THE LEVEL OF SEDATION

In the deeply sedated or chemically paralyzed patient, the brain is much like a "black box" with very few physiological parameters available for assessment of neurological function and the level of sedation. Tachycardia, hypertension, and diaphoreses may be the only signs of inadequate sedation, and these are nonspecific. Consequently, some researchers have investigated the utility of processed electroencephalogram (EEG) technology to evaluate the level of sedation in ICU patients. While this technology has shown some utility in the operating room in patients under general anesthesia, it has performed less well in the ICU. Most notably, clinical observation of the patient has been a more reliable indicator of the level of sedation than the EEG signal. Furthermore, this technology performs poorly when benzodiazepines and opiates are used for sedation and does not provide an indicator of the degree of anxiety or delirium. Therefore, clinical evaluation remains the only effective method of assessing sedation and neurological function in sedated ICU patients.

Ongoing clinical evaluation is the most effective method of assessing sedation. To provide a more consistent and objective means of assessing the degree of sedation, a number of sedation scales have been developed. The Glasgow Coma Scale was developed to assess the level of consciousness of trauma patients. This scale is commonly used in neurosurgical ICUs. The GCS, however, is essentially a measure of *pathologic obtundation* and cannot be recommended for monitoring the level of sedation in ICU patients. The Ramsey Sedation scale and variations of this scale are the most frequently used methods of assessing and documenting sedation in the ICU. The Ramsey scale was reported by Ramsey and colleagues in 1974 in a study that assessed the use of alphaxalone-alphadolone (Althesin) in 30 ICU patients. The Ramsey scale, however, has a number of significant limitations when used to assess the level of sedation in ICU patients: (1) The six levels of the scale are not mutually exclusive; for example, a patient may be agitated (level 1) yet poorly responsive (level 5). (2) The levels are not clearly defined, nor are they fully inclusive. (3) The scale cannot accurately document various degrees of agitation. (4) It is difficult to link the scale to sedation orders protocols. The scale is essentially a measure of the level of consciousness rather than reflecting the degree of agitation or hypnosis of ICU patients.

The ideal sedation scale should be simple to compute and record, should accurately describe the degree of sedation or agitation, and should be amenable to drug orders protocols. Riker and colleagues have developed the Sedation-Agitation Scale (SAS), which meets many of these requirements. Once the sedative/hypnotic agents are chosen, an order can be written to titrate to a specific SAS level. The nursing record should then record the SAS level (hourly).

Ramsey Sedation Score

I. Anxious and agitated

II. Cooperative, orientated, and tranquil

III. Drowsy, responds to verbal commands

IV. Asleep, responds briskly to light stimulation

V. Asleep, sluggish response to stimulation

VI. Asleep, no response to stimulation

The Sedation-Agitation Scale

1. *Unarousable:* Deep hypnosis, nonrousable, no spontaneous movement, no coughing
2. *Very sedated:* Rousable with strong tactile stimulus, occasional spontaneous and nonpurposeful movements, does not respond to commands
3. *Sedated:* Asleep/sedated but rousable with tactile stimulus and displays purposeful movements and follows simple commands
4. *Calm and cooperative:* Calm, awakens easily, follows commands
5. *Agitated:* Anxious or mildly agitated, attempts to sit up, calms down to verbal instructions
6. *Very agitated:* Does not calm despite frequent verbal remind; requires physical restraints, biting endotracheal tube
7. *Dangerous agitation:* Severe anxiety, diaphoresis, frequent vigorous movements, pulling on endotracheal tube, trying to remove catheters, climbing over bed rails, striking at staff, thrashing side to side

■ SEDATIVE/HYPNOTIC AND ANALGESIC AGENTS USED IN THE ICU

Lorazepam

- *Kinetics:* Half-life of 10 to 20 hours; less lipid-soluble than diazepam; slower onset of action (2 to 5 minutes) with peak effect at 30 minutes; metabolized in liver to inactive metabolites by glucuronide conjugation; least affected by liver and renal disease; longer duration of action due to smaller volume of distribution (10 to 20 hours)
- *Dose:* 1 to 2 mg q4–6h, intravenous (IV) administration. If poor response, change to an IV infusion of lorazepam at 2 mg/h and then titrate to effect, increasing by 1 to 2 mg/h, not more frequently than every 15 minutes.
- In patients with severe alcohol withdrawal syndrome, the starting dose of lorazepam may be increased to 10 mg/h depending on the degree of agitation.
- Lorazepam should be avoided in patients with liver failure.
- If end points cannot be achieved with lorazepam alone, add propofol.

Midazolam

- *Kinetics:* Half-life of 4 to 6 hours (shortest); hepatic transformation to active metabolite that is renally cleared; half-life (H/L) is prolonged in congestive heart failure, in the elderly, liver disease, renal disease, multiple organ failure. Rapid onset (1 to 3 minutes), peak 5 minutes, duration 1 to 2.5 hours. Accumulates with prolonged infusion.
- *Dose:* Boluses of 1 to 5 mg every 5 minutes until the desired effect is achieved. May be used in patients who are extremely restless and thrashing about in the bed and at risk of injuring/extubating themselves.
- Patients with alcohol withdrawal syndrome may require increased dosages with boluses of 2 to 5 mg every 5 minutes until the desired effect is achieved.

Propofol

- *Kinetics:* Half-life of 30 to 60 minutes. Onset 30 seconds; emergence few minutes (does not accumulate). Even when the drug is used for several days, the return to a conscious state occurs within 10 to 15 minutes. Propofol is metabolized by glucuronide and sulphate conjugation. Dose reduction is not required in patients with hepatic or renal disease.
- *Dose:* Produces stable and predictable levels of sedation. The starting dose of propofol is 5 μg/kg/min. The dose should be increased by 5 μg/kg/min every 15 minutes until the desired effect is achieved (SAS level). The normal dose range is between 15 and 100 μg/kg/min (depends on desired effect and co-administered drugs).
- The major drawback to the use of propofol is its excessive cost (now on the decline).
- Propofol should be used when adequate sedation cannot be achieved with lorazepam alone, or under the following conditions:
   Head injury, cerebrovascular event, post-neurosurgery
   Patients with liver failure
   As an adjunctive agent in patients requiring >10 to 15 mg/h of lorazepam
   When weaning a patient from long-term lorazepam
   To facilitate advanced modes of ventilation
- Propofol has no analgesic properties, and therefore analgesics may be required.
- The emulsion in which propofol is contained represents approximately 0.1 g of fat (1.1 Kcal) for every milliliter. This high lipid load may result in excessive CO_2 production as well as hyperlipidemia when used for prolonged periods of time in the ICU.

Significant elevation of serum triglyceride levels have been reported with prolonged infusions of propofol. It is currently recommended that the lipid profile be monitored closely if patients receive the drug for more than 72 hours and that appropriate adjustments be made to the enteral/parenteral nutritional formulations. Monitoring the serum triglyceride levels may be particularly important in patients with a history of alcohol abuse, as propofol-induced hypertriglyceridemia has been causally associated with pancreatitis.

- Propofol should not be used in nonintubated patients, as these patients may rapidly lose control of their airway.

Haloperidol

- *Kinetics:* Half-life 18 to 54 hours; onset 5 to 30 minutes; duration 4 to 8 hours.
- *Dose:* 5 mg IV is the drug of choice for delirium. The dose can be repeated with 5-mg increments every 15 minutes, up to 25 mg. *Avoid* in patients with prolonged QTc, i.e., procainamide, quinidine, amiodarone, etc.

Ketamine

- *Kinetics:* Onset 30 seconds, duration of action 20 minutes.
- *Dose:* Usual dose is 0.5 to 1 mg/kg.
- Ketamine is a dissociate anesthetic agent with potent analgesic properties. Unlike most anesthetic agents, ketamine is a respiratory and cardiovascular stimulant. This drug is useful when performing procedures in patients with chronic obstructive pulmonary disease (COPD) and for performing painful procedures, e.g., burn dressings. Ketamine maintains pharyngeal reflexes and increases salivation; it must be avoided in patients with upper airway problems and patients with poorly controlled hypertension. Emergence reactions (vivid dreams) may be avoided by predosing with a small dose of a benzodiazepine.

■ OPIATES

Fentanyl

- *Kinetics:* Half-life 2 to 4 hours; onset 1 to 2 minutes; duration 30 to 60 minutes. Fentanyl is a potent opiate that has a rapid time to onset, short duration of action (compared to morphine), is easily titratable, and has minimal hemodynamic effects. These properties make fentanyl the agent of choice for pain control in the ICU.

- *Dose:* 50- to 100-µg boluses q2–4h or an infusion starting at 50µg/ h titrate up to 200µg/h in 20-µg increments every 30 minutes.
- Transdermal fentanyl patches (which deliver 25/50/75 or 100µg/ h) may provide excellent pain control.

Morphine

- *Kinetics:* Half-life 2 to 3 hours; onset 1 to 2 minutes; peak effect 20 minutes; duration 1 to 2 hours.
- *Dose:* 2- to 5-mg boluses or an infusion starting at 2mg/h, titrate up to 10mg/h in 2-mg increments every 30 minutes.
- Morphine should be *Avoided* in patients with renal failure. Morphine has active metabolites (morphine 3-glucuronide and morphine 6-glucuronide), which are renally excreted; these accumulate in renal failure, causing "delayed" respiratory depression.

Meperidine

- *Meperidine should not be used in the ICU.* This drug has an active metabolite, normeperidine, which is a central nervous system (CNS) stimulant and causes seizures, particularly in patients with renal impairment and patients with a history of seizures.

■ DRUGS OF CHOICE FOR SEDATION (BASED ON COST, EFFICACY, TOLERANCE, SIDE EFFECTS, ETC.)

Long-term Sedation

Lorazepam is the drug of choice for nonintubated patients and patients who will require long-term sedation/hypnosis in the ICU (>48 hours). This is based on pharmacoeconomic and pharmacokinetic criteria. The dosage will depend upon whether the patient is ventilated, his/her age, ethanol use, level of consciousness and anxiety, etc. Benzodiazepines should be avoided in patients with liver disease. Lorazepam and propofol act synergistically; the addition of propofol should be considered to prevent oversedation and long waking time.

Short-Term Sedation, Neurological/Neurosurgical Patients

Propofol is the drug of choice for short-term sedation and in patients with neurological disorders. Propofol is highly lipophilic; this property results in rapid uptake and elimination from the CNS, resulting in rapid recovery from sedation.

Deep Hypnosis to Facilitate "Advanced Modes of Ventilation"

Patients requiring pressure-controlled ventilation or ventilation with high positive end-expiratory pressure (PEEP), or small tidal volumes, or inverse ratio ventilation have "traditionally" required neuromuscular blockade to facilitate these modes of ventilation. However, due to the severe potential complications of neuromuscular blockade (NMB), deep hypnosis without paralysis is preferable (see complications of NMB below). This may be achieved with propofol alone. However, propofol and lorazepam have synergistic effects, and the combination of both of these agents may achieve the desired level of hypnosis at a lower cost.

Treatment of Delirium or Sedation Without Respiratory Depression

Haloperidol is the drug of choice in patients with delirium. This drug is also useful in patients with COPD in whom anxiolysis without sedation is required.

Sedation for Invasive Procedures

Midazolam alone or in combination with fentanyl is/are the drugs of choice for supplemental short-lived sedation and analgesia.

■ SAS GOALS OF SEDATION

Nonventilated Patients

- SAS 3 to 4

Ventilated Patients

- Modes: Assist control, intermittent mandatory ventilation, pressure-support ventilation. Decrease movement and promote ventilator synchrony, prevent injury and self-extubation. SAS level 3 to 4.

- Modes: Inverse ratio ventilation or pressure-control ventilation. Deep sedation. SAS level 1 to 2.

■ EXAMPLE OF SEDATION ORDERS PROTOCOLS

Nonintubated Patients

Analgesia:	Fentanyl patch (25/50/75) or 25 to 50µg IV q2–4h.
Delirium:	Haldol 5mg, increasing by 5mg every 15 minutes up to 25mg.
Sedation:	Lorazepam 1 to 2mg q4–6h IV to achieve SAS level 3 to 4.
Delirium tremens:	Depending on degree of agitation, 5- to 10-mg bolus, followed by an infusion of lorazepam starting at 5- to 10-mg/h and titrated up to 30mg/h to achieve an SAS level of 3 to 4. If dose of 30mg/h does not control agitation, consider intubation and propofol. Haldol for delirium.

Intubated Patients

Analgesia:	Fentanyl patch (25/50/75), 25 to 50µg IV q2–4h or infusion 50 to 200µg/h.
Delirium:	Haldol 5mg, increasing by 5mg every 15 minutes up to 25mg.
Sedation:	1. Lorazepam

Level of Anxiety	Suggested Starting Dosages of Lorazepam
SAS level 5	Lorazepam 1 to 2mg q4–6h IV. If poor response, change to an IV infusion of lorazepam at 2mg/h and then titrate to desired SAS level, increasing by 1mg/h not more frequently than every 15 minutes.
SAS level 6	Lorazepam infusion: Start at 2mg/h and then titrate to desired SAS level, increasing by 2mg/h not more frequently than every 15 minutes.

| SAS level 7 | Lorazepam bolus of 4 mg. Lorazepam infusion: Start at 6 mg/h and then titrate to effect, increasing by 2 mg/h not more frequently than every 15 minutes. |

2. Propofol:
If adequate sedation (desired SAS level) is not achieved with lorazepam 10 mg/h (can use 15 mg/h), then add propofol starting at 5 µg/kg/min and increase by 5 µg/kg/min every 15 minutes until desired level of sedation is achieved.

Short-Term Sedation, Neurological/Neurosurgical Patients

For these patients, use propofol, starting at 5 µg/kg/min and increase by 5 µg/kg/min every 15 minutes until the desired level of sedation is achieved.

■ NEUROMUSCULAR BLOCKADE

Neuromuscular junction blocking agents have historically been used in the operating room to augment surgical anesthesia, where they have been found to be remarkably safe. These agents have, however, found their way into ICU's, where they have been used for prolonged periods of time to facilitate mechanical ventilation. The safety of these drugs has, however, been questioned, due to the increasing number of case reports of prolonged paralysis following their use. In particular, the concomitant use of nondepolarizing neuromuscular blocking agents and high-dose corticosteroids has been linked to the syndrome variously known as *acute quadriplegic myopathy*, *acute necrotizing myopathy*, and *thick-filament myopathy* (see Chapter 38). This syndrome may occur after use as short as 8 hours and without the concomitant use of corticoids. These agents, therefore, should be used only when absolutely indicated (and only when high-dose propofol has failed) and then only for the shortest possible period of time. NMB should *Never* be used for the treatment of anxiety or restlessness.

The major indication for neuromuscular blockage in the ICU is to facilitate ventilation in the following circumstances:

- When using high PEEP
- When peak airway pressures are high
- When using inverse-ratio or pressure-controlled inverse ratio-ventilation
- When using PEEP with low tidal volume ventilation

To prevent excessive and prolonged neuromuscular blockade, all patients receiving neuromuscular blocking agents should be monitored using a nerve stimulator. For practical purposes, the train of four (TOF) should be used to access the degree of neuromuscular blockade. The goal is to achieve one to two twitches (see below).

Neuromuscular Blocking Agents

Acute quadriplegic myopathy has been associated with the use of both steroid- and nonsteroid-based neuromuscular blocking agents and is probably a class-related phenomenon. Pancuronium is the most cost-effective agent. In patients in whom the vagolytic and histamine-releasing effects need to be avoided—e.g., in severe asthmatics and patients with a tachycardia—vecuronium or doxacurium can be used. In patients with hepatic/renal failure, atracurium (or doxacurium) should be used (pancuronium and vecuronium have active metabolites).

- Pancuronium: Duration 120 to 150 minutes
  Intubation: 0.06 to 0.08 mg/kg
  Maintenance: 4 to 8 mg/h
- Vecuronium: Duration 60 to 75 minutes
  Intubation: 0.07 to 0.1 mg/kg
  Maintenance: 4 to 10 mg/h
- Atracurium: Duration 45 to 60 minutes
  Intubation: 0.4 to 0.5 mg/kg
  Maintenance: 20 to 50 mg/h
- Doxacurium: Duration 30 to 160 minutes
  Intubation: 0.015 to 0.03 mg/kg
  Maintenance: 0.005 to 0.03 mg/kg/h
- Rocuronium: 0.6 to 1.2 mg/kg for intubation. Acts within 1 minute, with duration of action up to 30 minutes.
- Succinylcholine (*for intubation only*): Duration 5 to 15 minutes. 1 mg/kg. Beware bradycardia with repeated doses. *Contraindications to the use of succinylcholine include*
  Renal failure
  Burns
  Severe trauma with muscle injury
  Severe sepsis
  Ocular injuries

Train of Four Monitoring and Dosage Adjustments

The TOF (four stimuli 0.5 seconds apart) is a convenient way of monitoring the degree of NMB and roughly correlates with the degree of neuromuscular junction receptor occupation:

4 twitches	0 to 70% receptors occupied
3 twitches	70% to 80% receptors occupied
2 twitches	80% to 90% receptors occupied
1 twitch	>95% receptors occupied
0 twitches	100% receptors occupied

In principle, any superficially located peripheral motor nerve can be stimulated. The ulnar nerve, however, is the most popular site. The electrodes are best applied on the volar side of the wrist. The distal electrode should be placed about 1 cm proximal to the point at which the proximal flexion crease of the wrist crosses the radial side of the tendon to the flexor carpi ulnaris muscle. The proximal electrode should be placed 2 to 3 cm proximal to the distal electrode (Figure 48-1). With this placement of electrodes, electrical stimulation normally elicits finger flexion and thumb adduction.

Because different muscle groups have different sensitivities to neuromuscular blocking agents, results obtained for one muscle cannot be extrapolated automatically to other muscles. The diaphragm is the most resistant of all muscles to NMB. In general, the diaphragm requires 1.4 to 2 times as much muscle relaxant as the adductor pollicis muscle for an identical degree of blockade. From a practical point of view, 1 to 2 twitches (of TOF) of the adductor pollicis muscle will result in sufficient diaphragmatic paralysis to prevent the

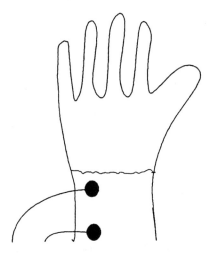

Figure 48-1. Placement of electrodes for TOF testing.

patient from coughing, hiccoughing, and breathing during mechanical ventilation.

Before paralysis, the supramaximal stimulation (SMS) must be determined. The SMS is defined as the level at which additional stimulation current does not increase the twitch response. It is important to note that each nerve may have a different SMS, and inadequate stimulation may lead the clinician to overestimate the degree of NMB present. The SMS is usually in the range of 20 to 60 mA.

Starting at 10 mA, increase the TOF current by 10 mA until four equal responses are obtained. Continue to increase the current until the intensity of the response does not increase any further. When this occurs, the prior setting will be the SMS for that nerve. Once the patient is paralyzed, the TOF is then performed using the SMS.

The TOF test should be performed hourly until the goal is achieved (1 to 2 twitches) and then every 6 hours. The rate of the infusion should be adjusted as follows:

0 Twitches: Stop infusion, restart when 2 twitches are present. Restart infusion rate at
      80% if 1 hour is required for 2 twitches
      75% if 2 hour is required for 2 twitches
      50% if 3 hour is required for 2 twitches
      25% if 4 hour is required for 2 twitches
1 Twitch: Reduce to 80% of present infusion rate.
2 Twitches: Maintain present infusion rate.
3 Twitches: Reload with 25% of loading dose; increase infusion rate by 25%.
4 Twitches: Reload with 50% of loading dose; increase infusion rate by 50%.

■ SELECTED REFERENCES

1. Boulain T. Unplanned extubations in the adult intensive care unit: a prospective multicenter study. Association des Reanimateurs du Centre-Ouest. *Am J Respir Crit Care Med*. 1998;157:1131–1137.
2. Chevron V, Menard JF, Richard JC, Girault C, Leroy J, Bonmarchand G. Unplanned extubation: risk factors of development and predictive criteria for reintubation. *Crit Care Med*. 1998;26:1049–1053.
3. Fischer JR, Baer RK. Acute myopathy associated with combined use of corticosteroids and neuromuscular blocking agents. *Ann Pharmacother*. 1996;30:1437–1445.
4. Kollef MH, Levy NT, Ahrens TS, Schaiff R, Prentice D, Sherman G. The use of continuous i.v. sedation is associated with prolongation of mechanical ventilation. *Chest*. 1998;114:541–548.
5. Kress JP, Pohlman AS, O'Connor MF, Hall JB. Daily interruption of sedative infusions in critically ill patients undergoing mechanical ventilation. *N Engl J Med*. 2000;342:1471–1477.

6. Osborne R, Joel S, Grebenik K, Trew D, Slevin M. The pharmacokinetics of morphine and morphine glucuronides in kidney failure. *Clin Pharmacol Ther*. 1993;54:158–167.
7. Ramsay MA, Savage TM, Simpson BR, Goodwin R. Controlled sedation with alphaxalone-alphadolone. *BMJ*. 1974;2:656–659.
8. Riker RR, Picard JT, Fraser GL. Prospective evaluation of the Sedation-Agitation Scale for adult critically ill patients. *Crit Care Med*. 1999;27:1325–1329.
9. Shapiro BA, Warren J, Egol AB, et al. Practice parameters for intravenous analgesia and sedation for adult patients in the intensive care unit: an executive summary. *Crit Care Med*. 1995;23:1596–1600.
10. Simmons LE, Riker RR, Prato BS, Fraser GL. Assessing sedation during intensive care unit mechanical ventilation with the Bispectral Index and the Sedation-Agitation. *Crit Care Med*. 1999;27:1499–1504.
11. Teasdale G, Jennett B. Assessment of coma and impaired consciousness: a practical scale. *Lancet*. 1974;2:81–84.
12. Treggiari-Venzi M, Borgeat A, Fuchs-Buder T, Gachoud JP, Suter PM. Overnight sedation with midazolam or propofol in the ICU: effects on sleep quality, anxiety and depression. *Intensive Care Med*. 1996;22:1186–1190.

49

Nutrition

During the last decade, the seemingly simple task of feeding critically ill patients has become exceedingly complex with much controversy. However, the two commandments of nutrition support still hold true, namely,

1. **If the bowel works, use it.**
2. **There is no disease process that benefits from starvation.**

The results of a number of randomized controlled clinical trials (and meta-analyses of these trials) have established the following principles on which to base nutritional support in critically ill patients:

1. No data indicates that total parenteral nutrition (TPN) is of any benefit in critically ill patients. The available evidence suggests that TPN increases complications and mortality rates. TPN should therefore be limited to patients who, after 5 to 7 days of starvation, are unable to tolerate even small volumes of enteral nutrition. Despite these data, patients with a functional gut continue to receive TPN!

2. Early enteral nutrition (within 24 hours of admission to the ICU) has been shown to reduce complications and improve the outcome of critically ill patients when compared to delayed enteral nutrition. No studies demonstrate an advantage to delaying nutritional support in seriously ill patients.

3. "Immune-enhancing" diets have been demonstrated to reduce complications and length of stay (LOS) in high-risk ICU patients.

4. Overfeeding patients is associated with significant complications including hyperglycemia, hepatic steatosis with hepatic dysfunction, elevated serum urea nitrogen, and excessive CO_2 production.

5. No data suggest that accurately measuring energy expenditure and nutritional requirements improves outcome.

From the above data it appears that the route, timing, and type of nutritional formulation is more important than the specific amounts of nutrients supplied, as long as overfeeding is avoided. This largely simplifies the approach to nutritional support in ICU patients: i.e., feed the bowel, do it early, do it slowly, and do it with an immune-enhancing diet (just *do it*).

During acute stress, the body mobilizes endogenous amino acid and energy stores. It is not possible to make catabolic patients anabolic. The role of nutritional support is to limit protein wasting and to supply essential and conditionally essential nutrients. Specialized *immune-enhancing* nutritional formulas have been developed based on experimental investigations; these formulas are generally peptide based (improved nitrogen absorption, less diarrhea, improved proteins synthesis) and contain arginine (enhanced protein synthesis and immune function), glutamine (maintain integrity of gastrointestinal tract), nucleotides (enhance immune function), and omega-3 fatty acids.

Recent studies have shown that dietary fatty acids can reduce the severity of inflammatory injury by altering the availability of arachidonic acid in tissue phospholipids. Animal and clinical studies have shown that nutritional intervention with dietary fish oil containing eicosapentaenoic acid (an omega-3 fatty acid) can favorably modulate proinflammatory eicosanoid production from arachidonic acid. Similarly, gamma-linolenic acid suppresses leukotriene biosynthesis and is further metabolized to the monoenoic prostaglandins, such as prostaglandin E_1. Prostaglandin E_1 is a potent vasodilator of pulmonary and systemic circulation and inhibits platelet aggregation, neutrophil chemotaxis, and oxygen radical release.

Over 20 randomized, double-blind, multicenter clinical trials have compared immune-enhancing diets with standard enteral formulas. These studies have consistently demonstrated that immune-enhancing diets decrease indices of inflammation, improve cell-mediated immunity, decrease organ failure and ICU complications, and reduce ventilator and ICU days. Immune-enhancing diets should therefore be given to all patients with acute lung injury or acute respiratory distress syndrome, sepsis, polytrauma, and other high-risk patients with an anticipated ICU stay in excess of 5 days.

The absence of bowel sounds does not mean that the bowel is not working. Bowel sounds result from air moving through the small intestine. The presence of bowel sounds requires gastric emptying and gastric air. Many seriously ill patients have gastroparesis and are being treated with nasogastric suctioning. These patients have little movement of air from the stomach to the small intestine and therefore have decreased bowel sounds. Furthermore, to declare the absence of bowel sounds, one should listen for 2 to 4 minutes in each of four quadrants (total of 10 to 16 minutes). Few clinicians listen for more than a few seconds. In addition, the quantity of bowel sounds (or volume of flatus) does not directly correlate with gut motility. Thus, bowel sounds are a poor indicator of small intestine function. The presence of bowel sounds is a better indicator of active gastric emptying.

Gastric feeding is delivered using nasogastric tubes, small-bore feeding tubes, or gastrostomy tubes. Larger-bore nasogastric tubes are preferred when feeding the stomach, as this allows for the monitoring of gastric residual volumes. Nasogastric tubes are generally easily placed (the oral route is preferred in intubated patients due to the lower risk of sinusitis). Gastric location must be confirmed before feeding (aspiration of gastric contents). In patients who fail gastric feeding (see below), postpyloric small-bore feeding tubes are recommended. While these feeding tubes can be placed at the bedside, endoscopic or radiographic placement is recommended. Some clinicians place feeding tubes into the stomach and wait until they migrate into the small intestine. This approach has little efficacy in critically ill patients with impaired gastric emptying. An aggressive approach to ensuring placement of small-bowel feeding tubes is necessary for the administration of early enteral nutrition.

Enteral feeding should be initiated within 12 to 48 hours of admission to the ICU. If oral feeds are not feasible, a gastric feeding tube should be placed and feeding attempted before placing a small bowel feeding tube. However, if a patient is at high risk for poor gastric emptying (i.e., severe multiple trauma, history of gastroparesis) or at high risk of aspiration, then a small bowel tube should be placed. The head of the bed should be elevated to 30 degrees to decrease the risk of aspiration. Feeding may be administered by boluses of 100 to 250 mL every 2 to 4 hours or by continuous infusion started at 25 to 30 mL/h and increased by 10 to 25 mL/h every 4 hours as tolerated (i.e., gastric residual volumes <150 mL) until caloric goal is achieved (25 to 30 kcal/day). Preliminary evidence suggests that bolus feeds that intermittently distend the stomach may result in better gastric emptying. Gastric residuals should be measured every 4 hours with continuous feeding or before each bolus. If the gastric residual is >150 mL and/or if the patient refluxes, the stomach should be emptied, feedings held for 2 hours, and then reinstated at one half the volume. *Erythromycin/metoclopramide* improves gastric emptying in critically ill patients and may prove useful in patients who have large residuals and/or tolerate tube feeding poorly. If the residual volumes remain high and/or the patient tolerates tube feeding poorly, postpyloric access should then be obtained.

The recommended average daily requirements are

- Nonprotein calories ±25 to 30 kcal/kg/day.
- CHO: MAX 4 mg/kg/day (±1600 cal). The body cannot utilize (oxidize) more than 4 mg/kg/day of glucose. Excess glucose administration will result in hyperglycemia and lipogenesis.
- Lipid: 4 to 12 kcal/kg/day.

- Protein ~1.5 g/kg/day.
- Water-soluble vitamins, fat-soluble vitamins, and trace elements.

Propofol emulsion contains approximately 0.1 g of fat (1.1 kcal) for every milliliter. An infusion of propofol may therefore provide a significant caloric load. In patients receiving high-dose propofol infusions, the enteral feeds need to be adjusted to take into account the added caloric load. A low-fat enteral formulation, such as Vivonex, may be used. The constituents of common enteral formulas are shown in Table 49-1.

■ NUTRITION IN SPECIFIC DISEASE STATES

Liver Failure (See Chapter 28)

Pancreatitis (See Chapter 27)

Renal Failure (See Chapter 32)

Most patients with acute renal failure (ARF) are hypercatabolic and require increased quantities of nutrients. Patients with ARF should receive protein in a minimum of 1 g/kg/day and optimal nonprotein calories. Protein intake in critically patients should not be limited in an attempt to avoid initiation of dialysis. In patients receiving TPN and continuous renal replacement therapy, the amino acid intake should be increased 30%. In patients with chronic renal failure, keto-analogs may be useful in patients with decreased protein intake for >1 week.

■ PARENTERAL NUTRITION

A small number of ICU patients may not tolerate enteral feeding due to a severe prolonged ileus, or enteral feeding may not be possible due to discontinuity of the bowel. In these patients, parenteral nutrition may be indicated. However, the concurrent administration of small volumes of enteral feeds (20 mL/h) may limit the gut mucosal atrophy that is seen in patients who receive TPN.

In most patients, a standard TPN formulation is adequate, with adjustments in the rate of infusion to meet patients' needs. The following is an example of a standard TPN formulation:

- 400 g CHO (dextrose; 1360 cal) +70 g protein in 1.5 to 2 L
- 250 ml of 20% fat solution (500 cal)

Table 49-1. Constituents of common enteral formulas (per 1000 cc).

Product	Calories	CHO (g)	Protein (g)	Fat (g)	Na (Meq)	K (Meq)	Osmol (mOsm/kg)
Ensure	1060	140	36	36	32	30	470
Ensure Plus	1500	197	54	53	50	60	690
Ensure Plus NH	1500	197	62	49	52	47	650
Promote	1000	130	63	26	40	51	330
Traumacal	1000	142	83	68	51	36	490
Perative	1300	177	67	38	45	44	385
Osmolite	1060	143	37	38	24	26	300
Osmolite HN	1060	139	43	36	40	40	300
Impact	1000	130	56	28	48	36	375
Jevity	1060	150	44	36	40	40	310
Hep Aid II	1180	170	40 (branch chain AA)	40	15	<5	560
Nepro	2000	215	70	95	36	27	635
AminoAid	2000	370	20 (essential AA)	50	0	0	850
Vivonex	1000	190	45	10	25	30	650

TPN should be initiated slowly; 50% of goal first day, 75% second day, 100% third to fourth day. In addition, TPN should not be suddenly stopped (may cause profound hypoglycemia).

TPN is associated with significant complications, including an increased incidence of infections (particularly, catheter-associated septicemia); metabolic disturbances such as hyperglycemia, hypophosphatemia, hypokalemia, and trace element deficiency; atrophy of the gastrointestinal mucosa, predisposing to bacterial translocation; immune suppression and hepatic dysfunction.

TPN frequently causes hepatic dysfunction. It is postulated that carbohydrate overload with increased lipid production may be contribute to the disorder. Hepatic dysfunction results in both biochemical and histologic changes in the liver. These include the following:

Biochemical

- Increase in transaminases usually 1 to 2 weeks after starting TPN. Transaminases usually normalize without stopping or changing TPN.
- Bilirubin and alkaline phosphatase may also increase.

Histologic

- Steatosis
- Lipidosis
- Cholestasis
- Steatohepatitis

Patients who develop hepatic dysfunction and require continuation of the TPN should receive 20% to 50% of nonprotein calories as fat, preferably in the form of medium chain triglycerides.

■ THE REFEEDING SYNDROME

Protein-calorie malnutrition has been shown to exist in up to 50% of hospitalized patients. Feeding malnourished patients, particularly after a period of starvation, may result in severe metabolic disturbances, most notably hypophosphatemia. Hypophosphatemia developing after initiating parenteral or enteral nutrition has been termed the *refeeding syndrome*. In addition to hypophosphatemia, changes in potassium, magnesium, and glucose metabolism occur during refeeding. Although classically described in cachectic patients after prolonged starvation, this syndrome has been reported to occur commonly in poorly nourished ICU patients who have been starved for as short as 48 hours.

The combination of total body phosphorus depletion and increased influx of phosphorus during refeeding leads to severe extracellular hypophosphatemia. Low serum phosphorus levels lead to depletion of high-energy phosphate bonds and adenosine triphosphate, altering cellular metabolism. Hypophosphatemia as an isolated metabolic abnormality has been found to impair organ function and may result in severe sequelae. In patients with poor baseline nutrition, refeeding should commence slowly and gradually. Serum levels of potassium, phosphate, and magnesium need to be determined before refeeding and monitored daily during the first week of refeeding.

The commercially available tube feed preparations contain between 50 and 60 mg/dL of phosphorus (the recommended daily allowance). However, in patients with high metabolic demands and in phosphorus-depleted patients, these formulas may not meet the requirements necessary to accommodate the massive transcellular shifts and possible whole-body depletion of phosphorus found in these patients.

■ SELECTED REFERENCES

1. Gadek JE, DeMichele SJ, Karlstad MD, et al. Effect of enteral feeding with eicosapentaenoic acid, gamma-linolenic acid, and antioxidants in patients with acute respiratory distress syndrome. Enteral Nutrition in ARDS Study Group. *Crit Care Med.* 1999;27:1409–1420.
2. Heyland DK, MacDonald S, Keefe L, Drover JW. Total parenteral nutrition in the critically ill patient: a meta-analysis. *JAMA.* 1998;280:2013–2019.
3. Marik PE, Bedigian MK. Refeeding hypophosphatemia in critically ill patients in an intensive care unit. A prospective study. *Arch Surg.* 1996;131: 1043–1047.
4. Moore EE, Jones TN. Benefits of feeding after major abdominal trauma—a prospective randomized study. *J Trauma.* 1986;26:874–881.
5. Perioperative total parenteral nutrition in surgical patients. The Veterans Affairs Total Parenteral Nutrition Cooperative Study Group. *N Engl J Med.* 1991;325:525–532.
6. Zaloga GP. Dietary lipids: ancestral ligands and regulators of cell signaling pathways. *Crit Care Med.* 1999;27:1646–1648.
7. Zaloga GP. Early enteral nutritional support improves outcome: hypothesis or fact? *Crit Care Med.* 1999;27:259–261.
8. Zaloga GP. Immune-enhancing enteral diets: where's the beef? *Crit Care Med.* 1998;26:1143–1146.

50

Hematology in the Intensive Care Unit

■ CRITICAL CARE ANEMIA

Anemia is a problem that commonly complicates the course of critically ill patients admitted to the ICU. Approximately 85% of patients admitted to the ICU with a length of stay of >1 week are transfused with at least 1 U of blood. Most of the transfusions in the ICU are *not associated with acute blood loss*; rather, ICU patients appear to have a constant transfusion requirement of 2 to 4 U/wk. The cause of the anemia is multifactorial, with the following factors playing a role: inappropriately low erythropoietin levels, a blunted response to erythropoietin, blood loss due to venesection, blood loss due to gastric stress ulceration, coagulopathy associated with systemic inflammation, and reduced red cell life span.

The use of recombinant erythropoietin has emerged as an alternative to blood transfusion. Corwin and co-workers demonstrated that the administration of recombinant erythropoietin to ICU patients resulted in a 45% reduction in the number of units of red blood cells (RBCs) transfused. The optimal dose and timing of recombinant erythropoietin administration remains to be determined. However, recent data suggest that a weekly dose of 600 U/kg/wk (~40,000) may be adequate. Considering the numerous complications associated with blood transfusion (see below) and the postulated association with increased morbidity and mortality, it would seem logical and cost-effective to treat all ICU patients with a projected ICU stay of >1 week with 40,000 U on the second or third ICU day (and then weekly). Patients receiving erythropoietin should receive oral iron supplementation (≥150 mg of elemental iron) with monitoring of the serum ferritin concentration. Parenteral iron should be considered in patients whose serum ferritin remains <100 ng/mL despite oral supplementation.

■ THE OPTIMAL HEMATOCRIT: HOW MUCH BLOOD IS ENOUGH?

Traditional wisdom in anesthesia has always held that patients should have a hemoglobin concentration >10 g/dL (hematocrit > 30) before the administration of anesthesia for surgery. Similarly, it has been taught that the hemoglobin of critically ill patients should be kept above 10 g/dL. The value of 10 g/dL is based on the theoretical premise that the arterial oxygen content should be greater than the oxygen extraction of tissue with the highest extraction, which for clinical purposes is the myocardium whose oxygen extraction is of the order of 12 mL/dL. This postulate was erroneously supported by a number of poorly designed clinical experiments. This simplistic view overlooks the physiologic adjustments seen in acute stress that serves to maintain adequate oxygen delivery and ignores the myriad deleterious effects associated with blood transfusion.

There are a lack of reliable data to define "*the ideal*" hemoglobin concentration in critically ill patients. A number of studies have failed to demonstrate an improvement in global and organ specific oxygenation when critically ill patients with a hemoglobin of less than 10 g/dL are transfused. Indeed, data suggest that the number of units of transfused blood may be an independent predictor of multisystem organ failure and death. The Canadian Critical Care Trials Group reported the results of a randomized study in which ICU patients were randomized to a conservative group (transfused if hemoglobin [Hb] < 7 g/dL, Hb maintained 7 to 9 g/dL) or liberal group (transfused if Hb < 10, and Hb maintained between 10 and 12 g/dL). The hospital mortality rate and incidence of complications were higher in the liberal group. Based on these data, a transfusion "trigger" of 7 to 8 g/dL may be a reasonable compromise. However, patients with coronary artery disease or "cardiac decompensation" may be at risk of silent ischemia at this level, and a transfusion trigger of 9 to 10 g/dL may be more appropriate in this group of patients.

■ BLOOD COMPONENT THERAPY (TABLE 50-1)

Indications

Red Cells

- Hb < 9 in patients with evidence of cardiac decompensation and/or history of coronary artery disease
- Acute gastrointestinal tract bleed with hematocrit < 30
- Hb < 7.5 in all other ICU

Table 50-1. Dosing guidelines for using blood components.

Blood component	Dose	Recommended infusion times
Fresh-frozen plasma	2–4 U (400–1000 mL)	1 h
Platelets	Use whatever dose is necessary to increase platelet count >50,000; 6 U are usually sufficient; or 1 U or random platelets per 10 kg	30 min
Cryoprecipitate	Desired increase in g/L = (0.2 × number bags)/plasma volume in liters; or use 1 bag/5 kg	IV push or 1000 U/10 min
Packed red blood cells	1 U increases hemoglobin by 1.0–1.5 g/dL	2–3 h

Platelets

- Platelets should generally be reserved for thrombocytopenic patients who are *bleeding* and thrombocytopenic patients undergoing invasive or operative procedures.
- Chronic thrombocytopenia (<5000) and patient bleeding.
- Acute or chronic thrombocytopenia (<10,000) and patient on chemotherapy.
- Acute thrombocytopenia (<50,000) and patient bleeding.
- Acute or chronic thrombocytopenia (<100,000) and operative bleeding.
- *Contraindicated in (TTP)* (see below).

Fresh-Frozen Plasma

- Replacement of clotting factors when prothrombin time (PT) and/or partial thromboplastin time (PTT) 1.5× control or greater *and patient bleeding or facing hemostatic challenge*
- Treatment of TTP
- Treatment of ATIII deficiency
- Rapid reversal of warfarin effect
- C1 esterase inhibitor deficiency

Cryoprecipitate

- Fibrinogen <100 mg/dL and patient bleeding
- Hemophilia A or von Willebrand's disease

Note

- Fresh-frozen plasma (FFP) contains all the stable and labile plasma constituents. One unit of FFP contains approximately 400 mg of fibrinogen and 1 U of clotting activity per milliliter.
- Cryoprecipitate is prepared from a cold-insoluble precipitate of plasma. It contains high levels of factor VIII (both procoagulant activity and von Willebrand's factor) and fibrinogen. Insufficient amounts of the other clotting factors are present to be of therapeutic value.

Risks and Adverse Effects Associated With Red Cell Transfusion

Infectious

Cytomegalovirus	Common
Non A, non B hepatitis	1:100 (before hepatitis C screening)
Hepatitis B	1:100 to 1:200
Human immune deficiency virus (HIV)	1:40,000 to 1:1,000,000
Bacterial sepsis	Rare

Immunologic

Fever, chills, urticaria	1:50 to 1:100
Acute hemolytic transfusion (t/f) reaction	1:12,000
Delayed hemolytic t/f reaction	1:1000
Fatal hemolytic t/f reaction	1:100,000
Anaphylaxis (IgA or IgG)	1:150,000
Graft vs. host reaction	Unknown
T/f-related acute lung injury	1:5000
Pulmonary leukoagglutination syndrome	
Passive transfer of leukocyte agglutinating or cytotoxic antibodies	
Febrile nonhemolytic reaction	1:100 to 1:200
Recipient antibodies to donor white blood cells	
Immunoparesis	
Impaired B- and T-cell function	

Other

An acute (transitory) neutrophilic leucocytosis
Increased blood viscosity

Microcapillary occlusion due to transfusion of poorly deformable RBCs

Hyperkalemia

Metabolic alkalosis

Hypothermia

The Effects of Massive Blood Transfusion

- A massive transfusion is defined as the administration of blood in excess of one blood volume within 24 hours (approximately 10 U blood).
- Dilutional coagulopathy: Prophylactic platelet transfusions and FFP are not recommended. The coagulopathy should be treated on an individual basis, dependent on the patient's clinical condition, the platelet count, and the PT and PTT.
- Citrate toxicity and hypocalcemia. Citrate toxicity is uncommon except in patients with underlying liver disease (citrate is metabolized to lactate and bicarbonate by the liver) and patients receiving in excess of 40 U blood. Calcium should be given only to patients with a low ionized serum calcium (<1 mmol/L).
- Electrolyte and acid–base. Hyperkalemia and alkalosis may develop after a massive transfusion.

■ DISSEMINATED INTRAVASCULAR COAGULATION

Diagnosis of Disseminated Intravascular Coagulation

Laboratory Features

- Peripheral blood smear will show fragmented RBCs and thrombocytopenia with large platelets.
- Prolonged PT and PTT.
- Thrombocytopenia.
- Decreased levels of fibrinogen.
- Decreased levels of anti-thrombin III.
- Increased levels of fibrin split products and D-dimer.
- Decreased levels of Protein C

Clinical Features Associated With Bleeding

Bleed from venipuncture sites, mucous membranes, hematuria, gastrointestinal bleeds, intracerebral bleeds

Petechia, purpura, and subcutaneous hematomas

Clinical Features of End Organ Damage Due to Thrombosis

- Acute lung injury syndrome
- Proteinuria and renal insufficiency
- Hepatocellular dysfunction
- Mental state changes and neurological deficits

Coagulation disorders are commonly encountered in the ICU. Many conditions including sepsis, malignancy, trauma, vasculitic disorders, and obstetrical accidents may give rise to a coagulopathy. In addition, patients may have medical conditions that predispose them to developing a coagulopathy: e.g., patients with liver disease, renal failure, lupus, leukemia, etc. Sepsis, however, is the single most common factor leading to a coagulopathy and disseminated intravascular coagulation (DIC). DIC has been reported in about 10% to 20% of patients with gram-negative bacteremia and 70% of patients with septic shock. DIC appears to be an important independent predictor of acute respiratory distress syndrome, multiple organ dysfunction syndrome, and death.

DIC results from the systemic activation of both the clotting and fibrinolytic systems, leading to the consumption of many coagulation factors and platelets. The initial activation of coagulation in sepsis is primarily dependent on activation of the extrinsic (tissue factor dependent) pathway. Tumor necrosis factor (TNF) plays an important role in the pathophysiology of DIC, as it induces the expression and release of tissue factor. In addition, TNF down-regulates thrombomodulin expression on endothelial cells, resulting in decreased protein C activity, thus further contributing to a procoagulant state. The systemic activation of the clotting system results in the widespread formation of fibrin thrombi. In patients with DIC, the fibrinolytic system is initially activated and subsequently inhibited. In the initial stages of DIC, there is an increase in both tissue-type plasminogen activator and urokinase-type plasminogen activator. This results in the increased conversion of plasminogen to plasmin with the breakdown of fibrin. However, within a few hours after the onset of sepsis, high levels of plasminogen activator inhibitor type 1 are found, with a rapid decline in plasminogen activator activity and plasmin generation. This imbalance between the activation of coagulation and the activation of fibrinolysis results in inadequate degradation of fibrin, resulting in widespread microcapillary thrombosis.

DIC is generally considered to be a systemic hemorrhagic syndrome. However, this is only because hemorrhage is obvious and often impressive. Less commonly appreciated is the formidable microvascular thrombosis that occurs. Fibrin deposition in the microcirculation is a frequent, if not invariable finding in patients with DIC. This microvascular thrombosis is closely related to the development of multiple organ dysfunction syndrome and is therefore closely linked to the prognosis of patients with DIC. This microvascular damage is especially pronounced in the lungs and kidneys.

The treatment of DIC remains controversial. This is primarily because very few studies have objectively examined various therapeutic strategies in patients with DIC. The essential therapeutic modality is to treat the triggering disease process. Since thrombosis is the process with the greatest impact on morbidity and mortality, low-dose heparin has been suggested by some authors to stop the intravascular process. There is, however, no conclusive evidence that heparin treatment reduces the morbidity or mortality associated with DIC. Low levels of anti-thrombin III (ATIII) are virtually a constant feature of DIC. Such a decrease in ATIII levels makes questionable the potential benefit of heparin therapy. In a small study comparing the infusion ATIII, heparin, and the combination of heparin and ATIII, Vinazzer demonstrated that the duration of DIC and the transfusion requirements were significantly greater in the patients receiving heparin alone and heparin together with ATIII than in those patients treated with ATIII alone. Antithrombin III is the most important physiological inhibitor of blood coagulation, as it interferes with the clotting process at various levels. In addition to its role in coagulation, ATIII has also been shown to have marked anti-inflammatory properties. This would suggest that ATIII may itself have a role in the treatment of sepsis. A small randomized study demonstrated that a high-dose infusion of ATIII in septic patients with DIC significantly reduced the duration of DIC with a reduction in mortality. However, the role of ATIII in sepsis remains to be determined.

DIC is frequently associated with a profound decrease in the plasma protein C (PC) levels. Moreover, patients dying of sepsis have substantially lower plasma PC levels than do surviving patients. PC is a vitamin-K dependent glycoprotein, which, after activation by the thrombomodulin/thrombin complex on the vascular endothelial surface, functions as a natural anticoagulant, limiting coagulation and augmenting fibrinolysis. It is assumed that administration of the PC concentrate during the early stages of DIC could help to maintain the regulatory control of PC, thereby arresting coagulation. A handful of case reports have demonstrated that infusions of PC attenuate the coagulopathy associated with sepsis, particularly purpura fulminans associated with meningococcal sepsis. However, at the present time, the limited clinical experience with PC in the treatment of sepsis does not allow firm recommendations to be made.

Blood component therapy is potentially hazardous in patients with DIC. Circulating plasmin will biodegrade most, if not all, of the coagulation factors supplied. Furthermore, the infused fibrinogen may become substrate for the creation of even higher levels of fibrinogen degradation products, which will further impair hemostasis. A case-controlled study of 336 patients with meningococcal septicemia suggested that the administration of FFP may actually increase mortality. The administration of FFP and platelets should be restricted to patients with active hemorrhage and severe decreases in prothrombin time and platelet count, respectively. Fibrinogen concentrates should be avoided, and the effects of replacement therapy on the coagulation profile should be closely monitored.

■ THROMBOCYTOPENIA IN THE ICU

Thrombocytopenia is an exceedingly common problem in ICU patients; the cause is often multifactorial. Sepsis is the most common cause of thrombocytopenia in the ICU. Thrombocytopenia is an early sign of sepsis and may occur in the absence of other features of DIC. Dilutional thrombocytopenia due to blood and fluid replacement is probably the second most common cause of thrombocytopenia in the ICU. Other causes include the following:

- Consumptive coagulopathy (DIC) due to liver failure, hemolysis, elevated liver enzymes, low platelets (HELLP) syndrome, abruptio placentae
- Microangiopathic hemolytic anemia, i.e., TTP, hemolytic uremic syndrome (HUS)
- Immune thrombocytopenias
  Idiopathic thrombocytopenic purpura
  Heparin (see below)
  Alloantibodies
  Collagen vascular diseases
  Malignancy
  Viral
  Drug induced (quinidine)
- Myelosuppressive chemotherapeutic agents

In addition, drugs are commonly implicated in the etiology of thrombocytopenia. Almost any drug can cause a thrombocytopenia. The commonly implicated drugs are listed below:

Antimicrobials

- Chloramphenicol
- Amphotericin
- Tetracyclines
- Sulfonamides
- Penicillins
- Cephalosporins

Anticonvulsants

- Phenytoin (Dilantin)
- Carbamazepine

Diuretics

- Furosemide
- Thiazides
- Ethacrynic acid

Others

- Alcohol
- Phenylbutazone
- Aspirin
- Gold salts
- Colchicine
- Chlorpromazine
- Chlordiazepoxide
- Cimetidine and other H_2 blockers

Thrombocytopenia in ICU patients is frequently attributed to the concurrent use of an H_2 blocker. However, the true incidence of this reaction is probably less than 0.1%. Furthermore, contrary to popular belief, there is no clear evidence that the rate of this reaction is higher with one H_2 blocker as compared with another.

■ THROMBOTIC THROMBOCYTOPENIC PURPURA

TTP, a disseminated thrombotic microangiopathy, is a fulminant, often lethal disorder that may be initiated by endothelial injury and subsequent release of von Willebrand's factor and other proco-agulant materials from the endothelial cell. A similar disorder occurs in children, the HUS. The two conditions are often regarded as variants of a single syndrome called thrombotic thrombocytopenic purpura-hemolytic-uremic syndrome. The syndrome is characterized by thrombocytopenia, microangiopathic hemolytic anemia, fever, renal abnormalities, and neurologic disturbances. The term *thrombotic thrombocytopenic purpura* is usually preferred for cases in adults in which neurologic dysfunction predominates, whereas cases involving predominantly glomerular damage, which occur mainly in children, are diagnosed as *hemolytic-uremic syndrome*. Different triggering factors may be involved, such as bacterial or viral infection, pregnancy, drug therapy, chemotherapy, and bone marrow transplantation.

A deficiency of von Willebrand's factor-cleaving protease has been implicated in patients with nonfamilial TTP (but not patients with HUS). In patients with acute TTP, inhibitory antibodies (IgG) to von Willebrand's factor-cleaving protease have been reported.

Platelet transfusion should be avoided at all costs in patients with TTP. Plasma exchange or infusion is considered the therapy of choice in patients with TTP. Presumably, patients with low titers of inhibitor would have a response to simple plasma infusion, whereas patients with high titers would require plasmapheresis to remove the inhibitory antibodies and supply normal protease. Plasmapheresis without plasma infusion is relatively ineffective in patients with TTP, perhaps because it does not increase the protease activity quickly.

■ HEPARIN-ASSOCIATED THROMBOCYTOPENIA

There are three different syndromes of heparin-induced thrombocytopenia:

- *Acute reversible thrombocytopenia.* This is seen immediately after an intravenous bolus injection of heparin. It is thought to be due to reversible clumping, trapping, and sequestration of platelets due to a direct effect of heparin. The acute reversible thrombocytopenia is mild and associated with no deleterious effects.
- *Mild thrombocytopenia,* with platelet counts between 100,000 and 150,000 developing 2 to 4 days after initiation of heparin therapy. The platelet count typically returns to normal within 1 to 5 days.
- *A delayed and persistent thrombocytopenia associated with heparin resistance, DIC, and thromboembolism.* The onset of the thrombocytopenia occurs between day 6 and 14, is usually severe, and platelet counts recover rapidly once the heparin is discontinued. The syndrome is independent of the dose of heparin and has been described with heparin-bonded catheters. This syndrome is associated with heparin-dependent platelet antibodies. Arterial and venous thrombosis and skin necrosis have been described in this syndrome, often called the *white clot syndrome.*

Immune-mediated heparin thrombocytopenia (HITS) is more common with unfractionated than fractioned heparin (low-molecular-weight heparin, LMWH). However, as the antibodies cross-react,

LMWH should not be used in patients with HITS. Heparinoids do not cross-react with heparin-associated antibodies and can be used if ongoing anticoagulation is required.

■ SELECTED REFERENCES

Critical Care Anemia

1. Fenwick JC, Cameron M, Naiman SC, et al. Blood transfusion as a cause of leucocytosis in critically ill patients. *Lancet*. 1994;344:855–856.
2. Goldberg MA, McCutchen JW, Jove M, et al. A safety and efficacy comparison study of two dosing regimens of epoetin alfa in patients undergoing major orthopedic surgery. *Am J Orthop*. 1996;25:544–552.
3. Goodnough LT, Brecher ME, Kanter MH, AuBuchon JP. Transfusion medicine. First of two parts—blood transfusion. *N Engl J Med*. 1999;340: 438–447.
4. Hebert PC, Wells G, Marshall J, et al. Transfusion requirements in critical care. A pilot study. Canadian Critical Care Trials Group. *JAMA*. 1995;273: 1439–1444.
5. Hebert PC, Wells G, Tweeddale M, et al. Does transfusion practice affect mortality in critically ill patients? Transfusion Requirements in Critical Care (TRICC) Investigators and the Canadian Critical Care Trials Group. *Am J Respir Crit Care Med*. 1997;155:1618–1623.
6. Krafte-Jacobs B, Levetown ML, Bray GL, Ruttimann UE, Pollack MM. Erythropoietin response to critical illness. *Crit Care Med*. 1994;22:821–826.
7. Purdy FR, Tweeddale MG, Merrick PM. Association of mortality with age of blood transfused in septic ICU patients. *Can J Anaesth*. 1997;44:1256–1261.

Disseminated Intravascular Coagulation

8. Bick RL, Arun B, Frenkel EP. Disseminated intravascular coagulation. Clinical and pathophysiological mechanisms and manifestations. *Haemostasis*. 1999;29:111–134.
9. Busund R, Straume B, Revhaug A. Fatal course in severe meningococcemia: clinical predictors and effects of transfusion therapy. *Crit Care Med*. 1993;21:1699–1705.
10. Fourrier F, Chopin C, Huart JJ, Runge I, Caron C, Goudemand J. Double-blind, placebo-controlled trial of antithrombin III concentrates in septic shock with disseminated intravascular coagulation. *Chest*. 1993;104:882–888.
11. Gando S, Nanzaki S, Sasaki S, Aoi K, Kemmotsu O. Activation of the extrinsic coagulation pathway in patients with severe sepsis and septic shock. *Crit Care Med*. 1998;26:2005–2009.
12. Lorente JA, Garcia-Frade LJ, Landin L, De Pablo R, Torrado C, Renes E. Time course of hemostatic abnormalities in sepsis and its relation to outcome. *Chest*. 1993;103:1536–1542.
13. Vinazzer H. Therapeutic use of antithrombin III in shock and disseminated intravascular coagulation. *Semin Thromb Hemost*. 1989;15:347–352.

Thrombotic Thrombocytopenic Purpura

14. Furlan M, Robles R, Galbusera M, et al. von Willebrand factor-cleaving protease in thrombotic thrombocytopenic purpura and the hemolytic-uremic syndrome. *N Engl J Med*. 1998;339:1578–1584.
15. Tsai HM, Lian EC. Antibodies to von Willebrand factor-cleaving protease in acute thrombotic thrombocytopenic purpura. *N Engl J Med*. 1998;339: 1585–1594.

51

Multiorgan Dysfunction Syndrome

With the widespread use of advanced technology for organ support, patients rarely die from their presenting disease but rather from its pathophysiological consequences; namely, the sequential dysfunction and failure of several organ systems. This syndrome has been called *multisystem organ failure*, *multiple organ system failure*, and more recently, *multiorgan dysfunction syndrome (MODS)*. MODS has an extraordinarily high mortality, and, for many patients, the support of this syndrome does not improve survival but rather prolongs the dying process. MODS is not an "all-or-nothing" condition but rather a continuum of dynamically changing organ failure.

Sepsis is the most common diagnosis leading to MODS in both nonoperative and operative patients. Patients may develop MODS as a consequence of a primary infection, or, as is more commonly the case, following nosocomial infections. However, in more than one third of patients with MODS, no focus of infection can be found on clinical examination or postmortem studies. Other well-recognized risk factors for the development of MODS include severity of disease, age >65 years, persistent deficit in oxygen delivery following resuscitation from circulatory shock, focus of devitalized tissue, severe trauma, major operations, and preexisting end-stage liver failure.

For over three decades, the goal of intensivists caring for patients with sepsis and organ dysfunction at the bedside has been to develop a paradigm that allows the physician to evaluate the pathophysiologic state of the individual at the cellular and tissue level. With the development of the pulmonary artery catheter, intensivists were able to ascertain global parameters of oxygenation. It was initially postulated that sepsis was associated with abnormalities in tissue oxygen utilization and that by increasing global oxygen delivery to supranormal levels one was able to improve clinical outcomes. This approach, however, has failed to consistently improve patient outcome.

Recently, local tissue dysoxia, particularly of the hepatosplanchnic circulatory bed, has been postulated to be important in fueling the continued pathophysiologic aberrations observed in critically ill patients. The gut hypothesis is currently the most popular theory to explain the development of MODS in critically ill patients. Splanchnic hypoperfusion is a common finding following trauma, sepsis, shock, or thermal injuries. Gut mucosal ischemia increases intestinal permeability with the translocation of bacteria, endotoxin, and other mediators into the systemic circulation. It is postulated that this results in activation of the proinflammatory cascade with local and systemic tissue injury leading to MODS. Increased intestinal mucosal permeability may therefore be central to the development of MODS. Indeed, Doig and colleagues demonstrated an excellent relationship between increased intestinal permeability on admission to the ICU and the subsequent development of MODS. While mesenteric hypoperfusion is common in critically ill patients, mucosal acidosis and increased permeability have been reported in the absence of mucosal hypoxia. Furthermore, increased intestinal permeability may occur without loss of cellular viability due to increased paracellular permeability.

■ DIAGNOSTIC CRITERIA AND SCORING SYSTEMS

At least 20 scoring systems have been described to diagnose and quantify the severity of MODS. These scoring systems differ appreciably, making it extremely difficult to compare the results from different research groups. In 1994, the European Society of Intensive Care Medicine organized a consensus meeting to create the Sepsis-related Organ Failure Assessment (SOFA) score, to describe and quantitate the degree of organ dysfunction/failure over time in groups of patients and individual patients. The SOFA score was constructed using simple physiologic measures of dysfunction in six organ systems. The elements of the SOFA scoring system are depicted in Table 51-1. The SOFA score was not designed to predict outcome but rather to describe and quantitate the sequence of complications in critically ill patients. Using similar physiological variables to those used in the SOFA score, Marshal and colleagues developed the Multiple Organ Dysfunction Score.

Table 51-1. The SOFA score.

Sofa Score	1	2	3	4
Respiration PaO_2/FiO_2 mm Hg	<400	<300	<200 with respiratory support	<100
Coagulation Platelets $\times 10^3/mm^3$	<150	<100	<50	<20
Liver Bilirubin mg/dL	1.2–1.9	2.0–5.9	6.0–11.9	>12
Cardiovascular Hypotension	MAP <70 mm Hg	Dopamine ≤5 or dobutamine any dose	Dopamine >5 or epinephrine ≤0.1 or norepinephrine ≤0.1	Dopamine >15 or epinephrine >0.1 or norepinephrine >0.1
Central nervous system Glasgow Coma Score	13–14	10–12	6–9	<6
Renal Creatinine mg/dL or urine output	1.2–1.9	2.0–3.4	3.5–4.9 or <500 mL/day	>5.0 or <200 mL/day

■ CURRENT MANAGEMENT STRATEGIES

The management of the patient with MODS remains a formidable problem. Despite advances in critical care therapeutics, the mortality of multiple organ failure remains unchanged since the syndrome was first characterized in the 1970s. At the present time, there are no modalities that can actively reverse established organ failure, hence, the treatment of these patients consists of metabolic and hemodynamic support until the process reverses itself or death occurs. An increasing emphasis is being placed on prevention of organ dysfunction, including maintenance of tissue oxygenation, nutrition, and infection control.

The primary goal in the management of any critically ill patient must be to prevent the occurrence of a single organ failure and when possible specific corrective therapy of all identifiable risk factors for the development of MODS. The importance of maintaining adequate tissue perfusion in high-risk patients has been increasingly recognized. The level of perioperative tissue oxygen debt has been related to the postoperative incidence of MODS and patient outcome. Failure of the gut barrier function is central to the gut hypothesis. Gastric intramucosal acidosis/hypercarbia may serve as a marker of the adequacy of splanchnic perfusion. Splanchnic resuscitation should be initiated early to prevent or reverse intramucosal acidosis/hypercarbia.

The preservation of gastrointestinal mucosal integrity may require a combination of therapeutic interventions, or so-called "total splanchnic resuscitation." The enterocyte requires glutamine for cell differentiation and division. The early institution of a glutamine-supplemented enteral diet may play an important role in maintaining the gut mucosal barrier function and preventing bacterial translocation. The toxic by-products of nitric oxide have been demonstrated to increase mucosal permeability, probably as a consequence of disruption of the cytoskeletal ring. In addition, oxidants are produced by ischemia–reperfusion and leukocyte-mediated inflammation. These oxidants damage cell membranes and subcellular structures. This suggests that antioxidant therapy may potentially reduce cellular damage (including enterocyte damage) in ischemia–reperfusion injuries and tissue inflamation. The list of potential therapeutic agents are myriad and include inhibitors of inducible nitric oxide synthetase, substances that contain free thiol groups such as reduced glutathione and *n*-acetylcysteine, which function as sacrificial antioxidants; mannitol (scavenges hydroxyl radicals); xanthine oxidase inhibitors (allopurinol); and selenium. One of the main scavenger systems responsible for cleavage of free radicals is the selenium-dependent glutathione peroxidase. Selenium deficiency has been reported in up to 40% of ICU patients and is correlated with mortality. Selenium replacement has been shown to improve several functions of the immunocompetent cells, including phagocytosis, natural killer cell activity, T cell proliferation, and immunoglobulin synthesis. In a small randomized, prospective pilot study, Angstwurm and colleagues demonstrated an improvement in clinical outcome in patients with SIRS who received selenium replacement. Further studies are required to determine the role of selenium and other oxidants in patients with systemic inflammatory response syndrome, trauma, and reperfusion injuries.

Fasting increases lipid peroxidation in experimental models. Fasting decreases the levels of vitamin C, zinc, and selenium and increases xanthine oxidase activity. Early enteral nutrition (particularly using immune-enhancing formula) may offer some protection against oxidative damage.

■ SELECTED REFERENCES

1. Angstwurm MW, Schottdorf J, Schopohl J, Gaertner R. Selenium replacement in patients with severe systemic inflammatory response syndrome improves clinical outcome. *Crit Care Med.* 1999;27:1807–1813.
2. Berrtleff MJOE, Bruining HA. How should multiple organ dysfunction syndrome be assessed? A review of the variations in current scoring systems. *Eur J Surg.* 1997;163:405–409.
3. Buchman AL. Glutamine: is it a conditionally required nutrient for the human gastrointestinal system? *J Am Coll Nutr.* 1996;15:199–205.
4. Doig CJ, Sutherland LR, Sandham JS, et al. Increased intestinal permeability is associated with the development of multiple organ dysfunction syndrome in critically ill ICU patiens. *Am J Respir Crit Care Med.* 1998;158:444–451.
5. Forceville X, Vitoux D, Gauzit R, et al. Selenium, systemic immune response syndrome, sepsis, and outcome in critically ill patients. *Crit Care Med.* 1998;26:1536–1544.
6. Gianotti L, Alexander JW, Gennari R, Pyles T, Babcock GF. Oral glutamine decreases bacterial translocation and improves survival in experimental gut-origin sepsis. *JPEN J Parenter Enteral Nutr.* 1995;19:69–74.
7. Marshall JC, Cook DJ, Christou NV, Bernard GR, Sprung CL, Sibbald WJ. Multiple Organ Dysfunction Score: a reliable descriptor of a complex clinical outcome. *Crit Care Med.* 1995;23:1638–1652.
8. Metnitz PG, Bartens C, Fischer M, et al. Antioxidant status in patients with acute respiratory distress syndrome. *Intensive Care Med.* 1999;25:180–185.
9. Moore EE, Jones TN. Benefits of feeding after major abdominal trauma—a prospective randomized study. *J Trauma.* 1986;26:874–881.
10. Singer M. Management of multiple organ failure: guidelines but no hard-and-fast rules. *J Antimicrob Chemother.* 1998;41(suppl A):103–112.
11. Vincent JL, Moreno R, Takala J, et al. The SOFA (Sepsis-related Organ Failure Assessment) score to describe organ dysfunction/failure. On behalf of the Working Group on Sepsis-Related Problems of the European Society of Intensive Care Medicine. *Intensive Care Med.* 1996;22:707–710.

52

Management of Alcohol Withdrawal Syndrome

Approximately 11 to 15 million people report heavy alcohol use or alcohol abuse and dependence in the United States. In patients hospitalized for alcohol withdrawal, but not treated with pharmacological agents, approximately 15% suffer from seizures and 15% progress to delirium tremens. Withdrawal manifests itself within hours of abstinence or reduction in the amount of alcohol consumed and can be classified as mild (tremors and minimal sympathetic symptoms), moderate (hallucinations and sympathetic symptoms), and severe (seizure activity, fever, change in mental status, and significant alteration in vital signs).

Delirium tremens (DTs), the most serious of the withdrawal spectrum, occurs in approximately 5% of hospitalized alcoholics and has a mortality rate approaching 15%. This disorder usually manifests itself on hospital day 3 to 5 and usually lasts <1 week, although prolonged DTs have been described. In one retrospective study, the risk of DTs was increased by the presence of one or more concurrent illnesses or patient abstinence for ≥2 days upon hospitalization.

The use of alcohol affects many of the regulatory systems in the body including an increase in the release of endogenous opiates, activation of the gamma-amino-butyric acid type A receptor (GABA-A), inhibition of the N-methyl-D-aspartate (NMDA) receptor, and interactions with both serotonin and dopamine receptors. Chronic exposure to the inhibitory GABA-A and excitatory NMDA receptors are thought to be involved in the pathogenesis of alcohol withdrawal.

Benzodiazepines form the cornerstone of therapy, whereas drugs such as beta-blockers and clonidine have been shown to be useful as adjunctive therapy. In cases of withdrawal refractory to standard therapy, propofol is very effective. Propofol's mechanism of action is thought to be similar to the action of alcohol on the central nervous system. Propofol directly activates the GABA-A receptor–chloride ionophore complex, increasing chloride conductance. In addition, propofol inhibits the NMDA subtype of glutamate receptor. In addition, propofol is associated with less cross-tolerance than the benzodiazepines, is easily titratable, and has a rapid metabolic clearance.

All the benzodiazepines have similar modes of action (bind to benzodiazepine receptors on the GABA receptor) and *all* are metabolized by the liver. They differ, however, in their pharmacokinetic profile and the presence of active metabolites. Lorazepam is the drug of choice for the treatment of alcohol withdrawal in the ICU. The dosage depends on the severity of the withdrawal syndrome; some patients require in excess of 80 mg/h. It is recommended that propofol be added to lorazepam once the dose of lorazepam exceeds 20 to 30 mg/h (in intubated patients). A beta-blocker (atenolol or metoprolol) and/or clonidine should be added in patients showing marked autonomic instability, i.e., tachycardia and hypertension. Haldol is the drug of choice for the management of severe delirium.

Lorazepam is the drug of choice in patients with alcohol withdrawal seizures. Lorazepam has been shown to reduce the risk of recurrent seizures. Phenytoin has no role in the management of withdrawal seizures.

Hypomagnesemia, hypokalemia, and hypophosphatemia are particularly common in chronic alcoholic patients; these electrolyte disorders may become life threatening after the initiation of nutrition (refeeding syndrome). These electrolytes should be routinely supplemented and closely monitored. In addition, alcoholic ketoacidosis may be seen in malnourished, nondiabetic alcoholic patients. Restoration of normal fluid balance with glucose-containing saline solution (with added thiamine) usually reverses this syndrome. Hypoglycemia may occur in the withdrawing alcoholic, since malnutrition and liver disease impair the storage of glycogen. This mandates monitoring the serum glucose in the withdrawing alcoholic.

Patients who abuse alcohol are at risk of developing acute pancreatitis, erosive gastritis, and acute alcoholic hepatitis. Hence, a serum amylase/lipase test and liver function tests should be performed in all acutely ill alcoholic patients. A cytoprotective agent such as sucralfate is indicated for the management of erosive gastritis.

■ SELECTED REFERENCES

1. Chiang WK, Goldfrank LR. Substance withdrawal. *Emerg Med Clin North Am.* 1990;8:613–631.
2. D'Onofrio G, Rathlev NK, Ulrich AS, et al. Lorazepam for the prevention of recurrent seizures related to alcohol. *N Engl J Med.* 1999;340:915–919.

3. Rathlev NK, D'Onofrio G, Fish SS, et al. The lack of efficacy of phenytoin in the prevention of recurrent alcohol-related seizures. *Ann Emerg Med.* 1994;23:513–518.
4. Turner RC, Lichstein PR, Peden JGJ, et al. Alcohol withdrawal syndromes: a review of pathophysiology, clinical presentation, and treatment. *J Gen Intern Med.* 1989;4:432–444.
5. Wolf KM, Shaughnessy AF, Middleton DB. Prolonged delirium tremens requiring massive doses of medication. *J Am Board Fam Pract.* 1993; 6:502–504.

53

Assessment of Tissue Oxygenation

Tissue hypoxia is common in critically ill patients and is likely a major factor leading to organ failure (multiorgan dysfunction syndrome, MODS) and death (see Chapter 51). Tissue hypoxia may result from (1) low arterial oxygen tension (hypoxic hypoxia), (2) microvascular hypoperfusion (stagnant hypoxia) due to shock and microvascular redistribution, (3) severe anemia (anemic hypoxia), and (4) inability to utilize oxygen (cytopathic hypoxia) due to derangements in cellular respiration. The expedient detection and correction of tissue hypoxia may limit organ dysfunction, reduce complications, and improve the outcome of patients treated in the ICU. It is probable that the earlier tissue hypoxia is detected and corrected, the greater the chance that outcome will be improved. Once cellular dysfunction has developed and organ failure has manifested clinically, it is likely that a cycle of irreversible and progressive organ dysfunction has been entered.

Tissue hypoxia is, however, exceedingly difficult to detect at the bedside; there are no specific clinical signs and no simple laboratory tests. Global indices of oxygen delivery (Do_2) and consumption ($\dot{V}o_2$) provide no useful information as to the adequacy of tissue oxygenation. Blood lactate concentration and mixed venous oxygen tension ($Pmvo_2$) (or saturation) are crude and insensitive indices of global oxygen balance (see below). The limitation of traditional ICU monitoring devices has driven the development of organ-specific monitors. Gastric tonometry and sublingual capnography are the only end-organ metabolic monitors that are clinically available at this time.

Gastric tonometry and sublingual capnography are based on the principle that tissue production of CO_2 rises sharply with tissue hypoxia. Present evidence indicates that the source of increased tissue CO_2 is intracellular buffering of excess hydrogen ions by bicarbonate. The increased hydrogen ions are, in turn, traced to anaerobic generation of excess lactic acid and degeneration of high-energy phosphate compounds during tissue hypoxia. Tissue partial pressure of carbon dioxide (Pco_2) tension is therefore an index of tissue energy status; tissue hypoxia, whether due to decreased oxygen availability (hypoxic, anemic, or stagnant hypoxia) or diminished ability to utilize oxygen (cytopathic hypoxia), results in an increase in tissue Pco_2 and an increase in the gradient between tissue and arterial Pco_2.

Tissue Pco_2 can be measured directly with CO_2-sensitive electrodes (sublingual capnography) or indirectly by tonometry. Tonometry is simply a method used to equilibrate gas tension between two compartments. Either gas (e.g., air) or fluid (e.g., normal saline) can be used as the solvent for equilibration of the gas in question (i.e., CO_2). A gastric tonometer is a standard nasogastric tube with a silicone balloon at its distal end. With conventional saline tonometry, the balloon of the tonometer is filled with normal saline and allowed to equilibrate (ideally for 90 minutes). Once equilibrated, the balloon is aspirated, and the Pco_2 of the fluid is determined using a standard blood gas analyzer. Air tonometry, particularly in conjunction with an automated system, has a number of advantages when compared with conventional saline tonometry. Unlike saline tonometry, in vitro studies have demonstrated that air tonometry has a very low bias with excellent precision. Furthermore, automated air tonometry has an equilibration time of <20 minutes and, being fully automated, may eliminate potential sources of error associated with saline tonometry.

Since tissue Pco_2 concentration is dependent upon the Pco_2 of the perfusing arterial blood, as well as tissue CO_2 production (and removal), tissue Pco_2 must be interpreted in conjunction with an arterial blood gas. Normally, the tissue Pco_2 is ~5 torr higher than arterial Pco_2. Hence, a tissue–arterial Pco_2 gap of >5 mm Hg (15 mm Hg for sublingual capnography) indicates the presence of tissue hypoxia.

Gastric tonometry is a monitor of gastric mucosal hypoxia. Measurement of the adequacy of the splanchnic circulation may be particularly important in the critically ill or injured patient. Splanchnic hypoperfusion occurs early in shock and may occur before the usual indicators of shock such as hypotension or lactic acidosis are present. Furthermore, the gut is highly susceptible to diminished tissue perfusion and oxygenation, as it has a higher critical Do_2 than the whole body and other vital organs, and the mucosal countercurrent microcirculation renders the villi particularly vulnerable to ischemia. Weil and colleagues have demonstrated that the very proximal gastrointestinal tract, namely, the tongue and/or sublingual mucosa, may serve as appropriate sites for measurement of tissue Pco_2. These authors have demonstrated an increase in sublingual Pco_2 that was closely related to decreases in arterial pressure and cardiac index during circulatory shock produced by hemorrhage and sepsis. Furthermore, the rise in sublingual P_{CO_2} closely paralleled the increase in gastric intra-mucosal CO_2. From a teleological point of view, it would therefore appear that during acute stressful situations, blood is diverted away from the entire gastrointestinal tract (don't need to chew and digest food during a fight-and-flight response). Gastrointestinal mucosal hypercarbia may thus be an early marker of tissue hypoperfusion.

The value of gastric intramucosal P_{CO_2} (or acidosis) as a predictor of morbidity and mortality in critically ill patients cannot be disputed. Furthermore, a number of prospective studies have suggested that maintaining the gastric intramucosal pH (or P_{CO_2} gap) in the normal range reduces the complications and improves the outcome of criti-cally ill and postoperative patients. At this time, however, titrating therapy to tissue P_{CO_2} levels is an attractive although unproven ther-apeutic approach.

■ LACTIC ACIDOSIS IN CRITICAL ILLNESS (SEE CHAPTER 29)

The normal blood lactate concentration in unstressed patients is $1.0 \pm 0.5\,mmol/L$. Patients with critical illness can be considered to have normal lactate concentrations of $<2\,mmol/L$. Hyperlactemia is defined as an increase in blood lactate concentration without metabolic aci-dosis, whereas lactic acidosis is characterized by an elevated lactate concentration in association with a metabolic acidosis.

Hyperlactemia occurs in situations in which tissues are well per-fused (no oxygen debt) and is characterized by a normal lactate/pyruvate ratio. Hyperlactemia commonly occurs in critical illnesses associated with hypermetabolic states, such as sepsis, burns, and trauma. It should be noted that the hyperlactemia associated with sepsis usually occurs in association with a normal lactate/pyruvate ratio and little evidence of a tissue oxygen debt. However, hyper-lactemia may cause an acidosis in the absence of tissue hypoxia; this is called type A lactic acidosis. Lactic acidosis resulting from tissue hypoxia is known as type B lactic acidosis. Type B lactic acidosis is associated with an increased lactate/pyruvate ratio.

In critically ill patients, an increased blood lactate concentration is associated with an increased mortality. However, lactate is an insen-sitive marker of tissue hypoxia, because

1. An elevated lactate may occur in the absence of tissue hypoxia.

2. The blood lactate concentration depends on the balance between tissue lactate production and hepatic removal. The liver has a large capacity for lactate removal, and therefore lactate production has to be substantially increased before the meta-

bolic threshold of the liver is exceeded, and increased blood concentrations occur.

3. Due to delayed hepatic clearance of lactate, tissue hypoxia may have resolved, yet the blood lactate concentration may remain elevated. Hepatic hypoperfusion, underlying liver disease, sepsis, and respiratory alkalosis reduce hepatic lactate clearance.

4. Other conditions interfere with lactate production, so that despite tissue hypoxia, blood lactate will be normal. In severe malnutrition, for example, glucose stores are insufficient to sustain glycolysis.

A large body of evidence has emerged dissociating lactate and tissue hypoxia. Blood lactate should therefore be regarded as "the poor man's test" for tissue hypoxia.

■ MIXED VENOUS O$_2$ MONITORING

True mixed venous blood is derived from a pool of venous blood entering the pulmonary artery via the great veins in the chest. It contains blood that has traversed all systemic capillary beds capable of extracting oxygen and is thoroughly mixed by the right ventricle, so that although its constituents from various sources have varying oxyhemoglobin saturations, it has a single oxyhemoglobin saturation. Due to inadequate mixing, blood drawn from a central venous catheter correlates poorly with the saturation of true mixed venous blood.

Mixed venous oxygen monitoring (mvo$_2$ (mixed venous oxygen tension) or Smvo$_2$ (mixed venous oxygen saturation)) is based on the principle that inadequate tissue oxygen delivery will be associated with a low mixed venous oxygen content:

Arterial O$_2$ content (Cao$_2$)	(Hb × 1.34 × Sat) + (0.031 × Pao$_2$)	17 to 20 mL/dL
Mixed venous O$_2$ content (Cvo$_2$)	(Hb × 1.34 × Sat) + (0.031 × Pvo$_2$)	12 to 15 mL/dL
Arteriovenous O$_2$ difference (avDo$_2$)	Cao$_2$ − Cvo$_2$	4 to 6 mL/dL
Oxygen delivery (Do$_2$)	(CO × Cao$_2$)/10	950 to 1150 mL/min

From the above, a low Smvo$_2$ (or Pmvo$_2$) may result from

1. Decreased hemoglobin (decreased Do$_2$)
2. Decreased arterial saturation (decreased Do$_2$)

3. Decreased cardiac output (decreased Do_2)

4. Increased systemic oxygen consumption (increased ($\dot{V}o_2$) with a high $avDo_2$

Mixed venous oxygen saturation is commonly used to assess the balance of total body oxygen delivery to oxygen demand. Given a stable metabolic rate and hemoglobin, an acute fall in $Smvo_2$ implies either a fall in cardiac output or a fall in arterial saturation. However, $Smvo_2$ monitoring has a number of major limitations, including the following:

1. There appears to be no clear-cut threshold that defines inadequate Do_2 and tissue hypoxia. Furthermore, the critical value of $Smvo_2$ is dependent on the type of hypoxia (anemic, stagnant, etc).

2. $Smvo_2$ correlates poorly with cardiac output, oxygen delivery, lactate, and intramucosal CO_2 gap. Only about 50% of the $Smvo_2$ changes represent anticipated changes in cardiac output.

3. $Smvo_2$ is insensitive to regional desaturation in organs whose venous blood comprises a small percentage of total mixed venous blood (e.g., brain and intestine).

The use of oximetric catheters that continuously monitor $Smvo_2$ has not been associated with a decrease in adverse hemodynamic events, length of ICU stay, complications, or mortality when compared to patients monitored with standard pulmonary artery catheters. It would therefore appear that oximetric pulmonary artery catheters have a limited role (if any) in monitoring critically ill ICU patients. Indeed, a "normal" $Smvo_2$ may erroneously lead to the conclusion that all the tissue beds are well oxygenated, while this clearly does not always hold true.

■ SELECTED REFERENCES

1. Gutierrez G, Palizas F, Doglio G, Wainzstein N, Gallesio A, Pacin J. Gastric intramucosal pH as a therapeutic index of tissue oxygenation in critically ill patients. *Lancet*. 1992;339:195–199.

2. Ivatury RR, Simon RJ, Islam S, Fueg A, Rohman M, Stahl WM. A prospective randomized study of end points of resuscitation after major trauma: global oxygen transport indices versus organ-specific gastric mucosal pH. *J Am Coll Surg*. 1996;183:145–154.

3. Jastremski MS, Chelluri L, Beney KM, Bailly RT. Analysis of the effects of continuous on-line monitoring of mixed venous oxygen saturation on patient outcome and cost-effectiveness. *Crit Care Med*. 1989;17:148–153.

4. Jin X, Weil MH, Sun S, et al. Decreases in organ blood flows associated with increases in sublingual PCO_2 during hemorrhagic shock. *J Appl Physiol*. 1998;85:2360–2364.
5. Mahutte CK, Jaffe MB, Sasse SA, et al. Relationship of thermodilution cardiac output to metabolic measurements and mixed venous oxygen saturation. *Chest*. 1993;104:1236–1242.
6. Marik PE. Gastric intramucosal pH. A better predictor of multiorgan dysfunction syndrome and death than oxygen-derived variables in patients with sepsis. *Chest*. 1993;104:225–229.
7. Maynard N, Bihari D, Beale R, Smithies M, Baldock G, Mason R. Assessment of splanchnic oxygenation by gastric tonometry in patients with acute circulatory failure. *JAMA*. 1993;270:1203–1210.
8. McDaniel LB, Zwischenberger JB, Vertrees RA, et al. Mixed venous oxygen saturation during cardiopulmonary bypass poorly predicts regional venous saturation. *Anesth Analg*. 1995;80:466–472.
9. Pernat A, Weil MH, Tang W, et al. Effects of hyper- and hypoventilation on gastric and sublingual PCO(2). *J Appl Physiol*. 1999;87:933–937.
10. Sato Y, Weil MH, Tang W. Tissue hypercarbic acidosis as a marker of acute circulatory failure (shock). *Chest*. 1998;114:263–274.
11. Vaughn S, Puri VK. Cardiac output changes and continuous mixed venous oxygen saturation measurement in the critically ill. *Crit Care Med*. 1988;16:495–498.
12. Weil MH, Nakagawa Y, Tang W, et al. Sublingual capnometry: a new noninvasive measurement for diagnosis and quantitation of severity of circulatory shock. *Crit Care Med*. 1999;27:1225–1229.

54

Brain Death and Management of the Heart-Beating, Brain-Dead Organ Donor

■ BRAIN DEATH

Brain death is defined as the permanent and irreversible loss of all brain function. Most states in the United States consider brain death to be synonymous with the death of the patient. *The patient who is brain dead is dead.* The determination of brain death is a clinical diagnosis. Confirmatory tests such as electroencephalogram (EEG) and blood flow studies are not required. The specific requirements for the determination of brain death vary from institution to institution and state to state. However, they all have a number of features in common:

1. The recognition of the irreversibility of the brain insult requires that
   a. The cause of brain death be established
   b. The insult be of a sufficient severity to account for the loss of the brain function

2. A period of reasonable observation (and treatment) is required before the determination of brain death, to ensure irreversibility of brain damage.
   a. At least 6 hours if structural brain damage is present.
   b. At least 12 hours if there is nonstructural brain damage.

    c. At least 24 hours post-cardiac arrest.

    d. When drugs are implicated, the blood levels of these agents must be below therapeutic levels before the determination of brain death.

    e. The patient's temperature must be >34°C.

    f. The patient must not be in shock.

3. Most institutions require that two physicians independently perform a clinical determination of brain death. The clinical findings must be clearly recorded in the patient's chart.

Clinical Determination of Brain Death

1. Absence of spontaneous movements, movements in response to pain, decerebrate or decorticate posturing

2. Absent brain stem responses

    a. Pupils fixed and nonresponsive to light

    b. Absent corneal reflex

    c. Absent cough and gag reflex

    d. Absent "doll's eyes"

    e. Negative caloric test; no response (nystagmus) to the instillation of 50 mL of ice saline in each auditory canal

    f. Positive apnea test: Preoxygenate the patient with 100% oxygen. Obtain blood gas. Disconnect the patient from the ventilator, and insert an oxygen catheter down the endotracheal tube. Observe for spontaneous respiratory movements. After 10 minutes, obtain a repeat blood gas (the $Paco_2$ increases by about 3 mm Hg/min). The patient is apneic if the Pco_2 > 60 mm Hg and there are no respiratory movements. If the patient's baseline $Paco_2$ is low (due to hyperventilation), it is prudent to allow this to normalize before performing the apnea test.

A number of ancillary tests can be performed to support the diagnosis of brain death. These tests are not required and in themselves are not sufficient to make the diagnosis of brain death. They are useful in the presence of toxic substances, sedative drugs, and cases of severe head/facial trauma.

- Cerebral angiography: No blood flow on a four-vessel angiogram establishes the irreversibility of coma.
- Cerebral radionuclide studies: Absent cerebral blood flow supports the diagnosis of brain death. Cerebral nuclide flow studies, however, are not as sensitive as four-vessel angiography for the determination of brain death.
- Brain stem evoked potentials: The absence of brain stem evoked potential establishes the irreversibility of coma.

- An isoelectric EEG, while compatible with brain death, may occur in patients with sedative overdose who subsequently recover.

In those states where brain-dead patients are considered legally dead, the physician does not require the permission of the family or other individuals to remove a dead patient from mechanical ventilation or other life support equipment. Organ donation should be considered in all brain-dead patients. When the patient is being evaluated for organ donation, this must be discussed with the family and their consent obtained.

■ MANAGEMENT OF THE HEART-BEATING, BRAIN-DEAD ORGAN DONOR

Recent advances in surgical technology, organ preservation, immunosuppressive therapy, and life support technology have allowed organ transplantation to play a major role in the treatment of patients with end-stage diseases that involve the thoracic and most of the abdominal viscera. Consequently, the demand for transplantable organs is increasing. Multiple organ retrieval from a single cadaver donor is an efficient means of procuring transplantable organs. In the United States alone, about 2 million people die each year, and of these, about 12,000 to 27,000 individuals are suitable to donate organs. The donor pool necessary to meet current transplantation needs has been projected to be between 10,000 and 15,000/year. Despite what seems to be an adequate donor pool, only 15% to 20% of potential donors become actual donors.

The refusal for organ donation by relatives and the unwillingness of health care providers to confront relatives with the diagnosis of brain stem death and to request permission to procure organs are major reasons for loss of potential transplantable organs. Neglecting the general routine care of potential donors before organ procurement will cause hemodynamic instability, infection, or unexpected cardiac arrest, leading to needless rejection of organs or tissues that otherwise would have been suitable for transplantation. Early donor recognition, rapid and accurate declaration of "brain death," physiological maintenance, and coordination with local organ procurement agency are all important aspects of organ donor management.

After a potential donor is identified and a consent is obtained or the patient has an organ donation card, the donor is evaluated for medical suitability and local organ procurement agency is contacted. It is important to assess the medical suitability of the donor and his/her organs. The various studies required for evaluation of the donor are listed in Table 54-1. All donors should, however, be evaluated on an individual basis.

A few absolute contraindications apply to all potential organ donors including infection with human immunodeficiency virus, other active viral infections (cytomegalovirus, hepatitis A, hepatitis B, systemic herpes), history of intravenous drug use, malignancy (except primary central nervous system tumors), and concurrent sepsis. The organ-specific contraindications for organ donation are listed in Table 54-2.

When the brain stem is dead, there is no possibility of recovery, since both the capacity and the ability to breathe have been lost irreversibly. The process of dying has started, and although not every cell in the body has yet ceased to function, the subsequent death of the organism is inevitable. In adults, irreversible cardiac arrest usually occurs within 48 to 72 hours of brain death despite all efforts to maintain the donor's circulation.

During the initial period of brain stem herniation, peripheral vasoconstriction is seen due to sympathetic outburst. This is followed by loss of vascular tone causing hypotension, venous pooling, and relative hypovolemia. Therapeutic dehydration (to decrease cerebral edema), incomplete fluid resuscitation, and diabetes insipidus may contribute to hypovolemia. Atrial and ventricular arrhythmias and

Table 54-1. Workup of the organ donor.

All donors	Height; weight; blood type; chem 7; ABG; CBC with platelets; PT; PTT; serology for HIV, CMV, EBV, toxoplasma, and hepatitis B. Blood cultures if infection suspected. Lymph node biopsy for tissue typing may be required.
Kidney	Urinalysis, BUN, creatinine, urine culture.
Heart	ECG, ECHO, chest x-ray, CPK-MB, cardiology consultation, cardiac catheterization (in selected case).
Lung	Chest x-ray, sputum Gram stain, and culture.
Liver	SGOT, SGPT, alkaline phosphatase, bilirubin
Pancreas	Amylase.
Small bowel	Amylase.

(ABG = arterial blood gas; BUN = serum urea nitrogen; CBC = complete blood count; CMV = cytomegalovirus; EBV = Epstein-Barr virus; CPK-MB = creatine phosphokinase-MB; ECG = electrocardiogram; ECHO = echocardiography; HIV = human immunodeficiency virus; PT = prothrombin time; PTT = partial thromboplastin time; SGOT = serum glutamate oxaloacetate transaminase; SGPT = serum glutamate pyruvate transaminase.)

Table 54-2. Organ-specific criteria.

	Age (Years)	Laboratory Parameters	Contraindications
Heart	Male <40 Female <45	Normal ECG, ECHO, CK-MB	Cardiomyopathy, valvular disease, congenital heart disease, chronic severe hypertension, severe chest trauma, open cardiac massage, prolonged (>20 min) cardiac massage, high-dose dopamine (>10 μg/kg), abnormal ECG, ECHO, cardiac catheter, CK-MB >5%, PaO_2 <50 mm Hg for 4 h
Kidney	>1 or <65	Urine output >0.5 mL/kg/h, BUN <30 mg%, serum creatinine <1.5 mg%, creatinine clearance >70 mL/min	Pyelonephritis, chronic renal disease, severe hypertension, pyuria, bacteriuria, diabetes mellitus, hematuria, DIC, abnormal sediment
Lung	Male <40 Female <45	PO_2 >110 on FiO_2 <0.3, normal chest x-ray, normal $A-aDO_2$, normal airway pressures	Pulmonary edema, infection, penetrating thoracic trauma, smoking history, chronic lung disease, >24 h mechanical ventilation, positive sputum culture, PO_2 <60 mm Hg at FiO_2 >0.4 and PEEP >5 cm H_2O.
Liver	6 months to 55	Normal SGOT, SGPT, alkaline phosphatase, bilirubin, PT/PTT	Penetrating abdominal injury, chronic liver disease, alcohol abuse, hepatobiliary sepsis, RUQ surgery, dopamine >10 μg/kg/min, abnormal LFT, PT, PTT, PO_2 <50 for 4 h
Pancreas	>2, <50	Normal amylase, lipase, glucose tolerance test	Pancreatitis, diabetes mellitus, gastric, duodenal or pancreatic surgery
Small bowel			Penetrating abdominal injury, elevated amylase
Heart valves	<60		Valvular heart disease, ECHO showing valvular deformity/dysfunction
Skin/bone			Local malignancies, local open injuries
Cornea	<90		Local injury, conjunctivitis

(DIC = disseminated intravascular coagulation; LFT = Liver function tests; PEEP = positive end-expiratory pressure; RUQ = right upper quadrant.)

various degrees of conduction block are not uncommon. They can be due to electrolyte imbalance, hypotension, myocardial ischemia, hypothermia, inotropic agents, myocardial contusion, and increased intracranial pressure. Despite all therapeutic efforts, all brain-dead patients will have terminal arrhythmias resistant to therapy. Electrolyte abnormalities are frequent in organ donor patients. Diabetes insipidus is seen commonly after brain death due to partial or complete loss of production of antidiuretic hormone.

Brain-dead patients are poikilothermic because they lack hypothalamic regulation of temperature. Hypothermia can lead to bradycardia, myocardial depression, arrhythmias, cold diuresis, coagulopathy, and left shift in oxygen dissociation curve.

■ SPECIFIC MANAGEMENT ISSUES

The successful donation of perfusable organs requires continued maintenance of the patient's cardiac function, the correction of all electrolyte and metabolic derangements, and the use of artificial respiration until the moment of the organ removal. The aims of management of the organ donor are to maintain body temperature, prevent infection, and optimize the condition of transplantable organs.

- Establish a cause of death.
- Minimum monitoring includes hourly measurements of temperature, pulse, blood pressure, and urine output. All patients will need wide-bore intravenous cannulazation and Foley catheterization. An arterial line is very helpful. Some may need a pulmonary artery catheter for fluid management.
- Check arterial blood gas; electrolytes including calcium, magnesium, and phosphate; complete blood count with platelets; prothrombin time and partial thromboplastin time frequently.
- Hypotension is best managed by fluid resuscitation to obtain systolic blood pressure of 90 to 100 mm Hg.
- A urine output of at least 0.5 mL/kg/h indicates adequate hemodynamics. If urine output is low despite adequate blood pressure, mannitol or furosemide may be used.
- Ventricular tachyarrhythmias, especially associated with hypothermia, respond best to bretylium tosylate.
- Bradyarrhythmias with hypotension are managed by dopamine infusion. This can be followed by an epinephrine infusion. Rarely, a transvenous pacemaker may be required. Atropine does help in this circumstance.
- Ventilation should achieve a normal pH, $Paco_2$, and O_2. CO_2 production falls after brain death, requiring a lower minute ventila-

tion. Maintain adequate oxygenation (Pao_2 > 70 mm Hg) on the lowest possible fraction of inspired oxygen (<0.4 if lungs are to be used) and minimal positive end-expiratory pressure (<5 cm).

- Use strictly aseptic techniques when performing invasive procedures and endotracheal suction. Some centers use prophylactic antibiotics.
- A high urine output (>4 mL/kg/h) can be managed by replacing urinary losses with intravenous fluid containing 0.45% saline with 30 mmol potassium phosphate per liter of fluid, on a volume-to-volume basis.
- Diabetes insipidus (urine output >5 to 7 mL/kg/h, urine specific gravity <1005) is managed by synthetic vasopressin infusion (0.5 to 15 U/h) to decrease urine output to 2 to 3 mL/kg/h.
- Control blood sugar (in range of 140 to 240 mg%) with intravenous insulin to keep serum glucose in the range of 140 to 240 mg/dL.
- Some centers routinely use replacement doses of triiodothyronine and cortisol.
- Keep body temperature >34°C.
- Keep hematocrit >25% and platelet count >30,000.

55

Accidental Hypothermia

Accidental hypothermia is defined as the unintentional decline in the core body temperature <35°C. The compensatory physiological responses to hypothermia are limited and fail below a temperature of 35°C. Usually, there is a history of obvious environmental exposure; however, subtle presentations are common in the elderly. Hypothermia is usually graded as mild, moderate, or severe (see Table 55-1).

In urban settings, hypothermia is most commonly associated with ethanol ingestion, underlying illness, and age. Elderly people have a decreased ability to sense cold and may thus fail to take appropriate adaptive action. The maladaptive response of paradoxical undressing is not uncommon. The elderly may exhibit confusion, become less communicative, and display lassitude or a peculiar "flat" affect. Subtle progression of mental deterioration may mimic senility. Symptoms such as slurred speech and ataxia may resemble those of a cerebrovascular accident. During a climbing expedition, the hypothermic individual may become uncooperative, uncoordinated, moody or apathetic.

■ CONDITIONS ASSOCIATED WITH HYPOTHERMIA

- Advanced age
- Hypothyroidism, hypoadrenalism
- Environmental exposure
- Chronic debilitating diseases, such as cardiac failure, renal failure, strokes

Table 55-1. Physiological changes associated with various degrees of hypothermia.

Severity	Body Temperature	Nervous	Cardiac	Other
Mild	32.2–35°C 90–95°F	Amnesia, dysarthria, apathy, confusion, shivering, ataxia	Tachycardia, then progressive bradycardia, vasoconstriction, increase in blood pressure	Tachypnea, then hypoventilation and bronchospasm Cold diuresis
Moderate	28–32.1°C 82.4–89.9°F	Decrease in level of consciousness, dilated pupils, hallucinations, hyporeflexia, rigidity	Decreased pulse and cardiac output, arrhythmias, J wave Cardiac conduction slows, with prolonged PR, QRS, and QT intervals, and ventricular irritability increases	Hypoventilation, decreased urine, coagulopathy (despite normal levels of clotting factors), lactic acidosis Depressed hepatic function
Severe	<28°C <82.4°F	Coma, loss of ocular reflexes, no movement, areflexia	Progressive fall in pulse and blood pressure, arrhythmias including atrial fibrillation and ventricular fibrillation, asystole	Pulmonary edema, apnea, oliguria, rhabdomyolysis, hemoconcentration, hyperglycemia, increased transaminases, hyperamylasemia

- An acute cerebrovascular accident, especially in the elderly, with immobility and poor thermoregulatory mechanisms
- Drugs
  Ethanol
  Phenothiazines
  Tricyclic antidepressants
  Barbiturates

■ MANAGEMENT

Laboratory Evaluation

- Frequent check of electrolytes. Hyperkalemia and hypokalemia are not uncommon; hypothermia masks the typical electrocardiographic changes of hyperkalemia.
- Acid–base evaluation:
  Arterial blood gas analyzers warm the blood to 37°C and report the values directly so that arterial blood gas values do not need to be corrected for the patient's lower body temperature. The use of uncorrected values permits reference to standard nomograms. The use of uncorrected arterial blood gas values as a guide to resuscitation is called the ectothermic strategy.
  When blood cools, the pH increases and the $Paco_2$ falls. The pH of neutrality is 7.5 and the $Paco_2$ is 30 mm Hg at a temperature of 30°C.
- A patient's hematocrit may be deceptively high as the result of a decreased plasma volume. As a rule of thumb, the hematocrit level should increase 2%/1°C fall in temperature. A normal hematocrit level in a moderate-to-severely hypothermic patient should raise the suspicion of blood loss or a preexisting anemia.
- Patients develop a coagulopathy, as the enzymatic nature of the activated clotting factors are depressed by the cold. Because the coagulation tests are performed at 37°C, the prothrombin time and partial thromboplastin time are frequently reported to be normal. However, a syndrome resembling disseminated intravascular coagulation (DIC) has been reported with hypothermia.
- A leukopenia and thrombocytopenia have been reported that reverse with rewarming.

Monitoring

- The core temperature should be continuously monitored: rectal, bladder, and/or esophageal. The tympanic temperature equili-

brates rapidly with core temperature and is closest to hypothalamic temperature.
- Bladder catheterization to monitor urine output.
- Continuous electrocardiographic monitoring.

Supportive Medical Therapy

- Endotracheal intubation is necessary unless the patient is alert with intact protective airway reflexes.
- Insertion of a nasogastric tube to prevent vomiting and aspiration; gastric dilatation is common.
- Toxicology screen.
- Due to cold-induced diuresis, decreased fluid intake, and "third-space" loss, patients usually have a decreased intravascular volume and require volume replacement (sometimes massive). Ringer's lactate should not be given to severely hypothermic patients, as the liver cannot convert lactate to bicarbonate. Five percent dextrose saline heated to 40° to 42°C is recommended. The fluid can be heated in a microwave; a 1-L bag requires an average of 2 minutes on high power.
- Insertion of a pulmonary artery catheter may incite ventricular ectopy and ventricular fibrillation and should be avoided. In hemodynamically unstable patients and/or patients with underlying cardiac disease, pulmonary artery catheterization should be delayed until the patient's core temperature is above 32°C.
- Rhabdomyolysis should always be excluded and aggressively managed if present (see Chapter 32).
- Vasoactive agents may precipitate severe arrhythmias. Low doses may be used in severely hypotensive patients who have failed to respond to fluids.
- Bretylium is the antiarrhythmic agent of choice.
- Pharmacological agents are usually ineffective below a temperature of 30°C.
- Myxedema and hypoadrenocorticism should be excluded. Patients should be treated with corticosteroids if there is a clinical suspicion of adrenal insufficiency (see Chapter 34). However, the empiric administration of parenteral levothyroxine to euthyroid patients with hypothermia is hazardous. An urgent serum thyroid-stimulating hormone level should almost always be performed and intravenous levothyroxine given in myxedematous patients.
- Exclude infection. Many of the signs and symptoms of infection, including fever and leukocytosis are obscured by hypothermia.
- Hypothermic patients have a coagulopathy with an increased tendency to bleed (inactivation of coagulation enzymes and platelet destruction by cold). Some patients, however may develop a DIC.

- The bradydysrhythmias are refractory to atropine (the brady-arrhythmias result from decreased spontaneous depolarization of the pacemaker cells).

Rewarming

The methods of rewarming (Figure 55-1) may be classified as (1) spontaneous rewarming, i.e., insulating to reduce heat loss without supplying heat; (2) active rewarming, i.e., supplying additional heat, either as surface heating or by central rewarming; and (3) a combination of different methods. There is no absolute temperature from which humans will not rewarm. However, the temperature from which any individual case will not rewarm will depend upon the patient's metabolic rate, age, the degree of hypothermia, drugs, concurrent illness or injury, and the effectiveness of insulation. In patients with subchronic hypothermia, if the rate of rewarming exceeds 0.5°C/h, there is a high risk of the patient's developing pulmonary and/or cerebral edema. It should be noted that the hands and feet should be kept cool; i.e., the hands should be placed down the side of the patient and not on the abdomen. Warm hands and feet reduce the stimulus for heat production and will allow reduction of vasoconstrictor tone, thus increasing heat loss.

Indications for Active Rewarming

- Cardiovascular instability
- Moderate or severe hypothermia (<32.2°C)
- Inadequate rate or failure to rewarm
- Endocrinologic insufficiency
- Traumatic (acute spinal cord transection) or toxicologic peripheral vasodilation
- Secondary hypothermia impairing thermoregulation

Active External Rewarming

- Involves direct exposure of the patient's skin to any exogenous heat source
- Includes immersion, radiant heat, forced air, and heating blankets
- Complications including thermal injury and peripheral vasodilation with core-temperature afterdrop

Active Core Rewarming

- Heated humidified air. Inhalation of air humidified and heated (via a mask or endotracheal tube) to a temperature of 40°C will raise the core body temperature by about 1° to 2°C/h.

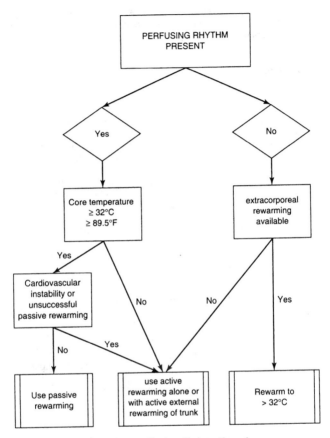

Figure 55-1. Approach to patients with hypothermia.

- Administration of intravenous fluids heated by countercurrent heat exchangers up to 42°C.
- Peritoneal lavage with 10 to 20 mL/kg of dialysate heated to 40°C at a rate of 6 L/h will raise core temperature by about 2° to 4°C/h.
- Gastric, colonic, and bladder irrigations should be avoided, as they may lead to unwanted complications.

- Mediastinal irrigation via chest tubes has been recommended by some investigators. This invasive procedure may be associated with many complications.
- Extracorporeal venovenous warming has been shown to be a very efficient and reasonably simple method of rewarming.
- Extracorporeal rewarming using the standard cardiopulmonary–bypass circuit. Femoral catheterization with flow rates of 2 to 3 L/min will raise the core temperature 1° to 2°C every 3 to 5 minutes. While cardiopulmonary bypass is the most rapid means of increasing the core body temperature, this procedure is impractical for most patients, as it requires specialized personnel and equipment and, usually, arterial and venous cutdowns, and it is usually restricted to the operating room.

56

Central Venous Catheterization

Central venous catheterization is frequently required in critically ill patients to facilitate fluid resuscitation; to administer vasoactive agents, sedative agents, antibiotics as well as myriad other medications; as well as to provide access for various dialytic approaches. The most common sites of venous access are the subclavian, internal jugular, and femoral veins. Central venous catheterization is not a benign procedure and may be associated with potentially life-threatening complications. Femoral venous catheterization is probably associated with the lowest incidence of periprocedural complications in the inexperienced operator. Furthermore, contrary to popular belief, the incidence of catheter-associated sepsis and thromboembolic complications may not be higher with femoral catheters. Femoral catheters, however, should be avoided in patients nursed in a chair or ambulating patients. The presence of a coagulopathy is not a contraindication to central vein catheterization; the rate of complications is related to the expertise of the operator rather than the ability of the patient's blood to clot. In the hands of the inexperienced, femoral vein catheterization is recommended in the coagulopathic patient. Catheter-associated sepsis is a serious complication in critically ill patients (see Chapter 44); central venous catheters should therefore be inserted under strict aseptic conditions; hand washing, gloves, gown, and extended drapes are mandatory. While the risk of infection is related to the number of ports and manipulations, triple-lumen catheters may limit the number of catheters required (and infections) and are therefore generally recommended. Furthermore, antibiotic-coated catheters and reduce the risk of infection are therefore recommended.

■ SUBCLAVIAN VEIN CATHETERIZATION

- *Advantages*: Consistent identifiable landmarks, easier long-term catheter maintenance, relatively high patient comfort.
- *Disadvantages*: Pneumothorax (1% to 2%) and subclavian artery puncture (1%). Subclavian puncture is a relative contraindication in patients with a coagulopathy and/or pulmonary compromise (dependent on the expertise of the operator).
- *Anatomy*: The subclavian vein is a continuation of the axillary vein, beginning at the outer border of the first rib, extending 3 to 4 cm along the undersurface of the clavicle, and joining the ipsilateral internal jugular vein behind the sternoclavicular joint (Figure 56-1).
- *Position* (most important): The patient is placed supine with arms at the side and head turned to the opposite side. The patient is placed in a 15- to 30-degree Trendelenburg's position, with a small bedroll placed between the shoulder blades.
- *Infraclavicular Approach*: Identify the clavicle, the suprasternal notch, and the acromium-clavicular junction. The operator's position is next to the patient's ipsilateral shoulder. Feel along the inferior border of the clavicle moving from medial to lateral, until you feel a give in the tissue resistance. This point is approximately at the junction between the medial and middle thirds of the clavicle and at the point of the first S bend in the clavicle. Infiltrate

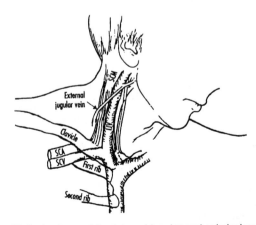

Figure 56-1. Anatomy of the internal jugular and subclavian veins. (IJV = internal jugular vein; SCA = Subclavian artery; SCM = Sterno-cleidomastoid muscle; SCV = Subclavian veiw.)

the skin and subcutaneous tissue with 1% lidocaine. Place the thumb of the left hand in the suprasternal notch, to serve as a landmark. Mount a 2 3/4-inch, 14-gauge needle on a syringe, and direct it cephalad from the point until the tip abuts under the clavicle. With the needle hugging the inferior edge of the clavicle, advance the needle toward the suprasternal notch (the thumb of your left hand). Advance the needle until the subclavian vein is entered.

■ INTERNAL JUGULAR VEIN CATHETERIZATION

- *Advantages*: Minimal risk for pneumothorax, preferred in patients with hyperinflation and those receiving mechanical ventilation.
- *Disadvantages*: Carotid artery puncture (2% to 10%), not recommended if platelet count <50,000 and elevated prothrombin time or partial thromboplastin time.
- *Anatomy*: The internal jugular vein emerges from the base of the skull through the jugular foramen, courses posterolateral to the internal carotid artery in the carotid sheath, and runs beneath the sternocleidomastoid muscle (see Figure 56-1).
- *Position*: The patient is placed supine in a 15-degree Trendelenburg's position with the head turned gently to the opposite side.
- *Central approach (recommended)*: Puncture the skin at the apex of the triangle formed by the two muscle bellies of sternocleidomastoid muscle and the clavicle, at a 30- to 45-degree angle with the frontal plane and directed at the nipple on the same side.
- *Anterior approach*: Insert the needle at the midpoint of the sternocleidomastoid muscle, approximately 5 to 6 cm from both the angle of the mandible and the sternal notch (four fingerbreadths), while feeling the carotid artery pulsation with the other hand and keeping the needle lateral to the pulsations. Introduce the needle at a 30 to 45-degree angle with the frontal plane, and direct it caudally parallel to the carotid artery toward the nipple on the same side. If the initial attempt is unsuccessful, direct the needle more laterally.
- *Finder needle*: A 22-gauge finder needle may be used to localize the internal jugular vein and avoid inadvertent internal carotid artery puncture with the wider bore needle. After venipuncture with the finder needle, either withdraw the finder needle and introduce a large-bore needle in the same plane, or leave it in place and introduce the larger needle directly above it.

■ FEMORAL VEIN CATHETERIZATION

- *Advantages*: Femoral vein catheterization is safe, easily accessible, and Trendelenburg's position is not needed. The risk of infection is not increased when compared to other sites. It is safe to perform in patients with a coagulopathy.
- *Disadvantages*: Limits flexion of leg at hip.
- *Anatomy*: The femoral vein is the continuation of the popliteal vein and becomes the external iliac vein at the inguinal ligament. It lies medial to the femoral nerve and femoral artery in the femoral sheath at the inguinal ligament.
- *Technique*: Clean and shave the area. Place the patient supine with the leg extended and slightly abducted at hip. Palpate for the femoral arterial pulsation; the site of puncture is 1 to 1.5 cm medial to the femoral arterial pulsation below the inguinal ligament. In a patient with no palpable femoral pulse, it is 1 to 1.5 cm medial to the junction of medial third and lateral two thirds of a line joining the anterior superior iliac spine and pubic tubercle. A 14-gauge needle is placed at the site of puncture and advanced at a 45- to 60-degree angle to the frontal plane with the tip pointed cephalad. After obtaining return of venous blood, the syringe and needle are depressed to the skin level and free aspiration of blood is reconfirmed.

■ POSTINSERTION CHEST FILM

Chest films (preferably upright in expiration) are recommended after all attempts at central venous catheterization (subclavian/internal jugular) to determine the position of the catheter tip, and to exclude a pneumothorax or hemothorax (see Chapter 16).

■ COMPLICATIONS OF CENTRAL VENOUS ACCESS

- Venous air embolism: Entry of air into the central venous system through the catheter can be fatal. It is best prevented by positioning patient in a 15-degree Trendelenburg's position during catheter insertion. It will manifest as tachypnea, wheezing, hypotension, and "mill wheel" murmur over precordium. The patient should be immediately turned onto his/her left side, in

Trendelenburg's position, and air should be aspirated after advancing the catheter into the right ventricle.

- Venous thrombosis: Common, usually of little clinical significance, mural thrombi occur in 10% to 20% of cases but are clinically significant in only 0% to 3% of patients.
- Local infection, and catheter-associated blood stream infection.
- Pneumothorax and/or hemothorax: Occurs due to injury to pleura and underlying lung; a small pneumothorax can be observed, but medium to large pneumothoraces will require chest tube insertion.
- Arterial puncture: If arterial puncture occurs, apply sufficient pressure for at least 10 minutes. Arterial puncture may be confirmed by pulsatile flow and high hydrostatic pressure.
- Catheter tip migration and perforation of the free wall of the cardiac chamber.
- Vascular erosions: Uncommon, typically occur 1 to 7 days after catheter insertion, cause sudden dyspnea with new pleural effusion or hydromediastinum on chest radiograph, more common with left-sided catheter placement.
- Occlusion of catheter: Common. Best treated by replacement of catheter.
- Retained catheter fragment: Catheter tips may get sheared off by traction on the beveled tip of an inserting needle or by fracture of the catheter due to improper fixation and excessive movement.
- Inadvertent venous catheter placement: Inadvertent placement into the internal jugular vein or opposite subclavian vein from the subclavian vein approach is not uncommon.

57

Obstetrical Problems Requiring Intensive Care Unit Management

■ PREECLAMPSIA/ECLAMPSIA

Diagnosis of Pregnancy-Induced Hypertension (American College of Obstetricians and Gynecologists)

- Blood pressure.
    Systolic blood pressure ≥140 mm Hg
    Diastolic blood pressure ≥90 mm Hg
    Or increase in systolic blood pressure of 30 mm Hg or diastolic of 15 mm Hg from baseline
- Proteinuria.
    More than 300 mg in a 24-hour period
    Urine protein concentration of at least 1 g/L in two random urine specimens collected at least 6 hours apart
- Edema and generalized weight gain of more than 5 lb in a week.
- These changes must have occurred after the 20th week of gestation.

Features of Severe Pregnancy-Induced Hypertension

- Blood pressure >160/110 mm Hg
- More than 5 g proteinuria in a 24-hour period or 3+ or 4+ proteinuria noted on semiquantitative assay
- Oliguria (<500 mL/day)

- Cerebral or visual disturbances
- Pulmonary edema
- Epigastric or right upper quadrant pain
- Deranged liver functions
- Thrombocytopenia

Factors Predisposing to Preeclampsia

- Occurs in about 5% of pregnancies
- Family history
- Nulliparity
- Diabetes
- Multiple gestation
- Renal disease
- Hydatiform mole
- Poor prenatal care

Other Features of Preeclampsia

- May have falsely high hematocrit due to hypovolemia and hemoconcentration.
- HELLP syndrome (hemolysis, elevated liver enzymes, low platelet) seen in 10%.
- Disseminated intravascular coagulation (DIC) uncommon.
- Pulmonary capillary wedge pressure usually low, cardiac index usually normal or low, and elevated mean pulmonary artery pressure.
- Preeclampsia typically regresses rapidly after delivery.
- Low doses of aspirin and dietary calcium supplementation may have some role in prevention of preeclampsia.

Features of Eclampsia

Eclampsia is presence of seizures in addition to preeclampsia criteria. Eclampsia occurs in about 1 in 700 pregnancies. The seizures may occur before, during, or after delivery. Postpartum eclampsia almost always occurs within 24 hours of delivery. Any seizure activity developing more than 48 hours postpartum merits further investigation.

■ MANAGEMENT OF PREECLAMPSIA/ECLAMPSIA

1. Hospitalize if preeclampsia is suspected.
2. Fluid therapy: cautious volume expansion with crystalloid or small volumes of high-molecular-weight solutions.

3. Prevent and control convulsions
    a. The data from the Collaborative Eclampsia Trial have clearly demonstrated that magnesium sulphate is superior to both diazepam and phenytoin in preventing recurrent seizures. Furthermore, both maternal and fetal outcome were better in those patients who received magnesium sulphate.
    b. Intravenous and intramuscular magnesium sulphate dosing regimen. Intravenous loading with 4 to 6 g of 20% solution at 1 g/min, and maintenance intramuscular dose of 5 g of 50% solution every 4 hours. Continue magnesium sulphate for 24 hours after all seizures have stopped. Intravenous magnesium sulphate dosing regimen: 6-g loading dose at 1 g/min, followed by 2-g/h maintenance dose.
    c. Aim for target serum level of 4 to 6 mEq/L. Monitor urine output, deep patellar reflex, and respiratory status. If the patient develops respiratory depression, may give 1 g of 10% calcium gluconate solution as antidote. If the patient develops respiratory failure, may need intubation and mechanical ventilation.
    d. Parenterally administered magnesium is cleared almost totally by renal excretion. In patients with renal impairment, the dosage must be adjusted according to calculated creatinine clearance.
    e. Patients may need additional magnesium sulphate (2 g of 20% solution intravenously) if seizures are not controlled. If still uncontrolled, may give 250 mg sodium amobarbital and monitor oxygenation and ventilation.
    f. Maintain airway, prevent tongue laceration, place the patient in the left lateral position to decrease aspiration risk, and maintain blood return from the inferior vena cava.

4. Control blood pressure (see also Chapter 20). The primary objective of treatment in women with severe hypertension and preeclampsia is to prevent cerebral complications such as encephalopathy and hemorrhage. The threshold for treatment is usually a sustained diastolic blood pressure of ≥110 mm Hg. Some experts recommend initiating treatment at diastolic blood pressure values of ≥105 mm Hg, whereas others use mean arterial pressure >125 mm Hg as the threshold. The aim of therapy is to keep the mean arterial pressure <126 mm Hg (but not <105 mm Hg) and the diastolic pressure <105 mm Hg (but not <90 mm Hg). The initial treatment of choice in women who have severe hypertension during the peripartum period is hydralazine given intravenously in 5-mg bolus doses. The dose may be repeated as needed every 20 minutes up to a cumulative total of 20 mg.

Labetalol and nicardipine (dihydropyridine calcium channel blocker) have been demonstrated to be efficacious and safe in hypertensive pregnant patients and may have advantages in patients treated in the ICU or in those patients who have not responded adequately to hydralazine. Angiotensin-converting enzyme (ACE) inhibitors should be avoided, as their use is associated with fetal death and hypotension in neonates. In addition, diuretics should be avoided, as they further compromise placental perfusion by reducing an already decreased intravascular volume.

5. Indications for pulmonary artery catheterization
   a. Pulmonary edema or acute respiratory distress syndrome (ARDS)
   b. Oliguria, unresponsive to initial volume expansion
   c. Severe hypertension unresponsive to vasodilator therapy
   d. Maternal cardiac disease
   e. Shock

6. Initiating delivery
   a. An expectant approach aimed at prolonging pregnancy is associated with high maternal morbidity and high perinatal mortality. Prompt delivery is indicated if near term and in the presence of severe hypertension persisting after 24 to 48 hours of treatment, low platelet count, liver/renal dysfunction, and premonitory signs of eclampsia (headache, hyperreflexia).
   b. Vaginal delivery is preferred, with amniotomy and induction of labor.
   c. Cesarean delivery in event of fetal compromise.

■ AMNIOTIC FLUID EMBOLISM

- Amniotic fluid embolism is characterized by a state of profound shock, developing suddenly and unexpectedly, during or shortly after delivery. It occurs due to embolization of amniotic fluid containing squamous cells, meconium, mucin, lanugo hair, and fat into maternal circulation.
- Exact incidence not known, probably 1 in 8000 to 80,000 live births.
- Very high maternal mortality (80% to 90%).
- Can be associated with abortion, amniocentesis, uncomplicated pregnancy, placental abruption, cesarean section, intrauterine death, violent labor, multiparity, and macrosomic fetus.
- Presents as abrupt cardiopulmonary collapse (hypotension and hypoxia) without a significant prodrome. Later pulmonary edema

develops due to left ventricular failure. Bronchospasm is unusual. About 10% to 15% patients may also develop seizures or DIC along with collapse.

- The manifestations of the syndrome are probably due to mechanical obstruction of pulmonary vasculature, alveolar capillary leak leading to ARDS, left ventricular dysfunction, and anaphylactic reaction to fetal antigens.
- Diagnosis is difficult. The physician needs high suspicion in the right setting.
- Pulmonary microvascular cytology (PMVC): Blood sample from the distal port of the pulmonary artery catheter in wedged position may show large number of fetal squames (flat, polygonal, keratinized, anucleate cells), mucin, and hair. PMVC showing squames with mucin and hair or squames coated with neutrophils strongly supports the diagnosis of amniotic fluid embolism.
- Management is supportive. Most patients will need intubation and mechanical ventilation with positive end-expiratory pressure. A pulmony artery catheter is needed for hemodynamic monitoring and PMVC. Hypotension should be corrected. Avoid fluid overloading. Replacement therapy with packed red cells and fresh-frozen plasma is indicated in event of severe coagulopathy and hemorrhage. There is no role for anticoagulants, corticosteroids, or empiric antibiotics in this disorder.

■ TOCOLYTIC-INDUCED PULMONARY EDEMA

- Beta-adrenergic agents (ritodrine, terbutaline, isoxsuprine) are widely used for inhibition of preterm labor.
- Maternal pulmonary edema is seen in 4% to 5% of such cases
- Pathophysiology is not clear, as both normal and high filling pressures have been seen on pulmonary artery monitoring.
- Typically, patients develop chest discomfort, dyspnea, chest pain, cough, tachypnea, crackles, and evidence of pulmonary edema on chest radiograph within 48 hours of starting tocolytic therapy.
- Hypotension and clotting abnormalities are uncommon
- Discontinue tocolytic therapy at first symptoms suggestive of pulmonary edema. Mechanical ventilation is rarely needed. Rarely, patients may need diuretics and pulmonary artery catheterization. Immediate delivery is not mandatory. First stabilize the patient, and then deliver the fetus.
- It can be prevented by proper patient selection. Avoid tocolytics in patients with preeclampsia, thyrotoxicosis, hypervolemia, and severe asthmatics on beta-agonists. Also avoid using tocolytics for more than 24 to 48 hours.

■ ABRUPTIO PLACENTA

- The incidence of abruptio placenta is about 1 in 120 deliveries.
- The cause is unknown, but it is associated with hypertensive disorders, parity, previous abruption, cocaine abuse, and trauma.
- The patient presents with abdominal pain, which may be associated with vaginal bleeding.
- Fetal condition depends upon the duration and degree of separation of the placenta.
- Management

    Establish adequate venous access, cross-match blood, perform coagulation studies, and monitor maternal hemodynamics and fetal heart rate.

    The decision to allow vaginal delivery or to proceed with cesarean section (if the fetus is alive) depends on the condition of both mother and fetus.

■ ACUTE FATTY LIVER OF PREGNANCY

- Acute fatty liver of pregnancy is acute hepatic dysfunction that develops late in pregnancy and is associated with microvesicular fat accumulation in hepatocytes.
- More common with twin pregnancies and is associated with preeclampsia in up to one half of cases.
- Occurs typically after the 30th week of gestation.
- The patient presents with nausea, vomiting, malaise, abdominal pain, and then hepatic failure, jaundice, and encephalopathy
- Incidence 1 in 13,000 deliveries; fetal mortality 23%, maternal mortality 18%.
- Death usually is a result of sepsis, hemorrhage, or hypoglycemia.
- Therapy is mainly supportive. Monitor for and treat bleeding, sepsis, and hypoglycemia. Immediate delivery is probably beneficial, as there are no reports of recovery before delivery.

■ PERIPARTUM CARDIOMYOPATHY

- Patients with peripartum cardiomyopathy present in the last month of pregnancy or the first 6 months after delivery (most patients present in the first 3 months postpartum). By definition, the patient has no preexisting heart disease, and there are no other identifiable causes of heart failure.

- It is seen in 1 in 3000 to 4000 deliveries. It is more common among black women, multiple gestation, toxemia, and presence of postpartum hypertension.
- Patients typically present with features of congestive heart failure (jugular venous distention, S3 gallop, cardiomegaly, edema, mitral regurgitation murmur). Chest radiograph demonstrates cardiomegaly and pulmonary edema and occasionally pleural effusions. Echocardiography shows global hypokinesia.
- Peripartum cardiomyopathy is a diagnosis of exclusion. Congenital and valvular heart disease and metabolic and toxic disorders causing heart failure must be excluded.
- Therapy involves the use of digoxin and diuretics. ACE inhibitors should be used in postpartum patients. Patients with intractable heart failure are candidates for cardiac transplantation. Systemic anticoagulation is indicated because of high risk of systemic and pulmonary emboli in these patients. Cases with severe decompensation occurring in the third trimester may require pulmonary artery catheter monitoring during labor and delivery.
- These patients have a high mortality: Up to 50% die in first 3 months postpartum. In survivors, it tends to recur in subsequent pregnancies, especially if heart size does not return to normal in 6 to 12 months after the initial episode.

58

Toxicology

This chapter provides a brief overview of the management of patients following an accidental or suicidal drug overdose. Readers are referred to toxicology texts and their local poison control center for information on the management of specific intoxications.

■ GENERAL MEASURES

1. Stabilize the patient, i.e., airway, breathing and circulation.
   a. Intubate obtunded and comatose patients and seizing patients
   b. Obtain intravenous (IV) access
   c. Treat hypotension initially with volume expansion

2. Comatose patients should be given naloxone 0.8 mg IV.

3. Flumazenil (a benzodiazepine antagonist) may be indicated in patients who present with obtundation or coma following the ingestion of benzodiazepines. Flumazenil is contraindicated in patients with mixed overdoses (tricyclic antidepressants and benzodiazepines) as well as patients with a history of seizures. An initial IV dose of 0.2 mg should be given over 30 seconds. Additional doses of 0.2 to 0.5 mg can be given up to a total of 3 mg.

4. Ipecac is not recommended for ingestions treated in hospital. It may be used at home for accidental ingestions in children. It should not be given after ingestion of caustic substances and acids.

5. Gastric lavage is indicated in the following circumstances:
   a. Recent ingestion (<1 hour) of a potentially life-threatening poison
   b. Ingestion of a substance that slows gastric emptying (e.g., anticholinergic medications)
   c. Ingestion of a poison that is slowly absorbed from the gastrointestinal tract
   d. Ingestion of a substance that does not bind well to activated charcoal (see below)
   e. Ingestion of specific life-threatening poisons (e.g., tricyclic antidepressants, theophylline, cyanide)
   f. Technique for performing gastric lavage
      i. Patients who cannot protect their airway must be intubated before gastric lavage is performed.
      ii. The patient is placed in a head-down lateral position.
      iii. Place a large-bore lavage tube through mouth.
      iv. Aspirate to empty stomach.
      v. Lavage with 150 to 300 mL tepid tap water.
      vi. Contraindicated in caustic ingestions.

6. Activated charcoal. This is the cornerstone of the management of most ingestions. Activated charcoal is administered in a dose of 50 to 100 g orally.
   a. Drugs not well bound to activated charcoal
      Bromides
      Caustics
      Cyanide
      Ethylene glycol
      Heavy metals
      Iron
      Isopropyl alcohol
      Lithium
      Methanol
   b. Drugs amenable to repeat-dose activated charcoal therapy
      Carbamazepine
      Diazepam
      Digitalis
      Phenobarbital
      Phenytoin
      Salicylates
      Theophylline
      Tricyclic antidepressants

7. Specific antidotes are available for a limited number of intoxications (Table 58-1).

8. Some drugs are cleared by hemodialysis/hemoperfusion; this technique should be instituted as clinical circumstances dictate.

a. Hemoperfusion
    Acetaminophen
    Theophylline
    Methotrexate
    Phenylbutazone
    Procainamide
    Quinidine
b. Hemodialysis
    Ammonium chloride
    Amphetamine
    Atenolol
    Meprobamate
    Methyldopa
    Nadolol
    Phenobarbital
    Procainamide
    Quinidine
    Sotalol
    Thallium
    Ethanol
    Methanol
    Ethylene glycol
    Isopropanol
    Aspirin
    Lithium
    Bromide
    Arsenic

Table 58-1. Toxic substances with specific antidotes.

Agent	Antidote
Acetaminophen	N-acetylcysteine
Anticholinergic poisoning	Physostigmine
Anticoagulants	Vitamin K, protamine
Benzodiazepines	Flumazenil
Beta-adrenergic antagonists	Glucagon, calcium salts, isoproterenol
Carbon monoxide	Oxygen, hyperbaric oxygen
Cholinergic syndrome	Atropine
Digoxin	FAB antibody, magnesium
Ethylene glycol	Ethanol, thiamine, fomepizole
Fluoride	Calcium and magnesium salts
Heavy metals	British anti-lewisite (BAL), dimercaptosuccinic acid, D-penicillamine
Iron	Desferoxime
Isoniazid	Gamma-aminobutyric acid agonists, pyridoxine
Methemoglobinemia	Methylene blue
Opioids	Naloxone

In the evaluation of the patient with a possible drug overdose, it is useful to look for symptom complexes, or toxidromes, that may help in identifying the type of drug ingested. The following toxidromes should be identified:

- *Depressed level of consciousness*: coma, stupor, lethargy, confusion
- *Anticholinergic signs*: mydriasis, increased blood pressure, tachycardia, warm dry skin, erythema, delirium, hallucination, urinary retention
- *Cholinergic signs*: salivation, lacrimation, urination, defecation (SLUD), miosis, bradycardia, sweating
- *Sympathetic signs:* high blood pressure, tachycardia, hyperthermia, mydriasis
- *Serotonin syndrome*: confusion, myoclonus, hyperreflexia, diaphoresis, tremor, flushing, diarrhea, fever
- *Neurological signs*: nystagmus, tremors, hyperreflexia, seizures, extrapyramidal signs, hallucinations

■ COMMON CAUSATIVE AGENTS

Depressed Level of Consciousness

- Alcohol
- Anticholinergics
- Anticonvulsants
- Antidepressants
- Antihistamines
- Antipsychotics
- Barbiturates
- Benzodiazepines
- Carbon monoxide
- Opiates
- Sulfonylureas

Seizures

- Phenytoin
- Beta-blockers
- Clonidine
- Theophylline
- Meperidine
- Amphetamines
- Cocaine

Anticholinergic Syndrome

- Antidepressants
- Antihistamines
- Antipsychotic
- Belladonna alkaloids
- Mushrooms

Cholinergic Syndrome

- Insecticides
- Mushrooms
- Nicotine

Sympathetic Syndrome

- Cocaine
- Amphetamines
- Phencyclidine

Serotonin Syndrome

- Selective serotonin reuptake inhibitor (SSRI): fluoxetine, etc.
- Isoniazid
- Meperidine
- Clomipramine

Extrapyramidal

- Antipsychotic

Nystagmus

- Alcohol
- Lithium
- Carbamazepine

Hallucinations

- Amphetamines
- Cocaine
- Phencyclidine
- Cannabinoids

■ COMMON INTOXICATIONS

Acetaminophen

Acetaminophen is an active ingredient of several hundred preparations and is the most common drug implicated in both accidental (children) and suicidal overdoses. The drug is well absorbed, with peak levels noted about 4 hours after an overdose. Although remarkably safe in therapeutic doses, ingestion of large doses (especially in alcoholics and malnourished persons) and overdosages can cause fatal hepatotoxicity. After therapeutic doses, approximately 90% of acetaminophen is conjugated by the liver to nontoxic inactive compounds, which are renally excreted. About 5% is excreted unchanged in the urine, and about 5% is oxidized by the P-450 mixed function oxidase enzyme to yield highly reactive toxic intermediates, which are detoxified by reduced glutathione. After overdosage, the amount of drug metabolized by the P-450 route is increased. The same process occurs in the kidney, and while renal toxicity may occur with acetaminophen overdose, it is far less common than hepatotoxicity. The hepatotoxicity may vary from asymptomatic elevation of liver enzymes to fatal liver failure. Pancreatitis and myocardial necrosis have also been described. It should be noted that stores of reduced glutathione are diminished in alcoholics and malnourished patients, predisposing them to hepatic toxicity at therapeutic dosages. Ingestions of >7.5 g in an adult should be considered potentially toxic.

Signs and Symptoms

- *Stage 1* (12 to 24 hours after ingestion): Asymptomatic or mild gastrointestinal (GI) symptoms.
- *Stage 2* (24 to 72 hours): Right upper quadrant pain, nausea and vomiting, liver enzymes begin to rise.
- *Stage 3* (72 to 96 hours): Maximal hepatic injury.
- *Stage 4* (4 days to 2 weeks): The patient either improves, with normalization of enzymes or progresses to acute hepatic necrosis with liver failure.

Management

Analyzing the serum acetaminophen concentration is essential in all cases of overdose (see Figure 58-1). A level before 4 hours is difficult to interpret. High potential for toxicity exists when the serum concentration is >200 μg/mL at 4 hours, 50 μg/mL at 12 hours, and 7 μg/mL at 24 hours after ingestion.

N-acetylcysteine should be administered as soon as possible within the first 24 hours of ingestion. However, antidotal therapy is optimal when given within 12 hours of acetaminophen ingestion. *N*-acetylcys-

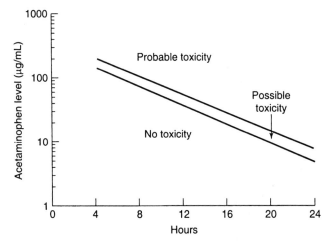

Figure 58-1. Acetaminophen treatment nomogram.

teine should be given if the patient has ingested more than 140 mg/kg (or 10 g) acetaminophen, if the serum level is >140 µg/ml, or if the serum level is in the toxic range (Figure 58-1). The dose of *N*-acetylcysteine is 140 mg/kg as an initial oral loading dose, followed by 70 mg/kg every 4 hours for a total of 17 doses.

It may be useful to measure a second level some time after starting *N*-acetylcysteine to determine the half-life of acetaminophen. A half-life greater than 4 hours is suggestive of hepatic toxicity. *N*-acetylcysteine should not be stopped as the level falls to zero, because it is not acetaminophen that is toxic but rather its metabolites.

Salicylates

Signs and Symptoms

The signs and symptoms of salicylate overdose are gastric upset, tinnitus, increased depth of breathing, headache, seizures, and coma. Anion gap metabolic acidosis and respiratory alkalosis also occur.

Management

- Serum salicylate levels are useful in confirming the diagnosis and assessing the severity of the toxicity but are, however, not used in directing therapy (Figure 58-2).

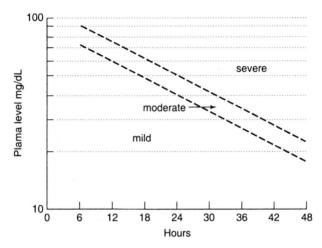

Figure 58-2. Assessment of severity of salicylate toxicity.

- Supportive measures, GI decontamination, and activated charcoal.
- Forced alkaline diuresis (ion trapping and increased elimination). In cases of severe toxicity, dialysis is useful. The decision to dialyze the patient is based on clinical grounds, i.e., seizures, altered level of consciousness. Blood level monitoring is useful to monitor drug elimination.

Tricyclic Antidepressants

The newer cyclic antidepressants (SSRI agents) are less toxic in overdose than the tricyclic drugs. Tricyclic antidepressants have anticholinergic and cardiac effects; however, they can cause seizures and altered mentation and level of consciousness, leading to coma in overdose. The most common antidepressants are listed in Table 58-2.

Signs and Symptoms

- Anticholinergic: mydriasis, blurred vision, dry mouth, tachycardia, hyperpyrexia, urinary retention, decreased GI motility.
- CNS: agitation, mental confusion, respiratory depression, seizures, coma.

Table 58-2. Antidepressant drugs.

	Sedative	Orthostatic	Anticholinergic	Conduction Disturbance or Arhythmia	Daily Dosage Range (mg)
Tricyclic					
Doxepin	High	Moderate	Moderate	Yes	25–400
Amitriptyline	High	Moderate	Highest	Yes	25–300
Imipramine	Mderate	High	Moderate	Yes	50–400
Trimipramine	High	Moderate	Moderate	Yes	50–300
Clomipramine	Moderate	High	High	Yes	75–300
Protriptyline	Lowest	Low	High	Yes	5–60
Nortriptyline	Moderate	Lowest	Moderate	Yes	25–150
Desipramine	Lowest	Low	Moderate	Yes	75–300
Other					
Amoxapine	Moderate	Low	Moderate	Very low	50–300
Maprotiline	Moderate	Low	Moderate	Very low	50–200
Trazodone	Moderate	Moderate	Very low	Very low	50–600
Fluoxetine	Low	Lowest	Low	Low	10–80
Sertraline	Low	Lowest	Low	Low	50–200
Paroxetine	Low	Lowest	Low	Low	10–20
Bupropion	Low	Lowest	Low	Low	75–300

- Cardiac: quinidine-like action on the heart; widened QRS, PR, and QT intervals, right bundle branch block, torsades de pointe. The best predictor of cardiac arrhythmias and seizures is a QRS complex >0.1 seconds or a prolonged QTc interval.

Management

- Antidepressants are highly tissue bound, and therefore serum concentrations do not correlate with toxicity and have little clinical value.
- Supportive measures, GI decontamination, and activated charcoal are essential.
- Alkalinization of the serum with bicarbonate to achieve an arterial pH of 7.5 to 7.55 should be instituted in patients with a prolonged QRS/QTc interval or cardiac arrhythmias. Alkalinization increases plasma protein binding (less free drug) and antagonizes the quinidine-like effects on the His-Purkinje system.
- Seizures are best treated with diazepam/midazolam or IV phenobarbital. Phenytoin is ineffective and may be dangerous.
- Lidocaine should be used for ventricular dysrhythmias.

Acute Ethanol Intoxication

Alcohol is the most common poison consumed by Americans; approximately a third of the population ingest this toxin on a chronic basis. The mechanism of action of alcohol is unclear; no specific ethanol receptors have been identified. It is postulated that ethanol influences multiple ion channels by causing alterations in their tertiary structure due to intercalation of ethanol into the bilipid cell membrane. Ethanol antagonizes the excitatory *N*-methyl-D-aspartate (NMDA) glutamate receptor and potentiates the inhibitory gamma-aminobutyric acid A receptor; these actions may explain the effect of alcohol on the central nervous system (CNS); ethanol is a CNS depressant.

Ethanol is readily absorbed from the GI tract, with 80% of the absorption occurring in the small intestine. Peak ethanol levels typically occur 30 to 60 minutes after ingestion. Metabolism occurs in the liver by first-order kinetics (i.e., at a constant rate unaffected by the serum level), predominantly by alcohol dehydrogenase. The clinical features and associated blood levels of ethanol intoxication are listed in Table 58-3. The blood alcohol level can be estimated by the following formula: EtOH level = osmolar gap × 4.3. Serum ethanol levels decline by about 15 to 30 mg/dL/h. The treatment of acute alcohol intoxication is largely supportive; with prevention and management of the associated complications. Hemodialysis may be helpful in severe cases.

Table 58-3. Features of acute alcohol intoxication.

Blood Ethanol Concentration (mg%)	Symptoms
50–150	Euphoria or dysphoria Uninhibited, impaired concentration and judgment
150–250	Slurred speech, ataxic gait, drowsiness, labile moods, antisocial behavior
250–400	Stupor, incoherent speech, vomiting
400–500	Coma
>500	Death

Medical complications associated with acute alcohol ingestion include the following:

- Acute myopathy with rhabdomyolysis
- Gastritis
- Esophagitis
- Mallory-Weiss lesion
- Thrombocytopenia
- Pancreatitis
- Alcoholic hepatitis
- Arrhythmias, especially atrial fibrillation
- Decreased myocardial contractility (synergistic with cocaine)
- Peripheral vasodilation and hypotension
- Alcohol withdrawal syndrome and delirium tremens
- Hypoglycemia
- Electrolyte disturbances, including hypokalemia, hyponatremia, hypophosphatemia, hypomagnesemia
- Wernicke's syndrome

Ethylene Glycol and Methanol Poisoning

Ethylene Glycol

Ethylene glycol is found in many de-icers, antifreezes, detergents, polishes, cosmetics, paints, and lacquers. It is colorless and odorless with a slightly sweet taste. Ethylene glycol initially causes an ethanol-like intoxication with little toxicity until it is metabolized in the liver to more harmful metabolites, including several aldehydes, carboxylic acids, and oxalic acid. These intermediates inhibit cellular respiration, protein synthesis, and RNA replication. Ethylene glycol initially undergoes oxidation by hepatic alcohol dehydrogenase to glycoaldehyde, which is then rapidly converted by aldehyde dehydrogenase to glycolic acid. Glycolic acid is converted to glyoxylic acid, whose most toxic metabolite is oxalic acid. Oxalic acid may crystalize as calcium oxalate in many tissues, causing hypocalcemia and tubular obstruction in the kidney. The anion gap acidosis results predominantly from elevated glycolic acid levels.

Classically, ethylene glycol poisoning has been divided into three stages.

- *Stage 1* (30 minutes to 12 hours) is characterized by CNS effects such as ethanol-like intoxication, stupor, coma, and convulsions.
- *Stage 2* (12 to 24 hours) is notable for cardiovascular and pulmonary effects such as tachypnea, cyanosis and pulmonary edema, and progressive CNS depression.
- *Stage 3* (48 to 72 hours) is characterized by the development of acute renal failure. In addition during this stage, prolonged generalized seizures may occur.

Methanol

Methanol is found in many cleaning materials, paints and varnishes, antifreeze, duplicating fluids, and gasoline. It is a colorless liquid with a distinct odor. Methanol is about half as potent as ethanol in its ability to cause CNS depression. Like ethylene glycol, it must undergo metabolic transformation before toxicity occurs. Alcohol dehydrogenase catalyzes the formation of formaldehyde, which is converted to formic acid. Formic acid is an inhibitor of mitochondrial cytochrome oxidase, causes histocytotoxic hypoxia, and is responsible for the metabolic acidosis and ocular toxicity seen with methanol. Lactic acidosis may be seen late in the course of methanol toxicity. Neurologic, ophthalmologic, and GI symptoms dominate the clinical features of methanol toxicity. Features of toxicity include blurred vision, scintillations, loss of sight, unreactive pupils, papilledema, vomiting, epigastric pain, convulsions, and coma. An anion gap metabolic acidosis (formate anions) is characteristic.

Treatment

The serum methanol and ethylene glycol levels should be measured; however, they can be estimated from the osmolar gap:

$$[\text{Methanol}] = 3.2 \times \text{osmolar gap}$$

$$[\text{Ethylene glycol}] = 6.2 \times \text{osmolar gap}$$

- Syrup of ipecac should be avoided, due to the risk of aspiration. The efficacy of activated charcoal is controversial.
- If pH <7.25, sodium bicarbonate should be given to maintain the pH >7.25. Large doses of bicarbonate may be required to control severe life-threatening metabolic acidosis. Unlike the metabolites

in lactic acidosis and ketoacidosis, the metabolites of ethylene glycol cannot be converted back to bicarbonate.

- *Ethanol.* Ethanol slows down the metabolism of both methanol and ethylene glycol, reducing their toxicity. Ethanol should be given to patients with ocular symptoms, acidosis, or a serum methanol or ethylene glycol level >20 mg/dL.

  Loading dose: 600 mg/kg IV

  Maintenance dose: 100 to 150 mg/h. The infusion should be titrated to maintain a serum ethanol level of 100 to 150 mg/dL.

- *Fomepizole.* Fomepizole is a potent inhibitor of alcohol dehydrogenase and is used as an alternative to ethanol. Fomepizole has been used successfully to treat methanol, ethylene glycol, and diethylene glycol poisoning in humans. The indications for fomepizole are the same as those for ethanol. The currently approved dose consists of a loading dose of 15 mg/kg IV over 30 minutes, followed by 10 mg/kg every 12 hours for four doses, then 5 mg/kg every 12 hours thereafter.

- *Hemodialysis.* Hemodialysis facilitates the removal of methanol, ethylene glycol, and their metabolites. Hemodialysis should be instituted in all patients with a serum level >50 mg/dL, in patients with ocular symptoms (methanol), and in patients with a significant metabolic acidosis. The ethanol infusion rate should be increased during dialysis, as it is also removed during dialysis.

- In methanol poisoning, folic/folinic acid (50 to 100 mg q4h) may mitigate the toxic effects of formate. Pyridoxine (100 mg) and thiamine 100 mg should be given daily in ethylene glycol poisoning.

Isopropyl Alcohol

In general, isopropyl alcohol is less toxic than either methanol or ethylene glycol. It is metabolized to acetone. Neither a metabolic acidosis nor an ion gap characteristically occur.

Signs and Symptoms

- Dizziness, confusion, slurred speech, headache, ataxia, stupor, and coma
- Nausea, vomiting, abdominal pain, hemorrhagic gastritis, diarrhea
- Hypotension, bradycardia, rhabdomyolysis, hemolysis

Management

Treatment is essentially supportive. Hemodialysis is recommended in severe poisoning, especially when accompanied by hypotension.

Theophylline

Signs and Symptoms

Nausea, vomiting, diarrhea, abdominal pain, tremors, headache, cardiac dysrhythmias, hypotension, seizures, coma, death.

Management

- Gastric lavage
- Activated charcoal
- Monitor blood levels
- Correct potassium, calcium, and magnesium
- Charcoal hemoperfusion
    Acute exposure
        Age <60 years plasma level >100 μg/mL
        Age >60 years plasma level >40 to 50 μg/mL
    Chronic exposure
        Age <60 years plasma level >60 μg/mL
        Age >60 years plasma level >30 to 40 μg/mL
    Any life-threatening poisoning regardless of level

For patients older than 60 years or patients with a history of respiratory failure, congestive heart failure, or liver disease, a theophylline concentration >40 μg/ml warrants consideration of hemoperfusion. A low threshold for hemoperfusion is recommended for patients taking theophylline chronically, since serum concentrations are not predictive of onset or severity of symptoms and because these patients have the potential to develop life-threatening complications at low serum concentrations.

Factors Affecting Serum Theophylline Level

- Drugs lowering theophylline levels
    Carbamazepine
    Phenobarbital
- Drugs raising theophylline levels
    Quinolone antibiotics
    Oral contraceptives
    Erythromycin
    H_2-antagonists
    Calcium channel blockers
    Phenytoin
    Propranolol
- Conditions lowering theophylline levels
    Cigarette smoking
    Cystic fibrosis
    Hyperthyroidism

- Conditions raising serum theophylline levels
    Hepatitis or cirrhosis
    Congestive heart failure
    Some viral infections

Digitalis

Signs and Symptoms

Signs and symptoms of digitalis toxicity are nausea, vomiting, diarrhea, fatigue, malaise, headache, confusion, delusions, hallucinations, blurred vision, disorder of green–yellow color perception, visualization of halos around objects and cardiac arrhythmias, including paroxysmal atrial tachycardia with 2:1 block, junctional tachycardia, varying degrees of heart block, ventricular and ectopy, ventricular tachycardia, and ventricular fibrillation.

Management

- Due to the high degree of tissue binding, serum drug levels do not accurately reflect tissue levels. Diagnosis of toxicity is a clinical diagnosis. The majority of patients who show signs of toxicity have a serum level >2 ng/mL; however, some patients may exhibit toxicity below this level. Similarly patients may have a level >2 ng/mL with no signs of toxicity.
- Gastric lavage and activated charcoal (acute ingestion).
- Continuous electrocardiograph (ECG) monitoring; evaluate old ECGs.
- Correction of electrolytes. Beware: K^+ may increase acutely with digoxin overdose.
- Atropine for conduction disturbances.
- Phenytoin or lidocaine for arrhythmias of impulse formation.
- Temporary pacemaker for arrhythmias that are resistant to atropine.
- Digoxin-specific antibodies (digoxin FAB fragment antibodies) for *serious arrhythmias and severe toxicity*: Digoxin FAB (Digibond) dosing:
    Use extreme caution if the patient is in renal failure.
    Serum levels are not useful once FAB is given.
    Dose is dependent on body load; each vial contains 40 mg FAB and binds 0.6 mg digoxin.

Body load of digoxin
= (serum digoxin concentration × 5.6 × weight in kg)/1000

Dose (vials) = body load/0.6

Phenytoin

Signs and Symptoms

The signs and symptoms of phenytoin toxicity are nystagmus, ataxia, slurred speech, confusion, seizures.

Management

Phenytoin is highly protein bound; therefore, serum levels do not correlate well with toxicity. Free levels are a better indicator of toxicity ($>2\,\mu g/mL$). Treatment includes gastric lavage and repeated activated charcoal.

Lithium

Signs and Symptoms

Mild to moderate toxicity occurs when the serum concentration of lithium is between 1.5 and 2.5 mEq/L, and severe toxicity occurs when the levels are between 2.5 and 3.5 mEq/L. Levels >3.5 mEq/L are life-threatening. Symptoms, however, do not necessarily correlate with lithium levels, and symptoms of toxicity may occur at therapeutic levels. Neurologic symptoms dominate the clinical picture of lithium toxicity. Symptoms include nausea, vomiting, diarrhea, polyuria, blurred vision, muscular weakness, confusion, vertigo, increased deep tendon reflexes, myoclonus, choreoathetoid movements, urinary and fecal incontinence, stupor, coma, seizures, cardiac arrhythmia, cardiovascular collapse, and death.

Predisposing Factors to Lithium Toxicity

- Infections
- Volume depletion
- Gastroenteritis
- Renal insufficiency
- Congestive cardiac failure
- Nonsteroidal anti-inflammatory drugs
- Diuretics
- Tetracycline

Management

Management of lithium toxicity is by gastric lavage and supportive therapy. Activated charcoal is not effective in removing lithium. Dehydrated patients should be actively rehydrated; however, forced saline diuresis is not recommended. Hemodialysis is indicated with levels >4 mEq/L or in patients with signs of serious toxicity and levels >2 mEq/L. The duration of dialysis should be guided by the serum levels. It is important to bear in mind that serum levels may rebound following dialysis and require repeat dialysis.

Opiates

Signs and Symptoms

The signs and symptoms of opiate toxicity are constricted pupils, bradycardia, hypotension, hypothermia, pulmonary edema, respiratory depression, and coma.

Management

Management of opiate toxicity includes supportive therapy and the administration of the opiate antagonist naloxone (Narcan). Naloxone should be given as an initial IV bolus of 0.4 mg. A bolus of from 0.4 mg up to 2 mg can be repeated every 3 to 5 minutes up to a total dose of 10 mg. Naloxone has a duration of action of about 45 to 60 minutes, which is considerably shorter than that of all the opiate agonists. Therefore, if the patient responds to the boluses of naloxone, a continuous infusion should be started, by placing 8 mg into 1000 mL 5% dextrose in water and infusing at a rate of 0.4 to 0.8 mg/h.

Calcium Channel Blockers

Signs and Symptoms

The signs and symptoms of calcium channel blocker toxicity are profound hypotension, conduction abnormalities (verapamil and diltiazem), bradyarrhythmia, decreased level of consciousness, lactic acidosis, hyperglycemia, and hypokalemia. Most cardiac effects occur within 6 hours of ingestion unless a sustained release preparation has been ingested, in which case toxicity may not be evident for 12 hours or more.

Management

Prophylactic pacemaker insertion should be considered. Management also may include administration of calcium chloride, 1 ampoule over 10 to 15 minutes; atropine, 0.5 mg IV every 5 minutes until the desired rate is achieved; or dopamine and glucagon, 5- to 10-mg IV bolus followed by a continuous infusion at 0.07 mg/kg/h.

Cocaine

Cocaine is an alkaloid derived from the coca plant, which is native to South America. Cocaine hydrochloride is a water-soluble powder that can be absorbed through the nasal mucosa or injected intravenously. Cocaine hydrochloride has a high melting point and decomposes when burned; this form of cocaine is therefore not suitable for smoking. Cocaine can be effectively smoked when it has been transformed into an alkaloid form, either "freebase" or "crack." Freebase and crack are the same chemical form of cocaine but are made using different techniques.

Cocaine acts by promoting the release and blocking the reuptake of neurotransmitters (norepinephrine, dopamine, and serotonin) at synaptic junctions, resulting in increased neurotransmitter concentrations. This results in sympathetic and central nervous stimulation. Cocaine, like other amide local anesthetic agents, blocks initiation and conduction of nerve impulses by decreasing axonal membrane permeability to sodium ions. At high doses, cocaine has Class 1 antiarrhythmic effects.

Cocaine can be smoked, nasally insufflated, or injected intravenously. Smoking crack cocaine is a popular and potentially dangerous route of administration. Due to the large absorptive surface area of the lung, very high serum levels can be achieved within seconds. Nasal insufflation produces euphoria in about 3 to 5 minutes, with peak cocaine levels being achieved in 30 to 60 minutes. The biological half-life in the blood is about 1 hour. Cocaine is metabolized to benzoylecgonine and ecgonine, which are excreted in the urine. Less than 5% of cocaine is excreted unchanged in the urine. Most urinary excretion occurs within 24 hours of administration. Most assays for detecting cocaine measure urinary benzoylecgonine levels. This assay will be positive for up to 6 days after a single use and for as long as 21 days with high-dose long-term use.

Alcohol enhances the euphoric effects of cocaine. Each year, approximately 12 million Americans use this drug combination. Cocaethylene is produced by the liver from the combination of cocaine and ethanol. Cocaethylene produces intense dopaminergic stimulation in the brain and myocardium. The risk of sudden death is 25 times greater in persons who abuse both alcohol and cocaine than in those who use only cocaine.

Complications Associated With the Use of Cocaine

Sudden Death

- Caused by arrhythmias, intracerebral bleeds, respiratory arrest, seizures, hyperthermia, and myocardial infarction

Psychiatric

- Cocaine use is associated with altered behavior and psychological, personality, and psychomotor alterations. Patients may have an underlying depression or personality disorder.

Cardiovascular

- Myocardial ischemia and infarction. The coronary arteries are usually normal; cocaine increases myocardial oxygen demand, induces coronary spasm, increases platelet aggregation, and has a procoagulant effect by depleting protein C and antithrombin III.
- Myocarditis and cardiomyopathy.
- Severe hypertension.
- Dissecting aortic aneurysm (often fatal).
- Arrhythmias, including supraventricular tachycardia, ventricular tachycardia, and fibrillation.

Pulmonary

- Asthma
- Thermal airway injury
- Noncardiogenic pulmonary edema
- Pulmonary hemorrhage
- BOOP (bronchiolitis obliterans with organizing pneumonia)
- Pneumothorax and pneumomediastinum
- Interstitial pneumonitis

Neurological

- Seizures
- Hemorrhagic strokes
- Cerebral infarctions
- Ruptured aneurysms

Renal

- Rhabdomyolysis and acute renal failure

Other

- Intestinal ischemia
- Gastroduodenal perforations
- Disseminated intravascular coagulation

- Placental abruption
- Hyperthermia

The Management of Cocaine Toxicity

- Agitation is best treated with benzodiazepines.
- Seizures: Solitary seizures usually do not require therapy. Status epilepticus, however, requires aggressive treatment with IV benzodiazepines followed by a loading dose of phenytoin.
- Hyperthermia must be treated immediately with cool-water washes and/or with cooling blankets.
- Hypertension is usually self-limiting. However, severe or sustained hypertension should be treated. Beta-blockers (including labetalol) may cause paradoxical worsening of hypertension as a result of unopposed alpha stimulation. Severe hypertension is best treated with a combination of benzodiazepines and calcium channel blockers (verapamil or nicardipine).
- Myocardial infarction: Administration of thrombolytic agents remains controversial. In cases of myocardial ischemia or impending infarction, calcium channel blockers, aspirin, and nitroglycerin are recommended. Beta-adrenergic blocking agents may exacerbate cocaine-induced coronary arterial vasoconstriction, thereby increasing the magnitude of myocardial ischemia. In contrast, nitroglycerin and verapamil reverse cocaine-induced hypertension and coronary arterial vasoconstriction; therefore, they are the agents of choice in treating patients with cocaine-associated chest pain.

Carbon Monoxide Poisoning

Carbon monoxide (CO) intoxication is the leading cause of death due to poisoning in the United States. Epidemics of CO poisoning commonly occur during winter months and sources include smoke from fires, fumes from heating systems, burning fuels, and exhaust fumes from motor vehicles. CO combines preferentially with hemoglobin to produce COHb, displacing oxygen and reducing systemic arterial oxygen (O_2) content. CO binds reversibly to hemoglobin with an affinity 200 to 230 times that of oxygen. Consequently, relatively minute concentrations of the gas in the environment can result in toxic concentrations in human blood. The history of exposure and carboxyhemoglobin levels should alert the physician to this diagnosis. In the absence of exposure history, CO poisoning should be considered when two or more patients are simultaneously sick with similar nonspecific symptoms.

Many victims of CO poisoning die or suffer permanent, severe neurological injury despite treatment. In addition, as many as 50%

of those who recover consciousness and survive may experience varying degrees of more subtle but still disabling neuropsychiatric sequelae. The features of acute CO poisoning are more dramatic than those resulting from chronic exposure. At low COHb levels, chronic cardiopulmonary problems, such as angina and chronic obstructive pulmonary disease, may be exacerbated, since cardiac myoglobin binds with great affinity and rapidly reduces myocardial O_2 reserve. Chest pain due to myocardial ischemia may occur, as can cardiac arrhythmias. Subacute or chronic CO poisoning presents with less severe symptoms (e.g., nausea, vomiting, headache), and patients may initially be misdiagnosed as having other illnesses.

The clinical presentation of acute CO poisoning is variable, but in general, the severity of observed symptoms correlates roughly with the observed level of COHb. However, in terms of diagnostic value, the nonspecificity of these presenting symptoms makes definitive diagnosis difficult. In addition, there have been several reports of levels near zero with patients showing neurologic deficits ranging from partial paralysis to coma. With levels less than 10%, the patient is usually asymptomatic. As COHb increases >20%, the patient may develop headache, dizziness, confusion, and nausea. Coma and seizures due to cerebral edema are common with levels >40%, and death is likely >60%. In reality, these symptom-level guidelines tend to be unreliable because of prehospital delays and early oxygen therapy and with concomitant poisoning from cyanide.

The mainstay of therapy for CO poisoning is supplemental O_2, ventilatory support, and monitoring for cardiac arrhythmias. There is general agreement that 100% oxygen should be administered before laboratory confirmation when CO poisoning is suspected. The goal of oxygen therapy is to improve the O_2 content of the blood by maximizing the fraction dissolved in plasma (Pao_2). Once treatment begins, O_2 therapy and observation must continue long enough to prevent delayed sequelae as carboxymyoglobin unloads. Unfortunately, there are no useful guidelines as to the length of the observation period.

The most controversial and widely debated topic regarding CO poisoning is the use of hyperbaric oxygen (HBO). There is little scientific evidence to support the clinical benefit of HBO. However, case reports, small case series, and retrospective studies have suggested that mortality and morbidity among patients treated with HBO appear improved beyond that expected with ambient pressure supplemental oxygen therapy. Currently, two prospective, randomized, blinded studies are being performed in patients with significant CO poisoning. In both these studies, patients are block randomized to normobaric (NBO) oxygen delivered in a hyperbaric chamber (sham control) and to a hyperbaric group. Interim analyses of both of these studies (with follow-up of 73 and 50 patients, respectively) have demonstrated no difference in outcome between the NBO- and HBO-treated groups. However, the role of HBO in CO poisoning will not be resolved until the final results of these studies are available.

59

End-of-Life Issues

End-of-life discussions play a central role in the management of critically ill ICU patients. The advanced life support technology that can be provided in the ICU is intended to provide temporary physiologic support for patients with potentially reversible organ failure or dysfunction. However, in many instances, the organ failures prove irreversible, with ICU care serving to merely prolong the dying process. In other instances, patients with clearly irreversible disease are admitted to the ICU, in the hope of a "miracle." It should be appreciated that death is the only certainty of life, and that the ICU is not a halfway station between life on earth and the hereafter. The function of the ICU is not to prolong death. According to Hippocrates, the purpose of medicine is to

> *"do away with the suffering of the sick, to lessen the violence of their diseases, and to refuse to treat those who are overmastered by their diseases, realizing that in such cases, medicine is powerless."*

It is essential that as health care providers in the ICU, we acknowledge the *limitations of our trade*, acknowledge that death is universal, and allow dying patients a dignified and comfortable death. Advanced life support technology should not be used to prolong death. In terminal or incurable illnesses, our aim should not be to preserve biological life, but to make the life that remains as comfortable and as meaningful as possible. The purpose of life support technology is not to prolong biological life without qualification. In circumstances where there is no realistic possibility of the patient returning to any semblance of cognitive or sapient life, our goal should be to allow the patient a good death.

Yet, the culture of our current health care system is highly invested in aggressive treatment of terminal disease with the notion that death represents medical failure. However, public interest in decisions regarding the use of medical technologies and pain control near the end of life is strong and growing. In addition, policy statements of national organizations such as the American Medical Association, the American Nurses Association, The American College of Physicians, and the Society of Critical Care Medicine/American College of Chest Physicians, recognize the right of competent patients to forgo treatment, even if refusal may lead to death. Increasingly, withholding and withdrawing life supportive measures, a practice that was once considered controversial, is now routine. However, recent studies document serious problems with medical care at the end of life. The Study to Understand Prognoses and Preferences for Outcomes and Risks of Treatments (SUPPORT) and other studies have demonstrated that physicians frequently attend to their patients without knowledge of their preferences with regard to end-of-life issues and that most patients suffer significant pain in their final days. The reasons that physicians fail to discuss and act upon their patients' desires regarding end-of-life issues are unclear. However, it is clear that many clinicians may lack a clear understanding of the benefits and limitations of our current advanced technologies and treatments. Others may avoid discussions of death and dying due to their own discomfort with the topic or fears that limitation of care at the end of life may imply that they are not providing the best care.

Nonmaleficence, the duty to do no harm to patients, is a basic principle of modern bioethics. If a therapeutic strategy has no hope of providing benefit to the patient but is likely to inflict pain, discomfort, or loss of dignity to the patient, it must be regarded as harmful and should therefore not be offered to the patient. We would consider a nonbeneficial medical intervention to be one that offers *no realistic expectation of leading to a cure or improvement of the medical condition or of providing meaningful palliation*. Physicians have no moral or ethical obligation to offer their patients a treatment that they believe will not be beneficial. Physicians do not offer nondying patients surgery or other intrusive forms of therapy that they believe will not benefit the patient. Furthermore, they do not get informed consent not to provide nonbeneficial therapy. So why should the care of a dying patient be any different from that of any other patient?

It is essential that the entire health care team be open and honest with each other and the patient and his/her surrogates when dealing with life-threatening illnesses. Conflict between members of the team *must* be resolved before discussions are held with the patient (surrogates) to avoid giving mixed messages. These discussion should focus on

1. *The patient's known wishes* or advance directives regarding life-support treatment

2. The patient's underlying disease(s) and physiologic function

3. The severity and reversibility of the patient's acute condition

In critically ill patients, an approach that focuses on realistic prognostic expectations and measures that ensure a dignified death is more likely to be accepted by patients and their surrogates than an approach that centers on medical interventions whose sole function is to prolong death. When dealing with dying patients, discussions should revolve around what will be done for the dying patient (i.e., treatment of pain and anxiety, etc.) rather than focusing on measures that will be withheld, such as cardiopulmonary resuscitation (CPR), dialysis, etc. The patients (and their surrogates) must not feel that they have been abandoned by the health care team.

■ DNR ORDERS IN THE ICU

Closed-chest massage, as first described by Kouwenhoven in 1960, was intended primarily to be administered to otherwise "healthy patients" with reversible conditions who experienced a sudden and unexpected cardiorespiratory arrest. A monograph on CPR written in 1965 states that CPR is intended to "resuscitate the victims of an acute insult, whether it be from drowning, electrical shock, untoward effects of drugs, anesthetic accident, heart block, acute myocardial infarction or surgery." At present, however, it is the current practice to attempt CPR on any patient who dies, regardless of the underlying illness, except in those circumstances where a specific do not resuscitate (DNR) order exists. Cardiac resuscitation, when applied to dying patients, may restore cardiac function, but it does not prevent death; it merely prolongs the dying process.

It is important to realize that all patients in the ICU are (should be) undergoing aggressive resuscitation (i.e., reversible conditions are being actively treated) and that in most instances cardiac arrest represents the natural progression of the patient's disease, rather than representing an unexpected event with clearly reversible causative factors. For this reason, CPR should be considered nonbeneficial for most ICU patients. However, this obviously excludes acute cardiorespiratory events related to reversible disease or procedures (e.g., acute myocardial infarction with ventricular fibrillation or tension pneumothorax during line insertion). Furthermore, it is essential to realize that a DNR order does not preclude the patient receiving highly aggressive care in an ICU. A DNR order merely instructs the medical team not to perform "chest acrobatics" (CPR) when the patient dies.

■ SELECTED REFERENCES

1. A controlled trial to improve care for seriously ill hospitalized patients: the Study to Understand Prognoses and Preferences for Outcomes and Risk Treatments (SUPPORT). *JAMA*. 1995;274:1591–1598.
2. American College of Physicians Ethics Manual. Fourth edition. *Ann Intern Med*. 1998;128:576–594.
3. American College of Chest Physicians/Society of Critical Care Medicine Consensus Panel. Ethical and moral guidelines for the initiation, continuation, and withdrawal of intensive care. *Chest*. 1990;97:946–958.
4. American Nurses Association Task Force on the Nurse's role in End of Life Decisions. *Position Statement on Forgoing Artificial Nutrition and Hydration*. Washington, DC: American Nurses Association; 1992.
5. Chadwick J, Mann WN. *The Medical Works of Hippocrates*. Boston: Blackwell Scientific; 1950.
6. *Current Opinions of the Council on Ethical and Judicial Affairs of the American Medical Association: Withholding or Withdrawing Life Prolonging Treatment*. Chicago, Ill: American Medical Association. 1992.
7. Kouwenhoven WB, Jude JR, Knickerbocker GG. Closed chest cardiac massage. *JAMA*. 1960;173:1064–1067.
8. Medical futility in end-of-life care: report of the Council on Ethical and Judicial Affairs. *JAMA*. 1999;281:937–941.
9. Talbott JH. Introduction. In: Jude JR, Elam JO, eds. *Fundamentals of Cardiopulmonary Resuscitation*. Philadelphia: FA Davis; 1965.

60

Marik's Evidence-Based Commonsense Critical Care Rules

With Wisdom comes Understanding.

(Proverbs 5:4)

- Don't assume the obvious.
- Common diseases occur commonly.
- When doing a procedure, remember nature always sides with the hidden flaw. *Corollary*: If something can go wrong, it will.
- Just when you thought things couldn't get any worse, they will.
- Never open a can of worms unless you plan to go fishing.
- Nothing in medicine stays constant.
- The Law of Subspecialization: If you are a hammer, the world looks like a nail.
- An acute surgical abdomen is when a good surgeon says it's an acute surgical abdomen. There is no test for it.
- Before ordering a test, decide what you will do if it is (a) positive or (b) negative. If both answers are the same, don't do the test. *Corollary*: If a test is unlikely to change your management, don't order it.
- There is no manifestation that cannot be caused by a given drug.
- If a drug is not working, stop it.
- The quality of patient care is inversely proportional to the number of consultants on any particular case.
- If it cannot be read, don't write it.
- Any order that can be misunderstood, will be misunderstood.
- Never ignore an ICU nurse's observation.
- Be kind to nurses, and they will be kind to you. Be unkind to nurses, and they will make your life miserable.

- When you don't know what to do, do nothing. *Corollary*: Doing something harmful is not better than doing nothing.
- No organ ever fails in isolation.
- Empty vessels make the most noise.
- He who thinks he knows everything knows nothing.
- A committee is the only life form that has twelve rectums and no brain.

Index